Physical Medicine and Rehabilitation

Physical Medicine and Rehabilitation

Edited by
Zayne Oliver

Larsen & Keller
www.larsen-keller.com

Physical Medicine and Rehabilitation
Edited by Zayne Oliver
ISBN: 978-1-63549-221-7 (Hardback)

Larsen & Keller
Published by Larsen and Keller Education,
5 Penn Plaza,
19th Floor,
New York, NY 10001, USA

Cataloging-in-Publication Data

Physical medicine and rehabilitation / edited by Zayne Oliver.
p. cm.
Includes bibliographical references and index.
ISBN 978-1-63549-221-7
1. Medicine, Physical. 2. Medical rehabilitation. 3. Medicine. 4. Physical therapy.
I. Oliver, Zayne.
RM700 .P49 2017
615.82--dc23

Printed and bound in China.

For more information regarding Larsen and Keller Education and its products, please visit the publisher's website www.larsen-keller.com

Table of Contents

Preface

Physical medicine and rehabilitation is that medicine which is used to restore the functional ability related to musculoskeletal disorders and quality of life for people suffering from disabilities. It is mainly used for patients dealing with issues of the nervous system, ligaments, muscles or bone injuries. This book is a valuable compilation of topics, ranging from the basic to the most complex theories and principles in the field of physical medicine and rehabilitation. While understanding the long-term perspectives of the topics, it makes an effort in highlighting their impact as a modern tool for the growth of the discipline. This textbook will provide comprehensive knowledge to the readers. For all those who are interested in physical medicine and rehabilitation, this book can prove to be an essential guide.

Given below is the chapter wise description of the book:

Chapter 1- Physical medicine and rehabilitation is a branch of medicine; its aim is to enhance the quality of life. Physiatrists specialize in treating patients with injuries to the bones, ligaments or nervous system. This chapter will provide an integrated understanding of physical medicine and rehabilitation.

Chapter 2- The branches of physical medicine and rehabilitation that have been explained in the section are cardiopulmonary rehabilitation, anaplastology and geriatric rehabilitation. Cardiopulmonary rehabilitation is the therapy that deals with the physical functions in patients with cardiac diseases. This section is a compilation of the various branches of physical medicine and rehabilitation that form an integral part of the broader subject matter.

Chapter 3- Physical therapy is a specialty in the field of physical medicine and rehabilitation and it uses mechanical force and movements and physical intervention. The topics elucidated in this section are neuromuscular medicine, sports medicine, pain management, spinal cord injury and postural restoration. Physical medicine is best understood in confluence with the major topics listed in the following chapter.

Chapter 4- Orthopedic surgery is the surgery that is performed or is concerned with the conditions involving the musculoskeletal system. The alternative types of rehabilitation medicine are aquatic therapy, hydrotherapy, medicine ball, stroke recovery, vocational rehabilitation and barthel scale. This section provides a plethora of the categories related to the subject matter for better comprehension of rehabilitation medicine.

Chapter 5- Audiology is a branch of science; it studies balance and also studies hearing. Those who practice audiology treat patients and prevent further damage related to hearing. Nursing, occupational therapist, orthotics, prosthetist and speech-language pathology are some of the topics discussed in the following chapter.

Chapter 6- The injuries cured by physical medicine and rehabilitation is head injury, sprain, tennis elbow, wound, cramp and bruise. Any damage done to the body is known as an injury, it can be caused by falls, hits or by accidents. Injuries can cause disability or death and some of the injuries can be cured by physical medicine and rehabilitation. This topic is of great importance as it helps the readers in broadening their existing knowledge on physical medicine.

At the end, I would like to thank all those who dedicated their time and efforts for the successful completion of this book. I also wish to convey my gratitude towards my friends and family who supported me at every step.

Editor

1

Introduction to Physical Medicine and Rehabilitation

Physical medicine and rehabilitation is a branch of medicine; its aim is to enhance the quality of life. Physiatrists specialize in treating patients with injuries to the bones, ligaments or nervous system. This chapter will provide an integrated understanding of physical medicine and rehabilitation.

Physical medicine and rehabilitation (PM&R), also known as physiatry or rehabilitation medicine, or physical and rehabilitation medicine (PRM) outside of the United States, is a branch of medicine that aims to enhance and restore functional ability and quality of life to those with physical impairments or disabilities. A physician having completed training in this field is referred to as a physiatrist. Physiatrists specialize in restoring optimal function to people with injuries to the muscles, bones, ligaments, or nervous system.

Scope of the Field

In the hospital setting, physiatrists commonly treat patients who have had an amputation, spinal cord injury, stroke, traumatic brain injury, and other debilitating injuries. In treating these patients, physiatrists lead an interdisciplinary team of physical, occupational, recreational and speech therapists, nurses, psychologists, and social workers. In outpatient settings, physiatrists also treat patients with muscle and joint injuries, pain syndromes, non-healing wounds, and other disabling conditions. Physiatrists are trained to perform intramuscular and interarticular injections as well as nerve conduction studies.

History

The specialty that came to be known as PM&R was officially established in 1947, when an independent board of Physical Medicine was established under the authority of the American Board of Medical Specialties. During the first half of the 20th century, two unofficial specialties, physical medicine and rehabilitation medicine, developed separately, but in practice both treated similar patient populations consisting of those with disabling injuries. Frank H. Krusen was a pioneer of physical medicine, which emphasized the use of physical agents, such as hydrotherapy and hyperbaric oxygen, at Temple University and then at Mayo Clinic and it was he that coined the term 'physiatry' in 1938. Rehabilitation medicine gained prominence during both World Wars in the treatment of injured soldiers and laborers. Howard A. Rusk, an internal medicine physician from Missouri, became a pioneer of rehabilitation medicine after being appointed to rehabilitate air force pilots during World War II. In 1943, the Baruch Committee, commissioned by philanthropist Bernard Baruch, defined the specialty as a combination of the two fields and laid the framework for its acceptance as an official medical specialty. The committee also distributed funds to establish training and research programs across the nation. In 1949, at the insistence of Dr. Rusk and others, the specialty incorporated rehabilitation medicine and changed its name to Physical Medicine and Rehabilitation.

Treatment

The major concern that PM&R deals with as a medical field is the ability of a person to function optimally within the limitations placed upon them by a disabling impairment or disease process for which there is no known cure. The emphasis is not on the full restoration to the premorbid level of function, but rather the optimization of the quality of life for those not able to achieve full restoration. A team approach to chronic conditions is emphasized to coordinate care of patients. Comprehensive Rehabilitation is provided by specialists in this field, who act as facilitators, team leaders, and medical experts for rehabilitation.

Training

In the United States, residency training for PM&R is four years long, including an intern year. There are 80 ACGME accredited programs in the United States across 28 states.

Subspecialties

Six formal sub-specializations are recognized by the field in the United States:

- Neuromuscular Medicine
- Pain Medicine
- Pediatric Rehabilitation Medicine
- Spinal Cord Injury Medicine
- Sports Medicine
- Brain Injury Medicine

Other subspecialties within the field that are recognized include the following:

- Hospice and palliative medicine
- Musculoskeletal pain management
- Intervention physiatry
- Surgical rehabilitation
- Rheumatological rehabilitation
- Obesity and other lifestyle disease modifications
- Cardiopulmonary rehabilitation
- Amputee care
- Electrodiagnostic medicine
- Cancer rehabilitation

References

- Verville, Richard (2009). War, Politics, and Philanthropy The History of Rehabilitation Medicine. Lanham, Maryland: University Press of America. ISBN 978-0-7618-4594-2.
- "A Step by Step Guide to Applying for a PM&R Residency". American Academy of Physical Medicine and Rehabilitation. Retrieved 13 May 2016.
- "Physical Medicine and Rehabilitation". Accreditation Council for Graduate Medical Education. Retrieved 13 May 2016.

2

Branches of Physical Medicine and Rehabilitation

The branches of physical medicine and rehabilitation that have been explained in the section are cardiopulmonary rehabilitation, anaplastology and geriatric rehabilitation. Cardiopulmonary rehabilitation is the therapy that deals with the physical functions in patients with cardiac diseases. This section is a compilation of the various branches of physical medicine and rehabilitation that form an integral part of the broader subject matter.

Cardiopulmonary Rehabilitation

Cardiac rehabilitation (CR) is a branch of rehabilitation medicine/Physical Therapy dealing with optimizing physical function in patients with cardiac disease or recent cardiac surgeries. CR services can be provided during hospitalization for the event or in an outpatient setting. While the "glue" of cardiac rehabilitation is exercise, programs are evolving to become comprehensive prevention centers where all aspects of preventive cardiology care are delivered. This includes nutritional therapies, weight loss programs, management of lipid abnormalities with diet and medication, blood pressure control, diabetes management, and stress management. CR exercise and prevention programs are supported by the American Heart Association and the American College of Cardiology.

Procedure

Patients typically enter cardiac rehabilitation in the weeks following an acute coronary event such as a myocardial infarction (heart attack), coronary artery bypass surgery, replacement of a heart valve, percutaneous coronary intervention (such as coronary stent placement), placement of a pacemaker, or placement of an implantable cardioverter defibrillator.

Inpatient Program

Patients receiving CR in the hospital after surgery are usually able to begin within a day or two. First steps include simple motion exercises that can be done sitting down, such as lifting the arms and legs. Heart rate is monitored and continues being monitored as the patient begins to walk.

Outpatient Program

Most patients wishing to participate in outpatient CR are able to begin within 4–6 weeks after surgery. In order to participate in an outpatient program, the patient must first obtain a physician's referral. Participation typically begins with an intake evaluation that includes measurement of cardiac risk factors such as lipid measures, blood pressure, body weight, and smoking status. An exercise stress test is usually performed both to determine if exercise is safe and to allow for the development of a custom exercise program. During exercise, the patient's heart rate and blood pressure are monitored to check the intensity of activity.

Short and long-term risk factors and goals are established, and patients are closely monitored by a "case-manager" who may be a cardiac-trained Registered Nurse, Physiotherapist, respiratory therapist, or an exercise physiologist. A dietitian helps create a healthy eating plan, and a counselor may help to alleviate stress or, for smokers, may give counseling on how to quit.

The duration of the program varies from patient to patient and can range from six months to several years. Even after CR is finished, there are long-term maintenance programs that should not be minimized, as benefits are maintained only with long-term adherence.

Underuse

Participation in cardiac rehabilitation is associated with a 25% decrease in overall mortality over three years.

Cardiac rehabilitation services are significantly underused in the United States, with only 19–29% of patients with eligible cardiac diagnoses participating. Underuse is related to many factors, including lack of available programs nearby and low referral rates by physicians, who often focus more attention on better reimbursed cardiac-intervention procedures than on long-term lifestyle treatments. With a contemporary focus on the cost-effectiveness of medical interventions, CR programs are well-positioned to assume a more prominent role in the long-term care of patients with coronary heart disease.

Benefits

The use of cardiac rehabilitation is well established in the scientific community. A Cochrane Review of 147 studies demonstrated that for myocardial infarction and heart failure patients, exercise-based cardiac rehabilitation improves quality of life and reduces readmission rates. However, there was no benefit in mortality. There appears to be no difference in outcomes between inpatient and outpatient programs. Rehabilitation programs that only have an educational or psychological component have not been shown to be effective.

Anaplastology

Anaplastology (*Gk.* ana-*again, anew, upon* plastos-*something made, formed, molded* logy-*the study of*) is a branch of medicine dealing with the prosthetic rehabilitation of an absent, disfigured or malformed anatomically critical location of the face or body. The term *anaplastology* was coined by Walter G. Spohn and is used worldwide.

An anaplastologist (also known as a maxillofacial prosthetist and technologist in the UK) is an individual who has the knowledge and skill set to provide the service of customizing a facial (craniofacial prosthesis), ocular or somatic prosthesis. In locations around the world where facial, ocular and somatic prostheses are not readily available, a dentist who specializes in maxillofacial prosthetics (prosthodontics), or a dental technician or an ocularist, may also be titled an anaplastologist. In urban or more developed locations, an individual referred to as an anaplastologist is one who solely works with facial, ocular or somatic prostheses. In such a setting, there are times the anaplastologist collaborates with prosthodontists and ocularists.

The studies of an anaplastologist consist of the arts and sciences. Visual arts are studied, namely photography, illustration, sculpture, and painting. Biology, behavioral sciences, materials science, and physics are the studied sciences with emphases in superficial anatomy and physiology of humans, polymer science, optics, dermatology, oral and maxillofacial surgery, otolaryngology, and oncology to name a few.

Certification in the field of anaplastology is provided by the Board for Certification in Clinical Anaplastology (BCCA). Professionals certified by the BCCA are designated as Certified Clinical Anaplastologists and denote their credential with the CCA title.

Geriatric Rehabilitation

Geriatric rehabilitation or geriatric physical therapy is the branch of medicine that studies rehabilitation and physical therapy issues in elderly.

Origins

Geriatric rehabilitation covers three areas – normal aging due to disuse and deconditioning, cardiovascular problems like vascular disease and stroke, and skeletal problems including osteoporosis and osteoarthritis conditions such as knee and hip replacements. Physical medicine physicians use rehabilitation to work toward the goal of returning the patient to a pre-injury quality of life and may use physical, occupational, and speech therapies.

With increased age, patients often face many physical and emotional changes that can affect level of function and well-being. Rehabilitation maintains functional independence in the elderly. Rehabilitation of geriatric patients is imperative for the patients' well-being and for society, so that we can thrive socially and economically. Essential to geriatric rehabilitation is communication, specifically improving any sensory impairment, including those related to vision and hearing. The prevention of falls and osteoporosis can improve the patient's health and longevity. Addressing malnutrition can promote healing and vitalize the patient to participate in a formal rehabilitation program. Depression is common in the older population if a functional loss of mobility and an inability to perform activities of daily living (ADLs) predominates. Cognitive impairment, such as delirium and dementia, can affect the patient's rehabilitation goals and outcomes. Finally, a driver's evaluation for an appropriate elderly candidate is an underutilized part of rehabilitation that has a considerable impact on society.

Geriatric rehabilitation also have a role in intermediate care, where patients are referred by a hospital or family doctor, when there is a requirement to provide hospital based short term intensive physical therapy aimed at the recovery of musculoskeletal function, particularly recovery from joint, tendon, or ligament repair and, or, physical medicine and rehabilitation care when elderly patients get out of sync with their medication resulting in a deterioration of their personal health which reduces their ability to live independently.

Finally, geriatric rehabilitation has a large influence on the growing life expectancy around the globe. The American Physical Therapy Association (APTA) surveyed 556 adults over 65 years old in order to gain an understanding on the factors that affect adherence to an exercise program. Adherence to an exercise program influences frailty, speed, ability to live independently, and best of all, life expectancy. The study compared two factors: exercise barriers and motivation. The study concluded that exercise barriers play the largest role in determining adherence to a home exercise program (HEP). According to APTA, motivators include self-efficacy, the ability to control behavior, and outcome expectation, the belief that consequences follow certain actions. APTA describes barriers as: insufficient time, lack of social support, no place to exercise, limited finances, no transportation, and the fear of falling. Researchers recently found that depression, stress levels, increased age, decreased health status and lack of pleasure while exercising contribute to exercise adherence.

3

Sub-Specialization of Physical Medicine

Physical therapy is a specialty in the field of physical medicine and rehabilitation and it uses mechanical force and movements and physical intervention. The topics elucidated in this section are neuromuscular medicine, sports medicine, pain management, spinal cord injury and postural restoration. Physical medicine is best understood in confluence with the major topics listed in the following chapter.

Physical Therapy

Physical therapy (PT), also known as physiotherapy, is a physical medicine and rehabilitation specialty that, by using mechanical force and movements, remediates impairments and promotes mobility, function, and quality of life through examination, diagnosis, prognosis, and physical intervention. It is performed by physical therapists (known as physiotherapists in many countries).

In addition to clinical practice, other activities encompassed in the physical therapy profession include research, education, consultation, and administration. Physical therapy services may be provided alongside, or in conjunction with, other medical services.

Overview

Physical therapy attempts to address the illnesses, or injuries that limit a person's abilities to move and perform functional activities in their daily lives. PTs use an individual's history and physical examination to arrive at a diagnosis and establish a management plan and, when necessary, incorporate the results of laboratory and imaging studies like X-rays, CT-scan, or MRI findings. Electrodiagnostic testing (e.g., electromyograms and nerve conduction velocity testing) may also be used. PT management commonly includes prescription of or assistance with specific exercises, manual therapy and manipulation, mechanical devices such as traction, education, physical agents which includes heat, cold, electricity, sound waves, radiation, rays, prescription of assistive devices, prostheses, orthoses and other interventions. In addition, PTs work with individuals to prevent the loss of mobility before it occurs by developing fitness and wellness-oriented programs for healthier and more active lifestyles, providing services to individuals and populations to develop, maintain and restore maximum movement and functional ability throughout the lifespan. This includes providing therapeutic treatment in circumstances where movement and function are threatened by aging, injury, disease or environmental factors. Functional movement is central to what it means to be healthy.

Physical therapy is a professional career which has many specialties including sports, neurology, wound care, EMG, cardiopulmonary, geriatrics, orthopedics, women's health, and pediatrics. Neurological rehabilitation is in particular a rapidly emerging field. PTs practice in many settings, such as private-owned physical therapy clinics, outpatient clinics or offices, health and wellness clinics, rehabilitation hospitals facilities, skilled nursing facilities, extended care facilities, private homes, education and research centers, schools, hospices, industrial and this workplaces or other occupational environments, fitness centers and sports training facilities.

Physical therapists also practise in the non-patient care roles such as health policy, health insurance, health care administration and as health care executives. Physical therapists are involved in the medical-legal field serving as experts, performing peer review and independent medical examinations.

Education varies greatly by country. The span of education ranges from some countries having little formal education to others having doctoral degrees and post doctoral residencies and fellowships.

History

Exercise to shoulder and elbow to increase motion following fracture and dislocation of humerus is being given by an Army therapist to a soldier patient.

Physicians like Hippocrates and later Galen are believed to have been the first practitioners of physical therapy, advocating massage, manual therapy techniques and hydrotherapy to treat people in 460 BC. After the development of orthopedics in the eighteenth century, machines like the Gymnasticon were developed to treat gout and similar diseases by systematic exercise of the joints, similar to later developments in physical therapy. The earliest documented origins of actual physical therapy as a professional group date back to Per Henrik Ling, "Father of Swedish Gymnastics," who founded the Royal Central Institute of Gymnastics (RCIG) in 1813 for manipulation, and exercise. The Swedish word for physical therapist is *sjukgymnast* = someone involved in gymnastics for those who are ill. In 1887, PTs were given official registration by Sweden's National Board of Health and Welfare. Other countries soon followed. In 1894, four nurses in Great Britain formed the Chartered Society of Physiotherapy. The School of Physiotherapy at the University of Otago in New Zealand in 1913, and the United States' 1914 Reed College in Portland, Oregon, which graduated "reconstruction aides." Since the profession's inception, spinal manipulative therapy has been a component of the physical therapist practice.

Modern physical therapy was established towards the end of the 19th century due to events that had an effect on a global scale, which called for rapid advances in physical therapy. Soon following American orthopedic surgeons began treating children with disabilities and began employing women trained in physical education, and remedial exercise. These treatments were applied and promoted further during the Polio outbreak of 1916. During the First World War women were recruited to work with and restore physical function to injured soldiers, and the field of physical therapy was institutionalized. In 1918 the term "Reconstruction Aide" was used to refer to individuals practicing physical therapy. The first school of physical therapy was established at Walter Reed Army Hospital in Washington, D.C., following the outbreak of World War I. Research catalyzed the physical therapy movement. The first physical therapy research was published in the United States in March 1921 in "The PT Review." In the same year, Mary McMillan organized the Physical Therapy Association (now called the American Physical Therapy Association (APTA). In 1924, the Georgia Warm Springs Foundation promoted the field by touting physical therapy as a treatment for polio. Treatment through the 1940s primarily consisted of exercise, massage, and traction. Manipulative procedures to the spine and extremity joints began to be practiced, especially in the British Commonwealth countries, in the early 1950s. Around this time when polio vaccines were developed, physical therapists have become a normal occurrence in hospitals throughout North America and Europe. In the late 1950s, physical therapists started to move beyond hospital-based practice to outpatient orthopedic clinics, public schools, colleges/universities health-centres, geriatric settings (skilled nursing facilities), rehabilitation centers and medical centers. Specialization for physical therapy in the U.S. occurred in 1974, with the Orthopaedic Section of the APTA being formed for those physical therapists specializing in orthopaedics. In the same year, the International Federation of Orthopaedic Manipulative Physical Therapists was formed, which has ever since played an important role in advancing manual therapy worldwide.

Education

Educational criteria for physical therapy providers vary from state to state and from country to country, and among various levels of professional responsibility. Most U.S. states have physical therapy practice acts that recognize both physical therapists (PT) and physical therapist assistants (PTA) and some jurisdictions also recognize physical therapy technicians (PT Techs) or aides. Most countries have licensing bodies that require physical therapists to be a member of before they can start practicing as independent professionals.

Physical Therapists

United States

The primary physical therapy practitioner is the Physical Therapist (PT) who is trained and licensed to examine, evaluate, diagnose and treat impairment, functional limitations and disabilities in patients or clients. Physical Therapist education curricula in the United States culminate in a Doctor of Physical Therapy (DPT) degree, but many currently practising PTs hold a Master of Physical Therapy degree, and some still hold a Bachelor's degree. Currently the education programs for physical therapy have changed. The Master of Physical Therapy and Master of Science in Physical Therapy degrees are no longer offered, and the entry-level degree is the Doctor of Physical Therapy degree, which typically takes 3 years. PTs who hold a Masters or bachelors in PT are encouraged to get their DPT because APTA's goal is for all PT's to be on a doctoral level. [WCPT recommends physical therapist entry-level educational programs be based on university or university-level studies, of a minimum of four years, independently validated and accredited. Curricula in the United States are accredited by the Commission on Accreditation in Physical Therapy Education (CAPTE). According to CAPTE, as of 2012 there are 25,660 students currently enrolled in 210 accredited PT programs in the United States. Updated CAPTE statistics list that for 2015-2016, there are 30,419 students enrolled in 233 accredited PT programs in the United States.

The physical therapist professional curriculum includes content in the clinical sciences (e.g., content about the cardiovascular, pulmonary, endocrine, metabolic, gastrointestinal, genitourinary, integumentary, musculoskeletal, and neuromuscular systems and the medical and surgical conditions frequently seen by physical therapists). Current training is specifically aimed to enable physical therapists to appropriately recognize and refer non-musculoskeletal diagnoses that may presently similarly to those caused by systems not appropriate for physical therapy intervention, which has resulted in direct access to physical therapists in many states.

Post-doctoral residency and fellowship education prevalence is increasing steadily with 219 residency, and 42 fellowship programs accredited in 2016. Residencies are aimed to train physical therapists in a specialty such as acute care, cardiovascular & pulmonary, clinical electrophysiology, faculty, geriatrics, neurology, orthopaedics, pediatrics, sports, women's health, and wound care, whereas fellowships train specialists in a subspecialty (e.g. critical care, hand therapy, and division 1 sports), similar to the medical model. Residency programs offer eligibility to sit for the specialist certification in their respective area of practice. For example, completion of an orthopaedic physical therapy residency, allows its graduates to apply and sit for the clinical specialist examination in orthopaedics, achieving the OCS designation upon passing the examination. Board certification of physical therapy specialists is aimed to recognize individuals with advanced clinical knowledge and skill training in their respective area of practice, and exemplifies the trend toward greater education to optimally treat individuals with movement dysfunction.

Canada

Canadian Physiotherapy programs are offered at 15 Universities, often through the university's respective college of medicine. In the past decade, each of Canada's physical therapy schools has transitioned from 3-year Bachelor of Science in Physical Therapy (BScPT) programs that required 2 years of pre-requisites university courses (5-year bachelor's degree) to 2-year Master's of Physical Therapy (MPT) programs that require pre-requisite bachelor's degrees. The last Canadian university to follow suit was the University of Manitoba who transitioned to the MPT program in 2012, making the MPT credential the new entry to practice standard across Canada. Existing practitioners with BScPT credentials are not required to upgrade their qualifications.

In the province of Quebec, prospective physiotherapists are required to have completed a college diploma in either health sciences, which lasts on average two years, or physical rehabilitation technology, which lasts at least three years, to apply to a physiotherapy program or program in university. Following admission, physical therapy students work on a bachelor of science with a major in physical therapy and rehabilitation. The B.Sc. usually requires three years to complete. Students must then enter graduate school to complete a master's degree in physical therapy, which normally requires one and a half to two years of study. Graduates who obtain their M.Sc. must successfully pass the membership examination to become member of the Ordre professionnel de la physiothérapie du Québec (OPPQ). Physiotherapists can pursue their education in such fields as rehabilitation sciences, sports medicine, kinesiology, and physiology.

To date, there are no bridging programs available to facilitate upgrading from the BScPT to the MPT credential. However, research Master's of Science (MSc) and Doctor of Philosophy (PhD) programs are available at every university. Aside from academic research, practitioners can upgrade their skills and qualifications through continuing education courses and curriculums. Continuing education is a requirement of the provincial regulatory bodies.

The Canadian Alliance of Physiotherapy Regulators (CAPR), or simply known as The Alliance, offers eligible program graduates to apply for the national Physiotherapy Competency Examination (PCE). Passing the PCE is one of the requirements in most provinces and territories to work as a licensed physiotherapist in Canada. The Alliance has members which are physiotherapy regulatory organizations recognized in their respective provinces and territories:

- Government of Yukon, Consumer Services
- College of Physical Therapists of British Columbia
- Physiotherapy Alberta College + Association
- Saskatchewan College of Physical Therapists
- College of Physiotherapists of Manitoba
- College of Physiotherapists of Ontario
- Ordre professionnel de la physiothérapie du Québec
- College of Physiotherapists of New Brunswick/Collège des physiothérapeutes

du Nouveau-Brunswick

- Nova Scotia College of Physiotherapists
- Prince Edward Island College of Physiotherapists
- Newfoundland & Labrador College of Physiotherapists

The Canadian Physiotherapy Association offers a curriculum of continuing education courses in orthopaedics and manual therapy. The program consists of 5 levels (7 courses) of training with ongoing mentorship and evaluation at each level. The orthopaedic curriculum and examinations takes a minimum of 4 years to complete. However, upon completion of level 2, physiotherapists can apply to a unique 1-year course-based Master's program in advanced orthopaedics and manipulation at the University of Western Ontario to complete their training. This program accepts only 16 physiotherapists annually since 2007. Successful completion of either of these education streams and their respective examinations allows physiotherapists the opportunity to apply to the Canadian Academy of Manipulative Physiotherapy (CAMPT) for fellowship. Fellows of the Canadian Academy of manipulative Physiotherapists (FCAMPT) are considered leaders in the field, having extensive post-graduate education in orthopaedics and manual therapy. FCAMPT is an internationally recognized credential, as CAMPT is a member of the International Federation of Manipulative Physiotherapists (IFOMPT), a branch of the World Confederation of Physical Therapy (WCPT) and the World Health Organization (WHO).

Physical Therapist Assistants

Physical therapist assistants may deliver treatment and physical interventions for patients and clients under a care plan established by and under the supervision of a physical therapist. Physical therapist assistants in the United States are currently trained under associate of applied sciences curricula specific to the profession, as outlined and accredited by CAPTE. As of August 2011, there were 276 accredited two-year (Associate degree) programs for physical therapist assistants In the United States of America. According to CAPTE, as of 2012 there are 10,598 students currently enrolled in 280 accredited PTA programs in the United States. Updated CAPTE statistics list that for 2015-2016, there are 12,726 students enrolled in 340 accredited PTA programs in the United States.

Curricula for the physical therapist assistant associate degree include:

- Anatomy & physiology
- Exercise physiology
- Human biology
- Physics

- Biomechanics
- Kinesiology
- Neuroscience
- Clinical pathology
- Behavioral sciences
- Communication
- Ethics
- Research
- Other coursework as required by individual programs.

Physical Therapy Technicians or Aides

Some jurisdictions allow physical therapists to employ technicians or aides or therapy assistants to perform designated routine tasks related to physical therapy under the direct supervision of a physical therapist. Some jurisdictions require physical therapy technicians or aides to be certified, and education and certification requirements vary among jurisdictions.

Canada

In the province of Quebec, physical rehabilitation therapists are health care professionals who are required to complete a three-year college diploma program in physical rehabilitation therapy and be member of the *Ordre professionnel de la physiothérapie du Québec* (OPPQ) in order to practise legally in the country.

Most physical rehabilitation therapists complete their college diploma at Collège Montmorency, Dawson College, or Cégep Marie-Victorin, all situated in and around the Montreal area.

After completing their technical college diploma, graduates have the opportunity to pursue their studies at the university level to perhaps obtain a bachelor's degree in physiotherapy, kinesiology, exercise science, or occupational therapy. The Université de Montréal, the Université Laval and the Université de Sherbrooke are among the Québécois universities that admit physical rehabilitation therapists in their programs of study related to health sciences and rehabilitation in order to credit courses that were completed in college.

United States

Job duties and education requirements for Physical Therapy Technicians or Aides may vary depending on the employer, but education requirements range from high school diploma or equivalent to completion of a 2-year degree program. O-Net reports that 64% of PT Aides/Techs have a high school diploma or equivalent, 21% have completed some college but do not hold a degree, and 10% hold an associate degree.

Employment

Physical therapy-related jobs in North America have shown rapid growth in recent years, but employment rates and average wages may vary significantly between different countries, states, provinces or regions.

United States of America

According to the United States Department of Labor's Bureau of Labor Statistics, there were approximately 198,600 Physical Therapists employed in the United States in 2010, earning an average $76,310 annually, or $36.69 per hour, with 39% growth in employment projected by the year 2020. The Bureau of Labor Statistics also reports that there were approximately 114,400 Physical Therapist Assistants and Aides employed in the United States in 2010, earning an average $37,710 annually, or $18.13 per hour, with 45% growth in employment projected by the year 2020. To meet their needs, many healthcare and physical therapy facilities hire "Travel physical therapists", who work temporary assignments between 8 and 26 weeks for much higher wages; about $113,500 a year. Bureau of Labor Statistics data on PTAs and Techs can be difficult to decipher, due to their tendency to report data on these job fields collectively rather than separately. O-Net reports that in 2011, PTAs in the United States earned a median wage of $51,040 annually or $24.54 hourly, and that Aides/Techs earned a median wage of $23,680 annually or $11.39 hourly in 2011.

Specialty Areas

The body of knowledge of physical therapy is large, and therefore physical therapists may specialize in a specific clinical area. While there are many different types of physical therapy, the American Board of Physical Therapy Specialties lists nine current specialist certifications, the ninth, Oncology, pending for its first examination in 2019. Most Physical Therapists practicing in a specialty will have undergone further training, such as an accredited residency program, although individuals are currently able to sit for their specialist examination after 2,000 hours of focused practice in their respective specialty population, in addition to requirements set by each respective specialty board.

Cardiovascular & Pulmonary Physiotherapy

Cardiovascular and pulmonary rehabilitation respiratory practitioners and physical therapists offer therapy for a wide variety of cardiopulmonary disorders or pre and post cardiac or pulmonary surgery. An example of cardiac surgery is coronary bypass surgery. Primary goals of this specialty include increasing endurance and functional independence. Manual therapy is used in this field to assist in clearing lung secretions experienced with cystic fibrosis. Pulminary disorders, heart attacks, post coronary bypass surgery, chronic obstructive pulmonary disease, and pulmonary fibrosis, treatments can benefit from cardiovascular and pulmonary specialized physical therapists.

Clinical Electrophysiology

This specialty area includes electrotherapy/physical agents, electrophysiological evaluation (EMG/NCV), physical agents, and wound management.

Geriatric

Geriatric physical therapy covers a wide area of issues concerning people as they go through normal adult aging but is usually focused on the older adult. There are many conditions that affect many people as they grow older and include but are not limited to the following: arthritis, osteoporosis, cancer, Alzheimer's disease, hip and joint replacement, balance disorders, incontinence, etc. Geriatric physical therapists specialize in providing therapy for such conditions in older adults.

Integumentary

Integumentary physical therapy includes the treatment of conditions involving the skin and all its related organs. Common conditions managed include wounds and burns. Physical therapists may utilize surgical instruments, wound irrigations, dressings and topical agents to remove the damaged or contaminated tissue and promote tissue healing. Other commonly used interventions include exercise, edema control, splinting, and compression garments. The work done by physical therapists in the integumentary specialty do work similar to what would be done by medical doctors or nurses in the emergency room or triage.

Neurological

Neurological physical therapy is a field focused on working with individuals who have a neurological disorder or disease. These can include stroke, chronic back pain, Alzheimer's disease, Charcot-Marie-Tooth disease (CMT), ALS, brain injury, cerebral palsy, l.g.b. syndrome, multiple sclerosis, Parkinson's disease, facial palsy and spinal cord injury. Common impairments associated with neurologic conditions include impairments of vision, balance, ambulation, activities of daily living, movement, muscle strength and loss of functional independence. The techniques involve in neurological physical therapy are wide ranging and often require specialized training.

Neurological physiotherapy is also called neurophysiotherapy or neurological rehabilitation.

Orthopedic

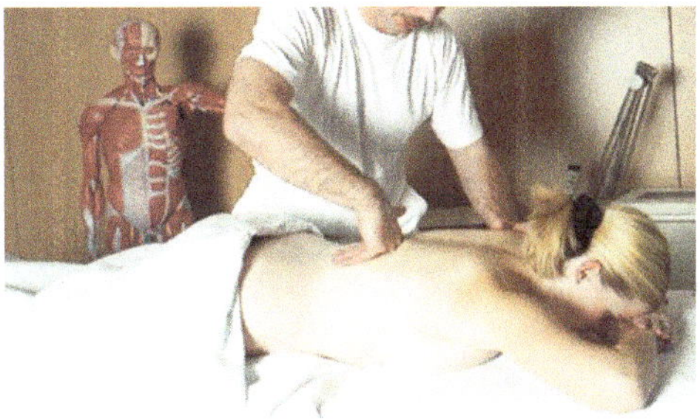

Treatment by orthopedic physical therapists

Orthopedic physical therapists diagnose, manage, and treat disorders and injuries of the musculoskeletal system including rehabilitation after orthopedic surgery. acute trauma such as sprains, strains, and injuries of insidious onset such as tendinopathy and bursitis. This speciality of physical therapy is most often found in the out-patient clinical setting. Orthopedic therapists are trained in the treatment of post-operative orthopedic procedures, fractures, acute sports injuries, arthritis, sprains, strains, back and neck pain, spinal conditions, and amputations.

Joint and spine mobilization/manipulation, dry needling (similar to acupuncture), therapeutic exercise, neuromuscular techniques, muscle reeducation, hot/cold packs, and electrical muscle stimulation (e.g., cryotherapy, iontophoresis, electrotherapy) are modalities employed to expedite recovery in the orthopedic setting. Additionally, an emerging adjunct to diagnosis and treatment is the use of sonography for diagnosis and to guide treatments such as muscle retraining. Those who have suffered injury or disease affecting the muscles, bones, ligaments, or tendons will benefit from assessment by a physical therapist specialized in orthopedics.

Pediatric

Pediatric physical therapy assists in early detection of health problems and uses a limited variety of modalities to provide physical therapy for disorders in the pediatric population. These therapists are specialized in the diagnosis, treatment, and management of infants, children, and adolescents with a variety of congenital, developmental, neuromuscular, skeletal, or acquired disorders/diseases. Treatments focus mainly on improving gross and fine motor skills, balance and coordination, strength and endurance as well as cognitive and sensory processing/integration.

Sports

Physical therapists are closely involved in the care and wellbeing of athletes including recreational, semi-professional (paid) and professional (full-time employment) participants. This area of practice encompasses athletic injury management under 5 main categories:

1. acute care - assessment and diagnosis of an initial injury;
2. treatment - application of specialist advice and techniques to encourage healing;
3. rehabilitation - progressive management for full return to sport;
4. prevention - identification and address of deficiencies known to directly result in, or act as precursors to injury, such as movement assessment
5. education - sharing of specialist knowledge to individual athletes, teams or clubs to assist in prevention or management of injury

Physical therapists who work for professional sport teams often have a specialized sports certification issued through their national registering organisation. Most Physical therapists who practice in a sporting environment are also active in collaborative sports medicine programs too

Women's Health

Women's health physical therapy mostly addresses women's issues related to the female reproductive system, child birth, and post-partum. These conditions include lymphedema, osteoporosis, pelvic pain, prenatal and post-partum periods, and urinary incontinence. It also addresses incontinence, pelvic pain, and other disorders associated with pelvic floor dysfunction. Manual physical therapy has been demonstrated in multiple studies to increase rates of conception in women with infertility.

Palliative Care

Physiotherapy in the field of oncology and palliative care is a continuously evolving and developing specialty, both in malignant and non-malignant diseases. Rehabilitation for both groups of patients is now recognized as an essential part of the clinical pathway, as early diagnoses and new treatments are enabling patients to live longer. it is generally accepted that patients should have access to an appropriate level of rehabilitation, so that they can function at a minimum level of dependency and optimize their quality of life, regardless of their life expectancy.

Effectiveness

A 2012 systematic review found evidence to support the use of spine manipulation by physical therapists as a safe option to improve outcomes for low back pain. A 2015 systematic review suggested that spine manipulation and therapeutic massage are effective interventions for neck pain; it also suggested, however, that electroacupuncture, strain-counterstrain, relaxation massage, heat therapy and ultrasound therapy are not effective and thus not recommended for the treatment of neck pain.

United States

Definitions and licensing requirements in the United States vary among jurisdictions, as each state has enacted its own physical therapy practice act defining the profession within its jurisdiction, but the American Physical Therapy Association (APTA) has also drafted a model definition in order to limit this variation, and the APTA is also responsible for accrediting physical therapy education curricula throughout the United States of America.

Neuromuscular Medicine

The field of neuromuscular medicine is subspecialty of neurology and physical medicine and rehabilitation. The field includes diseases that impact some part of the neuromuscular system such as the peripheral nerves (those in arms, legs, face and neck), muscle motor neurons, and neuromuscular junction – the spot where nerves and muscles come together. The field encompasses issues related to both diagnosis and medical treatment of these conditions, as well as relevant rehabilitation interventions to optimize the quality of life of individuals with these conditions. This field encompasses disorders that impact both adults and children. Many of the disorders are genetic. They however can also result from an abnormal immune response, a genetic mutation, and sometimes the cause is unknown. Because they frequently have no cure, the focus is on providing improvements in the patients quality of life by reducing symptoms. A formal educational process that includes one year of fellowship training following completion of residency training in neurology or physical medicine and rehabilitation was approved by the Accreditation Council for Graduate Medical Education.

Diagnostic Tools

The tools used by phyicians specializing in neuromuscular medicine to diagnose neuromuscular disorders include (nerve and muscle biopsy), needle and nerve conduction studytesting, and molecular and genetic tests.

Sports Medicine

Sports medicine, also known as sport and exercise medicine (SEM), is a branch of medicine that deals with physical fitness and the treatment and prevention of injuries related to sports and exercise. Although most sports teams have employed team physicians for many years, it is only since the late 20th century that sports medicine has emerged as a distinct field of health care.

Scope

Sport and exercise medicine doctors are specialist physicians who have completed medical school, appropriate residency training and then specialize further in sports medicine or 'sports and exercise medicine' (the preferred term). Specialization in sports medicine may be a doctor's first specialty (as in Australia, Netherlands, Norway, Italy). It may also be a sub-specialty or second specialisation following a specialisation such as physiatry or orthopedic surgery. The various approaches reflect the medical culture in different countries.

Specializing in the treatment of athletes and other physically active individuals, sports and exercise medicine physicians have extensive education in musculoskeletal medicine. SEM doctors treat injuries such as muscle, ligament, tendon and bone problems, but may also treat chronic illnesses that can affect physical performance, such as asthma and diabetes. SEM doctors also advise on managing and preventing injuries.

Specialists in SEM diagnose and treat any medical conditions which regular exercisers or sports persons encounter. The majority of an SEM physician's time is therefore spent treating musculoskeletal injuries, however other conditions include sports cardiology issues, unexplained underperformance syndrome, exercise-induced asthma, screening for cardiac abnormalities and diabetes in sports. In addition team physicians working in elite sports often play a role in performance medicine, whereby an athletes' physiology is monitored, and aberrations corrected, in order to achieve peak physical performance.

SEM consultants also deliver clinical physical activity interventions, negating the burden of disease directly attributable to physical inactivity and the compelling evidence for the effectiveness of exercise in the primary, secondary and tertiary prevention of disease.

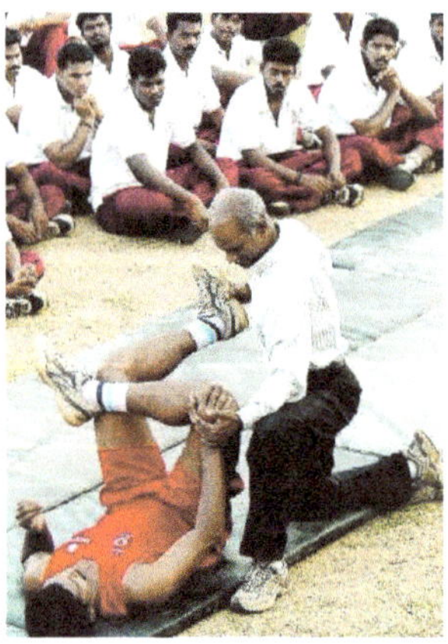

Exercise Medicine

The Foresight Report issued by the UK's Government Office for Science, 17 October

2007, highlighted the unsustainable health and economic costs of a nation that continues to be largely sedentary. It forecasts that the incremental costs of this inactivity will be $10 billion per year by 2050 and the wider costs to society and businesses $49.9billion. Physical inactivity inevitably leads to ill-health and it forecasts the cost of paying for this impact will be unsustainable in the future. No existing group of medical specialists is equipped with the skills and training to deal with this challenge.

Public Health

SEM physicians are frequently involved in promoting the therapeutic benefits of physical activity, exercise and sport for the individuals and communities. SEM Physicians in the UK spend a period of their training in public health, and advise public health physicians on matters relating to physical activity promotion. An example of published work includes the Royal College of Physicians publications.

Common Sports Injuries

Concussion – caused by severe head injury where the brain moves violently within the skull so that brain cells all fire at once, much like a seizure

Muscle cramps – a sudden tight, intense pain caused by a muscle locked in spasm. Muscle cramps are also recognized as an involuntary and forcibly contracted muscle that does not relax

ACL sprains – The anterior cruciate ligament (ACL) is a ligament involved in knee stabilization. An ACL rupture can occur when the foot is planted and the knee twists to change direction.

ACL tears – The anterior cruciate ligament; one of four major knee ligament necessary for comfortable knee movement, tears, causing major pain and causes the knee to “give out”. The knee ACL can tear for a number of reasons.

Ankle sprain – The ligaments that hold the ankle bones in place can easily be overstretched.

Shin splints – The tissue that attaches the muscles of your lower leg to the shin bone may be pulling away from the bone, or it may be inflamed from overuse.

Muscle strains – tears in muscle that cause pain and or loss of function

History

In recent years Western society has increasingly recognized the dangers of physical inactivity, and significant efforts have been made within the public health community to encourage the nation to become more physically active. To reflect this paradigm shift BASM has renamed itself BASEM (British Association of Sport and Exercise Medicine) and the speciality itself has rebranded from Sports Medicine to Sport & Exercise Medicine. Since 2007 several deaneries across the UK have established training programmes in SEM, and recurrent funding for 50 National Training Numbers (NTN's) is available.

Organizations

- American College of Sports Medicine (ACSM) Founded in 1954, the American College of Sports Medicine is the largest and most prominent sports medicine and exercise science organization in the world. ACSM has more than 45,000 International, National and Regional Chapter members.
- American Orthopaedic Society for Sports Medicine (AOSSM) The American Orthopaedic Society for Sports Medicine is a world leader in sports medicine education, research, communication, and fellowship. Founded in 1972, AOSSM is an international organization of orthopaedic surgeons and other allied health professionals dedicated to sports medicine. Essentially every professional and collegiate team has a team physician who is a member of the AOSSM.
- American Medical Society for Sports Medicine (AMSSM) Founded in 1991, AMSSM is a multi-disciplinary organization of physicians whose members are dedicated to education, research, collaboration and fellowship within the field of Sports Medicine. It now comprises over 2100 Sports Medicine Physicians whose goal is to provide a link between the rapidly expanding core of knowledge related to sports medicine and its application to patients in a clinical setting.
- National Athletic Trainers' Association(NATA) Founded in 1950, the mission of the National Athletic Trainers Association is to enhance the quality of health care provided by certified athletic trainers and to advance the athletic training profession.
- Canadian Athletic Therapists' Association(CATA) Founded in 1965. The Canadian Athletic Therapists Association (CATA) is an organization devoted to the comprehensive health care of an individual at any level of physical ability by Certified Athletic Therapists.
- American Medical Association(AMA) The American Medical Association recognized Athletic Training(AT) as an allied health profession in 1990.
- International Society of Arthroscopy, Knee Surgery and Sports Medicine (ISAKOS) The ISAKOS - International Society of Arthroscopy, Knee Surgery and Orthopaedic Sports Medicine is an international society with over 4,000 surgeons members, dedicated to advancing of education, research and patient care in arthroscopy, knee surgery and orthopaedic sports medicine around the world.
- International Association for Dance Medicine and Science (IADMS) The International Association for Dance Medicine & Science was formed in 1990 by an

international group of dance medicine practitioners, dance educators, dance scientists, and dancers. Membership is drawn equally from the medical and dance professions, and has grown from an initial 48 members in 1991 to over 900 members at present worldwide, representing 35 countries.

Hospice and Palliative Medicine

Hospice and palliative medicine is a formal subspecialty of medicine in the United States that focuses on symptom management, relief of suffering and end-of-life care.

In 2006, *hospice and palliative medicine* was officially recognized by the American Board of Medical Specialties, and is *co-sponsored* by

- the American Boards of Internal Medicine
- Anesthesiology
- Family Medicine
- Physical Medicine and Rehabilitation
- Psychiatry and Neurology
- Surgery
- Pediatrics
- Emergency Medicine
- Radiology
- Obstetrics and Gynecology.

Physicians who complete a residency in one of the *co-sponsoring* specialties are then eligible for further training in an ACGME-approved Hospice and Palliative Medicine fellowship program, after which they must pass the official examination to be board-certified in the subspecialty.

In 2007, the American Osteopathic Association Bureau of Osteopathic Specialists approved a Certificate of Added Qualifications (CAQ) in *hospice and palliative medicine*. By 2012 participants are the American Osteopathic Boards of

- Internal Medicine
- Family Medicine
- Neurology and Psychiatry

- Physical Medicine and Rehabilitation.

Candidates are eligible for CAQ certification after achieving board-certification following an American Osteopathic Association-approved residency.

Scope of the Subspecialty

Physicians in this subspecialty have advanced knowledge and skills to prevent and relieve the suffering experienced by patients with life-limiting, life-threatening and terminal illnesses. This specialist has expertise in the assessment of patients with advanced disease and catastrophic injury, the relief of distressing symptoms, the coordination of interdisciplinary patient and family-centered care in diverse settings, the use of specialized care systems including hospice, the management of the imminently dying patient; and legal and ethical decision making in end-of-life care. They work with an interdisciplinary hospice or palliative care team to maximize quality of life while addressing physical, psychological, social and spiritual needs of both patients and family members throughout the course of the disease, including through the dying process and subsequent bereavement. This carc can occur within or outside of a formal hospice or palliative care team.

Professional Organization

The American Academy of Hospice and Palliative Medicine (AAHPM) is the leading professional organization for physicians subspecializing in hospice and palliative medicine in North America. The International Association for Hospice and Palliative Care is the major professional organization devoted to the global spread of hospice and palliative medicine.

Pain Management

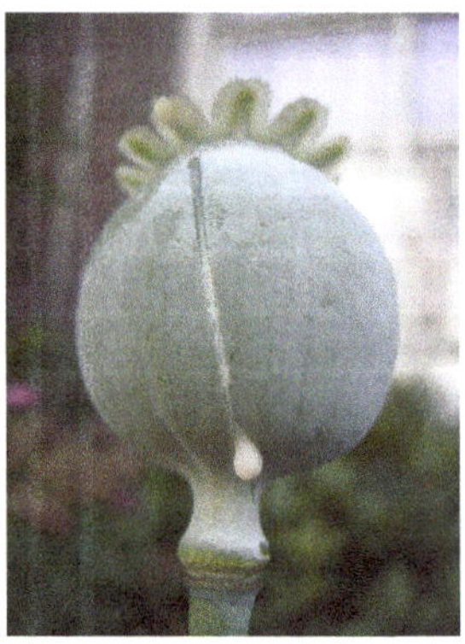

Opium poppies such as this one provide ingredients for the class of analgesics called opiates

Pain management, pain medicine, pain control or algiatry, is a branch of medicine employing an interdisciplinary approach for easing the suffering and improving the quality of life of those living with chronic pain The typical pain management team includes medical practitioners, pharmacists, clinical psychologists, physiotherapists, occupational therapists, physician assistants, nurse practitioners, and clinical nurse specialists. The team may also include other mental health specialists and massage therapists. Pain sometimes resolves promptly once the underlying trauma or pathology has healed, and is treated by one practitioner, with drugs such as analgesics and (occasionally) anxiolytics. Effective management of chronic (long-term) pain, however, frequently requires the coordinated efforts of the management team.

Medicine treats injury and pathology to support and speed healing; and treats distressing symptoms such as pain to relieve suffering during treatment and healing. When a painful injury or pathology is resistant to treatment and persists, when pain persists after the injury or pathology has healed, and when medical science cannot identify the cause of pain, the task of medicine is to relieve suffering. Treatment approaches to chronic pain include pharmacological measures, such as analgesics, antidepressants and anticonvulsants, interventional procedures, physical therapy, physical exercise, application of ice and/or heat, and psychological measures, such as biofeedback and cognitive behavioral therapy.

Uses

Pain can have many causes and there are many possible treatments for it. In the nursing profession, one common definition of pain is any problem that is "whatever the experiencing person says it is, existing whenever the experiencing person says it does". Different sorts of pain management address different sorts of pain.

Pain management includes patient communication about the pain problem. To define the pain problem, a health care provider will likely ask questions such as these:

- How intense is the pain?
- How does the pain feel?
- Where is the pain?
- What, if anything, makes the pain lessen?
- When did the pain start?

After asking questions such as these, the health care provider will have a description of the pain. Pain management will then be used to address that pain.

Adverse Effects

There are many types of pain management, and each of them have their own benefits, drawbacks, and limits.

A common difficulty in pain management is communication. People experiencing pain may have difficulty recognizing or describing what they feel and how intense it is. Health care providers and patients may have difficulty communicating with each other about how pain responds to treatments. There is a continuing risk in many types of pain management for the patient to take treatment which is less effective than needed or which causes other difficulty and side effects. Some treatments for pain can be harmful if overused. A goal of pain management for the patient and their health care provider to identify the amount of treatment which addresses the pain but which is not too much treatment.

Another problem with pain management is that pain is the body's natural way of communicating a problem. Pain is supposed to resolve as the body heals itself with time and pain management. Sometimes pain management covers a problem, and the patient might be less aware that they need treatment for a deeper problem.

Physical Approach

Physical Medicine and Rehabilitation

Physical medicine and rehabilitation employs diverse physical techniques such as thermal agents and electrotherapy, as well as therapeutic exercise and behavioral therapy, alone or in tandem with interventional techniques and conventional pharmacotherapy to treat pain, usually as part of an interdisciplinary or multidisciplinary program.

TENS

Transcutaneous electrical nerve stimulation has been found to be ineffective for lower back pain, however, it might help with diabetic neuropathy. Although there has not been adequate evidence based research on acute sensory TENS, chronic conditions are efficacious in relieving pain. TENS is indicated for any chronic musculoskeletal condition under the gate control theory of pain. Essentially, the gate control theory states that sensory fibers carry their signal faster than pain fibers, and thus make their way to the dorsal root ganglion of the spine (the gate) much faster. This in turn causes the pain signal to be blocked by the sensory TENS signal. This theory explains why rubbing a stubbed toe relieves pain. A study conducted by Oncel M and team compared the efficacy of TENS with a non-steroidal anti-inflammatory drug (NSAID, Naproxen sodium) in patients who had patients with uncomplicated minor rib fractures. The researchers found that TENS therapy given twice a day for 3 days resulted in significant pain reduction and was found to be more effective than NSAID or placebo.

Acupuncture

Acupuncture involves the insertion and manipulation of needles into specific points on the body to relieve pain or for therapeutic purposes. An analysis of the 13 highest quality studies of pain treatment with acupuncture, published in January 2009 in the *British Medical Journal*, was unable to quantify the difference in the effect on pain of real, sham and no acupuncture.

Acupuncture is believed to restore the energy balance in the body through stimulation of energy channels called the meridians. It is believed acupuncture therapy reduces pain signals through production of endorphins that are known to be the natural painkillers. Clinical studies suggest that acupuncture can reduce joint pain and so the therapy can be effective in reducing pain caused by knee osteoarthritis.

Light Therapy

Research has not found evidence that light therapy such as low level laser therapy is an effective therapy for relieving low back pain.

Interventional Procedures

Interventional procedures - typically used for chronic back pain - include epidural steroid injections, facet joint injections, neurolytic blocks, spinal cord stimulators and intrathecal drug delivery system implants.

Pulsed radiofrequency, neuromodulation, direct introduction of medication and nerve ablation may be used to target either the tissue structures and organ/systems responsible for persistent nociception or the nociceptors from the structures implicated as the source of chronic pain.

An intrathecal pump used to deliver very small quantities of medications directly to the spinal fluid. This is similar to epidural infusions used in labour and postoperatively. The major differences are that it is much more common for the drug to be delivered into the spinal fluid (intrathecal) rather than epidurally, and the pump can be fully implanted under the skin. Interestingly, it is suggested this approach allows a smaller dose of the drug to be delivered directly to the site of action, with fewer systemic side effects, which is thus therapeutically questionable due to the fact that the three main opioid receptors; chiefly the [μ-,Ϗ-,and δ (Mu-,Kappa-, and Delta- respectively] are limited in their anatomical locations. The 3 main receptors are found dominantly within the brain, CNS and Digestive tract.

A spinal cord stimulator is an implantable medical device that creates electric impulses and applies them near the dorsal surface of the spinal cord provides a paresthesia ("tingling") sensation that alters the perception of pain by the patient.

A small number of patients, especially those with severe pain from untreatable cancer, may benefit surgical treatment such as cordotomy.

Psychological Approach

Cognitive Behavioral Therapy

Cognitive behavioral therapy (CBT) for pain helps patients with pain to understand the relationship between one's physiology (e.g., pain and muscle tension), thoughts, emotions, and behaviors. A main goal in treatment is cognitive restructuring to encourage helpful thought patterns, targeting a behavioral activation of healthy activities such as regular exercise and pacing. Lifestyle changes are also trained to improve sleep patterns and to develop better coping skills for pain and other stressors using various techniques (e.g., relaxation, diaphragmatic breathing, and even biofeedback).

Studies have demonstrated the usefulness of cognitive behavioral therapy in the management of chronic low back pain, producing significant decreases in physical and psychosocial disability. A study published in the January 2012 issue of the *Archives of Internal Medicine* found CBT is significantly more effective than standard care in treatment of people with body-wide pain, like fibromyalgia. Evidence for the usefulness of CBT in the management of adult chronic pain is generally poorly understood, due partly to the proliferation of techniques of doubtful quality, and the poor quality of reporting in clinical trials. The crucial content of individual interventions has not been isolated and the important contextual elements, such as therapist training and development of treatment manuals, have not been determined. The widely varying nature of the resulting data makes useful systematic review and meta-analysis within the field very difficult.

In 2009 a systematic review of randomized controlled trials (RCTs) of psychological therapies for the management of adult chronic pain (excluding headache) found that "CBT and BT have weak effects in improving pain. CBT and BT [behavior therapy] have minimal effects on disability associated with chronic pain. CBT and BT are effective in altering mood outcomes, and there is some evidence that these changes are maintained at six months;"and a review of RCTs of psychological therapies for the management of chronic and recurrent pain in children and adolescents, by the same authors, found "Psychological treatments are effective in pain control for children with headache and benefits appear to be maintained. Psychological treatments may also improve pain control for children with musculoskeletal and recurrent abdominal pain. There is some evidence available to estimate effects on disability or mood."

Hypnosis

A 2007 review of 13 studies found evidence for the efficacy of hypnosis in the reduction of pain in some conditions, though the number of patients enrolled in the studies was small, bringing up issues of power to detect group differences, and most lacked credible controls for placebo and/or expectation. The authors concluded that "although the findings provide support for the general applicability of hypnosis in the treatment of chronic pain, considerably more research will be needed to fully determine the effects of hypnosis for different chronic-pain conditions."

Hypnosis has reduced the pain of some noxious medical procedures in children and adolescents, and in clinical trials addressing other patient groups it has significantly reduced pain compared to no treatment or some other non-hypnotic interventions. However, no studies have compared hypnosis to a convincing placebo, so the pain reduction may be due to patient expectation (the "placebo effect"). The effects of self hypnosis on chronic pain are roughly comparable to those of progressive muscle relaxation.

Mindfulness Meditation

A meta-analysis of studies that used techniques centered around the concept of mindfulness, concluded, "Findings suggest that MBIs decrease the intensity of pain for chronic pain patients."

Medications

The World Health Organization (WHO) recommends a *pain ladder* for managing analgesia. It was first described for use in cancer pain, but it can be used by medical professionals as a general principle when dealing with analgesia for any type of pain. In the treatment of chronic pain, whether due to malignant or benign processes, the three-step WHO Analgesic Ladder provides guidelines for selecting the kind and stepping up the amount of analgesia. The exact medications recommended will vary with the country and the individual treatment center, but the following gives an example of the WHO approach to treating chronic pain with medications. If, at any point, treatment fails to provide adequate pain relief, then the doctor and patient move onto the next step.

Common types of pain and typical drug management		
Pain type	**typical initial drug treatment**	**comments**
headache	paracetamol /acetaminophen, NSAIDs	doctor consultation is appropriate if headaches are severe, persistent, accompanied by fever, vomiting, or speech or balance problems; self-medication should be limited to two weeks
migraine	paracetamol, NSAIDs	triptans are used when the others do not work, or when migraines are frequent or severe
menstrual cramps	NSAIDs	some NSAIDs are marketed for cramps, but any NSAID would work
minor trauma, such as a bruise, abrasions, sprain	paracetamol, NSAIDs	opioids not recommended
severe trauma, such as a wound, burn, bone fracture, or severe sprain	opioids	more than two weeks of pain requiring opioid treatment is unusual
strain or pulled muscle	NSAIDs, muscle relaxants	if inflammation is involved, NSAIDs may work better; short-term use only
minor pain after surgery	paracetamol, NSAIDs	opioids rarely needed

severe pain after surgery	opioids	combinations of opioids may be prescribed if pain is severe
muscle ache	paracetamol, NSAIDs	if inflammation involved, NSAIDs may work better.
toothache or pain from dental procedures	paracetamol, NSAIDs	this should be short term use; opioids may be necessary for severe pain
kidney stone pain	paracetamol, NSAIDs, opioids	opioids usually needed if pain is severe.
pain due to heartburn or gastroesophageal reflux disease	antacid, H2 antagonist, proton-pump inhibitor	heartburn lasting more than a week requires medical attention; aspirin and NSAIDs should be avoided
chronic back pain	paracetamol, NSAIDs	opioids may be necessary if other drugs do not control pain and pain is persistent
osteoarthritis pain	paracetamol, NSAIDs	medical attention is recommended if pain persists.
fibromyalgia	antidepressant, anti-convulsant	evidence suggests that opioids are not effective in treating fibromyalgia

Mild Pain

Paracetamol (acetaminophen), or a non-steroidal anti-inflammatory drug (NSAID) such as ibuprofen.

Mild to Moderate Pain

Paracetamol, an NSAID and/or paracetamol in a combination product with a weak opioid such as tramadol, may provide greater relief than their separate use. Also a combination of opioid with acetaminophen can be frequently used such as Percocet, Vicodin, or Norco.

Moderate to Severe Pain

When treating moderate to severe pain, the type of the pain, acute or chronic, needs to be considered. The type of pain can result in different medications being prescribed. Certain medications may work better for acute pain, others for chronic pain, and some may work equally well on both. Acute pain medication is for rapid onset of pain such as from an inflicted trauma or to treat post-operative pain. Chronic pain medication is for alleviating long-lasting, ongoing pain.

Morphine is the gold standard to which all narcotics are compared. Semi-synthetic derivatives of morphine such as hydromorphone (Dilaudid), oxymorphone (Numorphan, Opana), nicomorphine (Vilan), hydromorphinol and others vary in such ways as duration of action, side effect profile and milligramme potency. Fentanyl has the benefit of less histamine release and thus fewer side effects. It can also be administered via transdermal patch which is convenient for chronic pain management. In addition to the intrathecal patch and injectable Sublimaze, the FDA has approved various immediate release fentanyl products for breakthrough cancer pain (Actiq/OTFC/Fentora/Onsolis/Subsys/Lazanda/Abstral). Oxycodone is used across the Americas and Europe for relief of serious chronic pain; its main slow-release formula is known as OxyContin, and short-acting tablets, capsules, syrups and ampules are available making it suitable for acute intractable pain or breakthrough pain. Diamorphine, methadone and buprenorphine are used less frequently. Pethidine, known in North America as meperidine, is not recommended for pain management due to its low potency, short duration of action, and toxicity associated with repeated use. Pentazocine, dextromoramide and dipipanone are also not recommended in new patients except for acute pain where other analgesics are not tolerated or are inappropriate, for pharmacological and misuse-related reasons. In some countries potent synthetics such as piritramide and ketobemidone are used for severe pain, and tapentadol is a newer agent introduced in the last decade.

For moderate pain, tramadol, codeine, dihydrocodeine, and hydrocodone are used, with nicocodeine, ethylmorphine and propoxyphene and dextropropoxyphene less commonly.

Drugs of other types can be used to help opioids combat certain types of pain, for example, amitriptyline is prescribed for chronic muscular pain in the arms, legs, neck and lower back with an opiate, or sometimes without it and/or with an NSAID.

While opiates are often used in the management of chronic pain, high doses are associated with an increased risk of opioid overdose.

Opioids

From the Food and Drug Administration's website: "According to the National Institutes of Health, studies have shown that properly managed medical use of opioid analgesic compounds (taken exactly as prescribed) is safe, can manage pain effectively, and rarely causes addiction."

Opioid medications can provide short, intermediate or long acting analgesia depending upon the specific properties of the medication and whether it is formulated as an extended release drug. Opioid medications may be administered orally, by injection, via nasal mucosa or oral mucosa, rectally, transdermally, intravenously, epidurally and intrathecally. In chronic pain conditions that are opioid responsive a combination of a long-acting (OxyContin, MS Contin, Opana ER, Exalgo and Methadone) or extended release medication is often prescribed in conjunction with a shorter-acting medication (oxycodone, morphine or hydromorphone) for breakthrough pain, or exacerbations.

Most opioid treatment used by patients outside of healthcare settings is oral (tablet, capsule or liquid), but suppositories and skin patches can be prescribed. An opioid injection is rarely needed for patients with chronic pain.

Although opioids are strong analgesics, they do not provide complete analgesia regardless of whether the pain is acute or chronic in origin. Opioids are efficacious analgesics in chronic malignant pain and modestly effective in nonmalignant pain management. However, there are associated adverse effects, especially during the commencement or change in dose. When opioids are used for prolonged periods drug tolerance, chemical dependency, diversion and addiction may occur.

Clinical guidelines for prescribing opioids for chronic pain have been issued by the American Pain Society and the American Academy of Pain Medicine. Included in these guidelines is the importance of assessing the patient for the risk of substance abuse, misuse, or addiction; a personal or family history of substance abuse is the strongest predictor of aberrant drug-taking behavior. Physicians who prescribe opioids should integrate this treatment with any psychotherapeutic intervention the patient may be receiving. The guidelines also recommend monitoring not only the pain but also the level of functioning and the achievement of therapeutic goals. The prescribing physician should be suspicious of abuse when a patient reports a reduction in pain but has no accompanying improvement in function or progress in achieving identified goals.

Commonly-used long-acting opioids and their parent compound:

- OxyContin (oxycodone)
- Hydromorph Contin (hydromorphone)
- MS Contin (morphine)
- M-Eslon (morphine)
- Exalgo (hydromorphone)
- Opana ER (oxymorphone)
- Duragesic (fentanyl)
- Nucynta ER (tapentadol)
- Metadol/Methadose (methadone)*
- Hysingla ER (hydrocodone bitartrate)
- Zohydro ER (hydrocodone bicarbonate)

*Methadone can be used for either treatment of opioid addiction/detoxification when taken once daily or as a pain medication usually administered on an every 12-hour or 8-hour dosing interval.

Non-steroidal Anti-inflammatory Drugs

The other major group of analgesics are non-steroidal anti-inflammatory drugs

(NSAID). Acetaminophen/paracetamol is not always included in this class of medications. However, acetaminophen may be administered as a single medication or in combination with other analgesics (both NSAIDs and opioids). The alternatively prescribed NSAIDs such as ketoprofen and piroxicam have limited benefit in chronic pain disorders and with long-term use are associated with significant adverse effects. The use of selective NSAIDs designated as selective COX-2 inhibitors have significant cardiovascular and cerebrovascular risks which have limited their utilization.

Antidepressants and Antiepileptic Drugs

Some antidepressant and antiepileptic drugs are used in chronic pain management and act primarily within the pain pathways of the central nervous system, though peripheral mechanisms have been attributed as well. These mechanisms vary and in general are more effective in neuropathic pain disorders as well as complex regional pain syndrome. Drugs such as gabapentin have been widely prescribed for the off-label use of pain control. The list of side effects for these classes of drugs are typically much longer than opiate or NSAID treatments for chronic pain, and many antiepileptics cannot be suddenly stopped without the risk of seizure.

Cannabinoids

Chronic pain is one of the most commonly cited reasons for the use of medical marijuana.A 2012 Canadian survey of participants in their medical marijuana program found that 84% of respondents reported using medical marijuana for the management of pain.

Evidence of medical marijuana's pain mitigating effects is generally conclusive. Detailed in a 1999 report by The Institute of Medicine, "the available evidence from animal and human studies indicates that cannabinoids can have a substantial analgesic effect." In a 2013 review study published in Fundamental & Clinical Pharmacology, various studies were cited in demonstrating that cannabinoids exhibit comparable effectiveness to opioids in models of acute pain and even greater effectiveness in models of chronic pain.

Other Analgesics

Other drugs are often used to help analgesics combat various types of pain, and parts of the overall pain experience, and are hence called adjuvant medications. Gabapentin — an anti-epileptic — not only exerts effects alone on neuropathic pain, but can potentiate opiates. While perhaps not prescribed as such, other drugs such as Tagamet (cimetidine) and even simple grapefruit juice may also potentiate opiates, by inhibiting CYP450 enzymes in the liver, thereby slowing metabolism of the drug. In addition, orphenadrine, cyclobenzaprine, trazodone and other drugs with anticholinergic properties are useful in conjunction with opioids for neuropathic pain. Orphenadrine and cyclobenzaprine are also muscle relaxants, and therefore particularly useful in painful musculoskeletal conditions. Clonidine has found use as an analgesic for this same purpose, and all of the mentioned drugs potentiate the effects of opioids overall.

Society and Culture

Undertreatment

Undertreatment of pain is the absence of pain management therapy for a person in pain when treatment is indicated.

Consensus in evidence-based medicine and the recommendations of medical specialty organizations establish the guidelines which determine the treatment for pain which health care providers ought to offer. For various social reasons, persons in pain may not seek or may not be able to access treatment for their pain. At the same time, health care providers may not provide the treatment which authorities recommend.

In Children

Acute pain is common in children and adolescents as a result of injury, illness, or necessary medical procedures. Chronic pain is present in approximately 15–25% of children and adolescents, and may be caused by an underlying disease, such as sickle cell anemia, cystic fibrosis, rheumatoid arthritis, or cancer or by functional disorders such as migraines, fibromyalgia, or complex regional pain.

Assessment

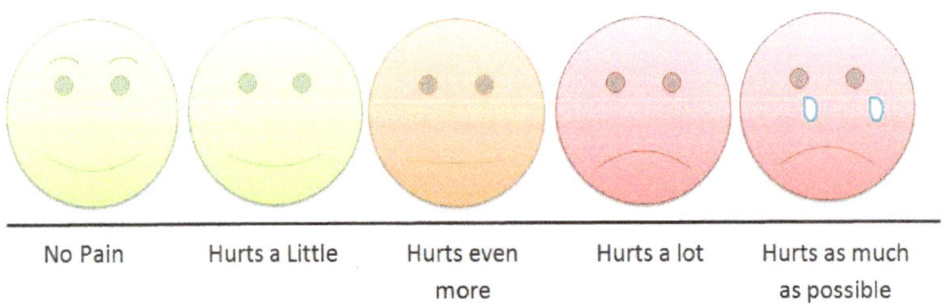

Young children can indicate their level of pain by pointing to the appropriate face on a children's pain scale.

Pain assessment in children is often challenging due to limitations in developmental level, cognitive ability, or their previous pain experiences. Clinicians must observe physiological and behavioral cues exhibited by the child to make an assessment. Self-report, if possible, is the most accurate measure of pain; self-report pain scales developed for young children involve matching their pain intensity to photographs of other children's faces, such as the Oucher Scale, pointing to schematics of faces showing different pain levels, or pointing out the location of pain on a body outline. Questionnaires for older children and adolescents include the Varni-Thompson Pediatric Pain Questionnaire (PPQ) and the Children's Comprehensive Pain Questionnaire, which are often utilized for individuals with chronic or persistent pain.

Nonpharmacologic

Caregivers may provide nonpharmacological treatment for children and adolescents because it carries minimal risk and is cost effective compared to pharmacological treatment. Nonpharmacologic interventions vary by age and developmental factors. Physical interventions to ease pain in infants include swaddling, rocking, or sucrose via a pacifier, whereas those for children and adolescents include hot or cold application, massage, or acupuncture. Cognitive behavioral therapy (CBT) aims to reduce the emotional distress and improve the daily functioning of school-aged children and adolescents with pain through focus on changing the relationship between their thoughts and emotions in addition to teaching them adaptive coping strategies. Integrated interventions in CBT include relaxation technique, mindfulness, biofeedback, and acceptance (in the case of chronic pain). Many therapists will hold sessions for caregivers to provide them with effective management strategies.

Pharmacologic

Acetaminophen, nonsteroidal anti-inflammatory agents, and opioid analgesics are commonly used to treat acute or chronic pain symptoms in children and adolescents, but a pediatrician should be consulted before administering any medication.

Professional Certification

Pain management practitioners come from all fields of medicine. In addition to medical practitioners, a pain management team may often benefit from the input of pharmacists, physiotherapists, clinical psychologists and occupational therapists, among others. Together the multidisciplinary team can help create a package of care suitable to the patient.

Pain physicians are often fellowship-trained board-certified anesthesiologists, neurologists, physiatrists or psychiatrists. Palliative care doctors are also specialists in pain management. The American Board of Anesthesiology, the American Osteopathic Board of Anesthesiology (recognized by the AOABOS), the American Board of Physical Medicine and Rehabilitation, and the American Board of Psychiatry and Neurology each provide certification for a subspecialty in pain management following fellowship training which is recognized by the American Board of Medical Specialties (ABMS) or the American Osteopathic Association Bureau of Osteopathic Specialists (AOABOS). As the field of pain medicine has grown rapidly, many practitioners have entered the field, some non-ACGME board-certified.

Spinal Cord Injury

A spinal cord injury (SCI) is damage to the spinal cord that causes changes in its function, either temporary or permanent. These changes translate into loss of muscle function, sensation, or autonomic function in parts of the body served by the spinal cord below the level of the lesion. Injuries can occur at any level of the spinal cord and can be classified as *complete injury*, a total loss of sensation and muscle function, or *incomplete*, meaning some nervous signals are able to travel past the injured area of the cord. Depending on the location and severity of damage along the spinal cord, the symptoms can vary widely, from pain or numbness to paralysis to incontinence. The prognosis also ranges widely, from full recovery in rare cases to permanent tetraplegia (also called quadriplegia) in injuries at the level of the neck, and paraplegia in lower injuries. Complications that can occur in the short and long term after injury include muscle atrophy, pressure sores, infections, and respiratory problems.

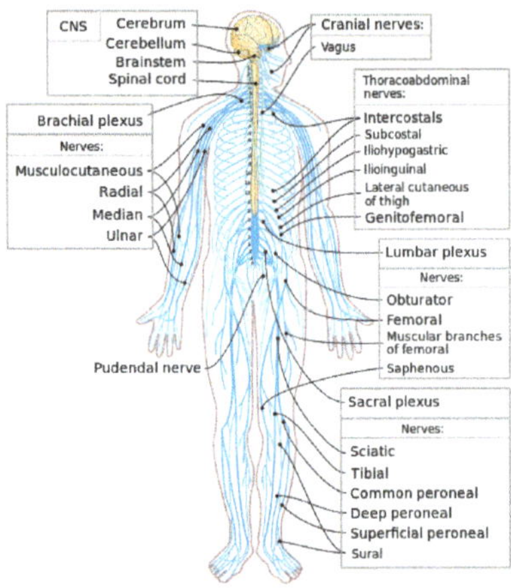

The spinal cord relays messages between the brain and the peripheral nerves.

In the majority of cases the damage results from physical trauma such as car accidents, gunshots, falls, or sports injuries, but it can also result from nontraumatic causes such as infection, insufficient blood flow, and tumors. Efforts to prevent SCI include individual measures such as using safety equipment, societal measures such as safety regulations in sports and traffic, and improvements to equipment. Known since ancient times to be a catastrophic injury and long believed to be untreatable, SCI has seen great improvements in its care since the middle of the 20th century. Treatment of spinal cord injuries starts with stabilizing the spine and controlling inflammation to prevent further damage. Other interventions needed can vary widely depending on the location and extent of the injury, from bed rest to surgery. In many cases, spinal cord injuries require substantial, long-term physical and occupational therapy in rehabilitation, especially if they interfere with activities of daily living. Research into new treatments for spinal cord injuries includes stem cell implantation, engineered materials for tissue support, and wearable robotic exoskeletons.

Classification

Spinal cord injury can be traumatic or nontraumatic, and can be classified into three types based on cause: mechanical forces, toxic, and ischemic (from lack of blood flow).

The damage can also be divided into primary and secondary injury: the cell death that occurs immediately in the original injury, and biochemical cascades that are initiated by the original insult and cause further tissue damage. These secondary injury pathways include the ischemic cascade, inflammation, swelling, cell suicide, and neurotransmitter imbalances. They can take place for minutes or weeks following the injury.

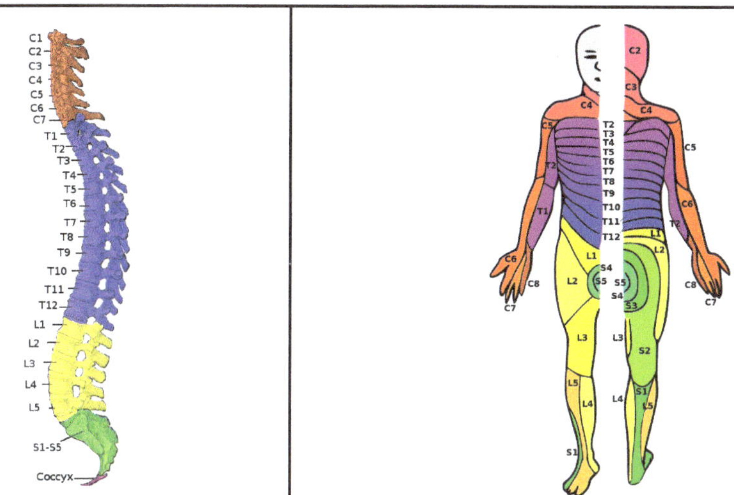

The effects of injury depend on the level along the spinal column (left). A dermatome is an area of the skin that sends sensory messages to a specific spinal nerve (right).

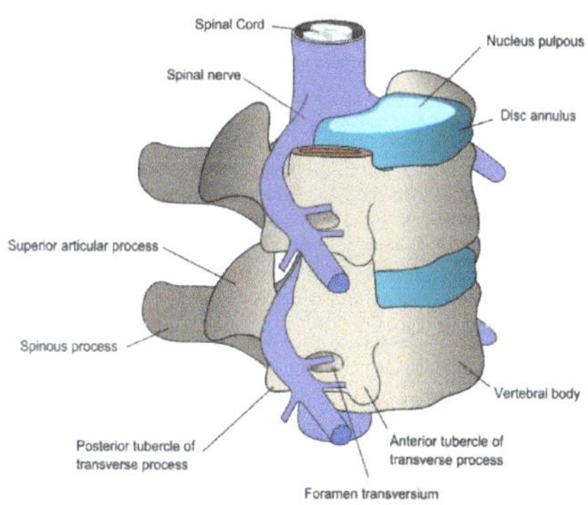

Spinal nerves exit the spinal cord between each pair of vertebrae.

At each level of the spinal column, spinal nerves branch off from either side of the spinal cord and exit between a pair of vertebrae, to innervate a specific part of the body. The area of skin innervated by a specific spinal nerve is called a dermatome, and the group of muscles innervated by a single spinal nerve is called a myotome. The part of the spinal cord that was damaged corresponds to the spinal nerves at that level and below. Injuries can be cervical 1–8 (C1–C8), thoracic 1–12 (T1–T12), lumbar 1–5 (L1–L5), or sacral (S1–S5). A person's level of injury is defined as the lowest level of full sensation and function. Paraplegia occurs when the legs are affected by the spinal cord damage (in thoracic, lumbar, or sacral injuries), and tetraplegia occurs when all four limbs are affected (cervical damage).

SCI is also classified by the degree of impairment. The *International Standards for Neurological Classification of Spinal Cord Injury* (ISNCSCI), published by the American Spinal Injury Association (ASIA), is widely used to document sensory and motor impairments following SCI. It is based on neurological responses, touch and pinprick sensations tested in each dermatome, and strength of the muscles that control key motions on both sides of the body. Muscle strength is scored on a scale of 0–5 according to the table on the right, and sensation is graded on a scale of 0–2: 0 is no sensation, 1 is altered or decreased sensation, and 2 is full sensation. Each side of the body is graded independently.

Muscle strength		ASIA Impairment Scale for classifying spinal cord injury	
Grade	**Muscle function**	**Grade**	**Description**
0	No muscle contraction	A	**Complete injury**. No motor or sensory function is preserved in the sacral segments S4 or S5.
1	Muscle flickers	B	**Sensory incomplete**. Sensory but not motor function is preserved below the level of injury, including the sacral segments.
2	Full range of motion, gravity eliminated	C	**Motor incomplete**. Motor function is preserved below the level of injury, and more than half of muscles tested below the level of injury have a muscle grade less than 3.
3	Full range of motion, against gravity	D	**Motor incomplete**. Motor function is preserved below the level of injury and at least half of the key muscles below the neurological level have a muscle grade of 3 or more.
4	Full range of motion against resistance	E	**Normal**. No motor or sensory deficits, but deficits existed in the past.
5	Normal strength		

Complete and Incomplete Injuries

Level and completeness of injuries		
	Complete	**Incomplete**
Tetraplegia	18.3%	34.1%
Paraplegia	23.0%	18.5%

In a "complete" spinal injury, all functions below the injured area are lost, whether or not the spinal cord is severed. An "incomplete" spinal cord injury involves preservation of motor or sensory function below the level of injury in the spinal cord. To be classed as incomplete, there must be some preservation of sensation or motion in the areas innervated by S4 to S5, e.g. voluntary external anal sphincter contraction. The nerves in this area are connected to the very lowest region of the spinal cord, and retaining sensation and function in these parts of the body indicates that the spinal cord is only partially damaged. Incomplete injury by definition includes a phenomenon known as sacral sparing: some degree of sensation is preserved in the sacral dermatomes, even though sensation may be more impaired in other, higher dermatomes below the level of the lesion. Sacral sparing has been attributed to the fact that the sacral spinal pathways are not as likely as the other spinal pathways to become compressed after injury due to the lamination of fibers within the spinal cord.

Spinal Cord Injury Without Radiographic Abnormality

Spinal column injury is trauma that causes fracture of the bone or instability of the ligaments in the spinal column; this can coexist with or cause injury to the spinal cord, but each injury can occur without the other. Spinal cord injury without radiographic abnormality (SCIWORA) exists when SCI is present but there is no evidence of spinal column injury on radiographs. Abnormalities might show up on magnetic resonance imaging (MRI), but the term was coined before MRI was in common use.

Central Cord Syndrome

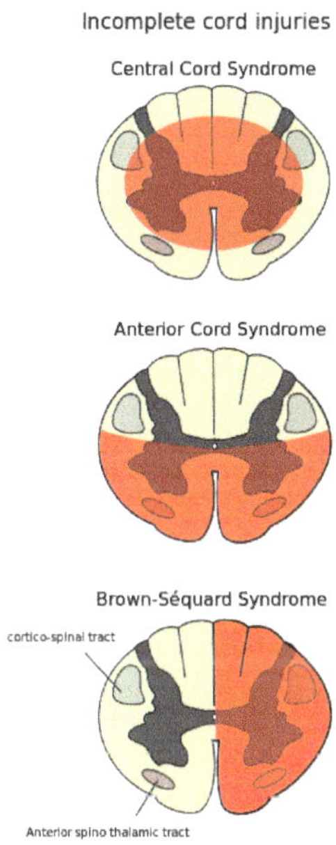

Incomplete lesions of the spinal cord: Central cord syndrome (top), Anterior cord syndrome (middle), and Brown-Séquard syndrome (bottom).

Central cord syndrome, almost always resulting from damage to the cervical spinal cord, is characterized by weakness in the arms with relative sparing of the legs, and spared sensation in regions served by the sacral segments. There is loss of sensation of pain, temperature, light touch, and pressure below the level of injury. The spinal tracts that serve the arms are more affected due to their central location in the spinal cord, while the corticospinal fibers destined for the legs are spared due to their more external location. The most common of the incomplete SCI syndromes, central cord syndrome usually results from neck hyperextension in older people with spinal stenosis. In younger people, it most commonly results from neck flexion. The most common causes are falls and vehicle accidents; however other possible causes include spinal stenosis and impingement on the spinal cord by a tumor or vertebral disk.

Anterior Cord Syndrome

Anterior cord syndrome, due to damage to the front portion of the spinal cord or reduction in the blood supply from the anterior spinal artery, can be caused by fractures or dislocations of vertebrae or herniated disks. Below the level of injury, motor function, pain sensation, and temperature sensation are lost, while sense of touch and proprioception (sense of position in space) remain intact. These differences are due to the relative locations of the spinal tracts responsible for each type of function.

Brown-Séquard Syndrome

Brown-Séquard syndrome occurs when the spinal cord is injured on one side much more than the other. It is rare for the spinal cord to be truly hemisected (severed on one side), but partial lesions due to penetrating wounds (such as gunshot or knife wounds) or fractured vertebrae or tumors are common. On the ipsilateral side of the injury (same side), the body loses motor function, proprioception, and senses of vibration and touch. On the contralateral (opposite side) of the injury, there is a loss of pain and temperature sensations.

Posterior Cord Syndrome

Posterior cord syndrome, in which just the dorsal columns of the spinal cord are affected, is usually seen in cases of chronic myelopathy but can also occur with infarction of the posterior spinal artery. This rare syndrome causes the loss of proprioception and sense of vibration below the level of injury while motor function and sensation of pain, temperature, and touch remain intact. Usually posterior cord injuries result from insults like disease or vitamin deficiency rather than trauma. Tabes dorsalis, due to injury to the posterior part of the spinal cord caused by syphilis, results in loss of touch and proprioceptive sensation.

Conus Medullaris and Cauda Equina Syndromes

Conus medullaris syndrome is an injury to the end of the spinal cord, located at about the T12–L2 vertebrae in adults. This region contains the S4–S5 spinal segments, responsible for bowel, bladder, and some sexual functions, so these can be disrupted in this type of injury. In addition, sensation and the Achilles reflex can be disrupted. Causes include growths, physical trauma, and ischemia.

Cauda equina syndrome (CES) results from a lesion below the level at which the spinal cord splits into the cauda equina, at levels L2–S5 below the conus medullaris. Thus it is not a true spinal cord syndrome since it is nerve roots that are damaged and not the cord itself; however it is common for several of these nerves to be damaged at the same time due to their proximity. CES can occur by itself or alongside conus medullaris syndrome. It can cause low back pain, weakness or paralysis in the lower limbs, loss of sensation, bowel and bladder dysfunction, and loss of reflexes. Unlike in conus medullaris syndrome, symptoms often occur on only one side of the body. The cause is often compression, e.g. by a ruptured intervertebral disk or tumor. Since the nerves damaged in CES are actually peripheral nerves because they have already branched off from the spinal cord, the injury has better prognosis for recovery of function: the peripheral nervous system has a greater capacity for healing than the central nervous system.

Signs and Symptoms

Actions of the spinal nerves	
Level	**Motor Function**
C1–C6	Neck flexors
C1–T1	Neck extensors
C3, C4, C5	Supply diaphragm (mostly C4)
C5, C6	Move shoulder, raise arm (deltoid); flex elbow (biceps)
C6	externally rotate (supinate) the arm
C6, C7	Extend elbow and wrist (triceps and wrist extensors); pronate wrist
C7, T1	Flex wrist; supply small muscles of the hand
T1–T6	Intercostals and trunk above the waist
T7–L1	Abdominal muscles
L1–L4	Flex thigh
L2, L3, L4	Adduct thigh; Extend leg at the knee (quadriceps femoris)
L4, L5, S1	abduct thigh; Flex leg at the knee (hamstrings); Dorsiflex foot (tibialis anterior); Extend toes
L5, S1, S2	Extend leg at the hip (gluteus maximus); Plantar flex foot and flex toes

Signs (observed by a clinician) and symptoms (experienced by a patient) vary depending on where the spine is injured and the extent of the injury. A section of skin innervated through a specific part of the spine is called a dermatome, and injury to that part of the spine can cause p

n, numbness, or a loss of sensation in the related areas. Paraesthesia, a tingling or burning sensation in affected areas of the skin, is another symptom. A person with a lowered level of consciousness may show a response to a painful stimulus above a certain point but not below it. A group of muscles innervated through a specific part of the spine is called a myotome, and injury to that part of the spinal cord can cause problems with movements that involve those muscles. The muscles may contract uncontrollably (spasticity), become weak, or be completely paralysed. Spinal shock, loss of neural activity including reflexes below the level of injury, occurs shortly after the injury and usually goes away within a day.

The specific parts of the body affected by loss of function are determined by the level of injury.

Lumbosacral

The effects of injuries at or above the lumbar or sacral regions of the spinal cord (lower back and pelvis) include decreased control of the legs and hips, genitourinary system, and anus. People injured below level L2 may still have use of their hip flexor and knee extensor muscles. Bowel and bladder function are regulated by the sacral region. It is common to experience sexual dysfunction after injury, as well as dysfunction of the bowel and bladder, including fecal and urinary incontinence. It is also possible for the bladder to fail to empty, leading to a potentially harmful buildup of urine. One sign of spinal cord injury that emergency providers may find is priapism, an erection of the penis.

Thoracic

In addition to the problems found in lower-level injuries, thoracic (chest height) spinal lesions can affect the muscles in the trunk. Injuries at the level of T1 to T8 result in inability to control the abdominal muscles. Trunk stability may be affected; even more so in higher level injuries. The lower the level of injury, the less extensive its effects. Injuries from T9 to T12 result in partial loss of trunk and abdominal muscle control. Thoracic spinal injuries result in paraplegia, but function of the hands, arms, and neck are not affected.

One condition that occurs typically in lesions above the T6 level is autonomic dysreflexia (AD), in which the blood pressure increases to dangerous levels, high enough to cause potentially deadly stroke. It results from an overreaction of the system to a stimulus such as pain below the level of injury, because inhibitory signals from the brain cannot pass the lesion to dampen the excitatory sympathetic nervous system response. Signs and symptoms of AD include anxiety, headache, nausea, ringing in the ears, blurred vision, flushed skin, and nasal congestion. It can occur shortly after the injury or not until years later.

Other autonomic functions may also be disrupted. For example, problems with body temperature regulation mostly occur in injuries at T8 and above. Another serious complication that can result from lesions above T6 is neurogenic shock, which results from an interruption in output from the sympathetic nervous system responsible for maintaining muscle tone in the blood vessels. Without the sympathetic input, the vessels relax and dilate. Neurogenic shock presents with dangerously low blood pressure, low heart rate, and blood pooling in the limbs—which results in insufficient blood flow to the spinal cord and potentially further damage to it.

Cervical

Spinal cord injuries at the cervical (neck) level result in full or partial tetraplegia (also called quadriplegia). Depending on the specific location and severity of trauma, limited function may be retained.

Function after complete cervical spinal cord injury		
Level	**Motor Function**	**Respiratory function**
C1–C4	Full paralysis of the limbs	Cannot breathe without mechanical ventilation
C5	Paralysis of the wrists, hands, and triceps	Difficulty coughing, may need help clearing secretions
C6	Paralysis of the wrist flexors, triceps, and hands	
C7–C8	Some hand muscle weakness, difficulty grasping and releasing	

Additional signs and symptoms of cervical injuries include low heart rate, low blood pressure, problems regulating body temperature, and breathing dysfunction. If the injury is high enough in the neck to impair the muscles involved in breathing, the person may not be able to breathe without the help of an endotracheal tube and mechanical ventilator.

Causes

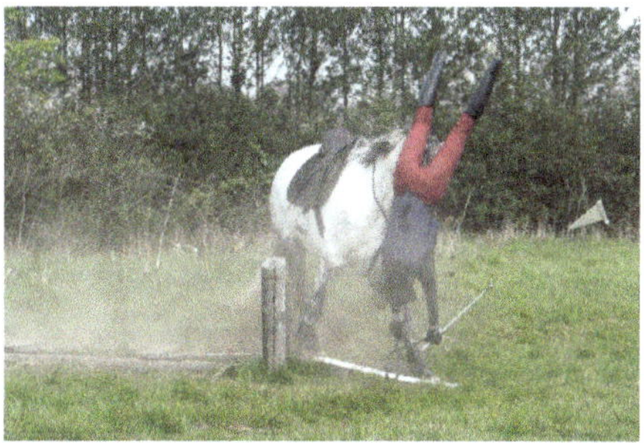

Falling as a part of recreational activities can cause spinal cord injuries.

Spinal cord injuries are most often caused by physical trauma. Forces involved can be hyperflexion (forward movement of the head); hyperextension (backward movement); lateral stress (sideways movement); rotation (twisting of the head); compression (force along the axis of the spine downward from the head or upward from the pelvis); or distraction (pulling apart of the vertebrae). Traumatic SCI can result in contusion, compression, or stretch injury.

In the US, Motor vehicle accidents are the most common cause of SCIs; second are falls, then violence such as gunshot wounds, then sports injuries. In some countries falls are more common, even surpassing vehicle crashes as the leading cause of SCI. The rates of violence-related SCI depend heavily on place and time. Of all sports-related SCIs, shallow water dives are the most common cause; winter sports and water sports have been increasing as causes while association football and trampoline injuries have been declining. Hanging can cause injury to the cervical spine, as may occur in attempted suicide. Military conflicts are another cause, and when they occur they are associated with increased rates of SCI. Another potential cause of SCI is iatrogenic injury, caused by an improperly done medical procedure such as an injection into the spinal column.

SCI can also be of a nontraumatic origin. Nontraumatic lesions cause anywhere from 30 to 80% of all SCI; the percentage varies by locale, influenced by efforts to prevent trauma. Developed countries have higher percentages of SCI due to degenerative conditions and tumors than developing countries. In developed countries, the most common cause of nontraumatic SCI is degenerative diseases, followed by tumors; in many developing countries the leading cause is infection such as HIV and tuberculosis. SCI may occur in intervertebral disc disease, and spinal cord vascular disease. Spontaneous bleeding can occur within or outside of the protective membranes that line the cord, and intervertebral disks can herniate. Damage can result from dysfunction of the blood vessels, as in arteriovenous malformation, or when a blood clot becomes lodged in a blood vessel and cuts off blood supply to the cord. When systemic blood pressure drops, blood flow to the spinal cord may be reduced, potentially causing a loss of sensation and voluntary movement in the areas supplied by the affected level of the spinal cord. Congenital conditions and tumors that compress the cord can also cause SCI, as can vertebral spondylosis and ischemia. Multiple sclerosis is a disease that can damage the spinal cord, as can infectious or inflammatory conditions such as tuberculosis, herpes zoster or herpes simplex, meningitis, myelitis, and syphilis.

Prevention

Vehicle-related SCI is prevented with measures including societal and individual efforts to reduce driving under the influence of drugs or alcohol, distracted driving, and drowsy driving. Other efforts include increasing road safety (such as marking hazards and adding lighting) and vehicle safety, both to prevent accidents (such as routine maintenance and antilock brakes) and to mitigate the damage of crashes (such as head restraints, air bags, seat belts, and child safety seats). Falls can be prevented by making changes to the environment, such as nonslip materials and grab bars in bathtubs and showers, railings for stairs, child and safety gates for windows. Gun-related injuries can be prevented with conflict resolution training, gun safety education campaigns, and changes to the technology of guns (such as trigger locks) to improve their safety. Sports injuries can be prevented with changes to sports rules and equipment to increase safety, and education campaigns to reduce risky practices such as diving into water of unknown depth or head-first tackling in association football.

Diagnosis

A radiographic evaluation using an X-ray, CT scan, or MRI can determine if there is damage to the spinal column and where it is located. X-rays are commonly available and can detect instability or misalignment of the spinal column, but do not give very detailed images and can miss injuries to the spinal cord or displacement of ligaments or disks that do not have accompanying spinal column damage. Thus when X-ray findings are normal but SCI is still suspected due to pain or SCI symptoms, CT or MRI scans are used. CT gives greater detail than X-rays, but exposes the patient to more radiation, and it still does not give images of the spinal cord or ligaments; MRI shows body structures in the greatest detail. Thus it is the standard for anyone who has neurological deficits found in SCI or is thought to have an unstable spinal column injury.

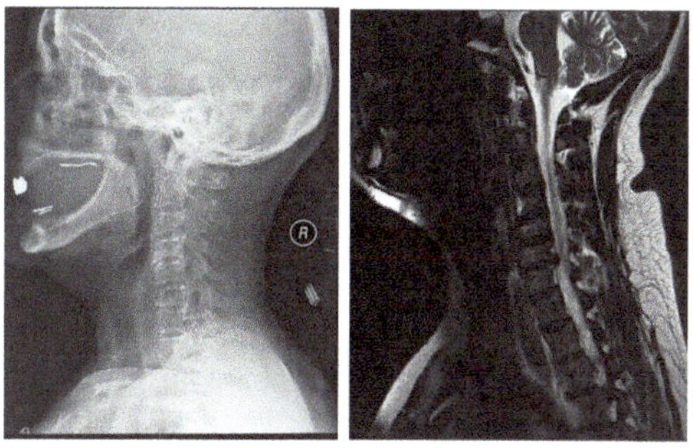

X-rays (top) are more available, but can miss details like herniated disks that MRIs can show (bottom).

Neurological evaluations to help determine the degree of impairment are performed initially and repeatedly in the early stages of treatment; this determines the rate of improvement or deterioration and informs treatment and prognosis. The ASIA Impairment Scale outlined above is used to determine the level and severity of injury.

Management

Prehospital Treatment

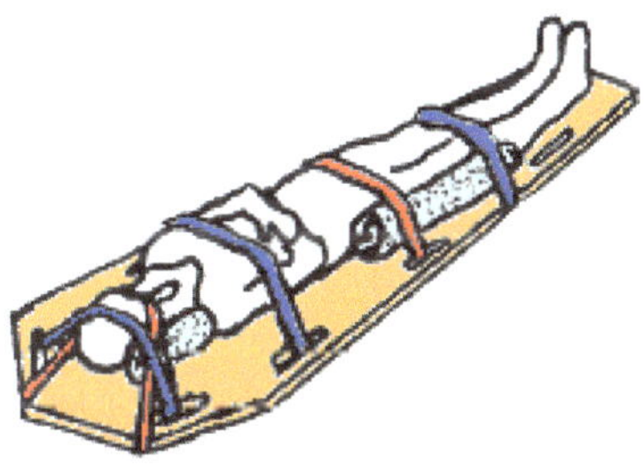

Spine immobilization with a long spine board

The first stage in the management of a suspected spinal cord injury is geared toward basic life support and preventing further injury: maintaining airway, breathing, and circulation and immobilizing the spine. In the emergency setting, anyone who has been subjected to forces strong enough to cause SCI is treated as though they have instability in the spinal column and is immobilized to prevent damage to the spinal cord. Injuries or fractures in the head, neck, or pelvis as well as penetrating trauma near the spine and falls from heights are assumed to be associated with an unstable spinal column until it is ruled out in the hospital. High-speed vehicle crashes, sports injuries involving the head or neck, and diving injuries are other mechanisms that indicate a high SCI risk. Since head and spinal trauma frequently coexist, anyone who is unconscious or has a lowered level of consciousness as a result of a head injury is immobilized. A rigid cervical collar is applied to the neck, and the head is held immobile with blocks on either side and the person is strapped to a backboard. Extrication devices are used to move people without moving the spine if they are still inside a vehicle or other confined space.

Modern trauma care includes a step called clearing the cervical spine, ruling out spinal cord injury if the patient is fully conscious and not under the influence of drugs or alcohol, displays no neurological deficits, has no pain in the middle of the neck and no other painful injuries that could distract from neck pain. If these are all absent, no immobilization is necessary. If an unstable spinal column injury is moved, damage may occur to the spinal cord. Between 3 and 25% of SCIs occur not at the time of the initial trauma but later during treatment or transport. While some of this is due to the nature of the injury itself, particularly in the case of multiple or massive trauma, some of it reflects the failure to immobilize the spine adequately.

SCI can impair the body's ability to keep warm, so warming blankets may be needed.

Early Hospital Treatment

Initial care in the hospital, as in the prehospital setting, aims to ensure adequate airway, breathing, cardiovascular function, and spinal immobilization. Imaging of the spine to ascertain presence of SCI may need to wait if emergency surgery is needed to stabilize a life-threatening injury. Acute SCI merits treatment in an intensive care unit, especially injuries to the cervival spinal cord. Patients with SCI need repeated neurological assessments and treatment by neurosurgeons.

If the systolic blood pressure falls below 90 mmHg within days of the injury, blood supply to the spinal cord may be reduced, resulting in further damage. Thus it is important to maintain the blood pressure using a central venous catheter, intravenous fluids, and vasopressors, and to treat cases of shock. Mean arterial blood pressure is measured and kept at 85 to 90 mmHg for seven days after injury. The treatment for shock from blood loss (hypovolemic shock) is different from that for neurogenic shock, and could harm people with the latter type, so it is necessary to determine why someone is in shock. However it is also possible for both causes to exist at the same time. Another important aspect of care is prevention of hypoxia (insufficient oxygen in the bloodstream), which could deprive the spinal cord of much-needed oxygen. People with cervical injuries may experience a dangerously slowed heart rate; treatment to speed it up include atropine and electrical cardiac pacing.

Swelling can cause further damage to the spinal cord by reducing the blood supply and causing ischemia, which can give rise to an ischemic cascade with a release of toxins that damages neurons. Thus treatment is often geared toward limiting this secondary injury. People are sometimes treated with drugs to reduce swelling. The corticosteroid drug methylprednisolone is commonly used within eight hours of the injury, but its use is controversial because of side effects. Studies have shown high dose methylprednisolone may improve outcomes if given within 6 hours of injury. However, the improvement shown by clinical trials has been inconclusive, and comes at the cost of increased risk of serious infection or sepsis, gastrointestinal bleeding, and pneumonia. Thus organizations that set clinical guidelines have increasingly stopped recommending methylprednisolone in the treatment of acute SCI.

Surgery may be necessary, e.g. to relieve excess pressure on the cord, to stabilize the spine, or to put vertebrae back in their proper place. In cases involving instability or compression, failing to operate can lead to worsening of the condition. Surgery is also necessary when something is pressing on the cord, such as bone fragments, blood, material from ligaments or intervertebral discs, or a lodged object from a penetrating injury. Although the ideal timing of surgery is still debated, studies have found that earlier surgical intervention (within 24 hours of injury) is associated with better outcomes. Sometimes a patient has too many other injuries to be a surgical candidate this early. Surgery is controversial because it has potential complications (such as infection), so in cases where it is not clearly needed (e.g. the cord is being compressed), doctors must decide whether to perform surgery based on aspects of the patient's condition and their own beliefs about its risks and benefits. In cases where a more conservative approach is chosen, bed rest, cervical collars, immobilizing devices, and optionally traction are used. Surgeons may opt to put traction on the spine to remove pressure from the spinal cord by putting dislocated vertebrae back into alignment, but herniation of intervertebral disks may prevent this technique from relieving pressure. *Gardner-Wells tongs* are one tool used to exert spinal traction to reduce a fracture or dislocation and to immobilize the affected areas.

Rehabilitation

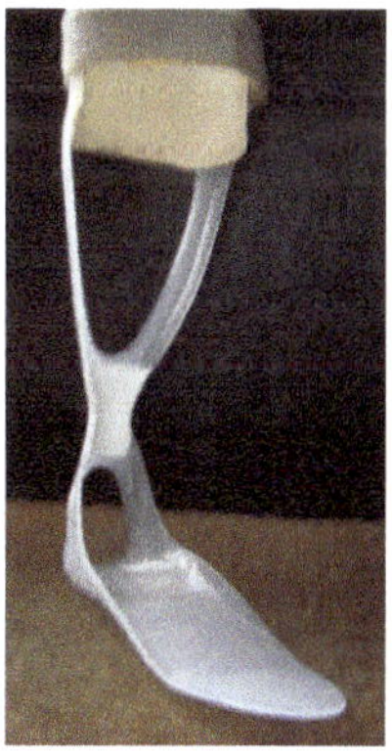

Orthopedic devices such as ankle-foot orthoses can aid in walking.

SCI patients often require extended treatment in specialized spinal unit or an intensive care unit. The rehabilitation process typically begins in the acute care setting. Usually the inpatient phase lasts 8–12 weeks and then the outpatient rehabilitation phase lasts 3–12 months after that, followed by yearly medical and functional evaluation. Physical therapists, occupational therapists, recreational therapists, nurses, social workers, psychologists and other health care professionals work as a team under the coordination of a physiatrist to decide on goals with the patient and develop a plan of discharge that is appropriate for the person's condition.

In the acute phase physical therapists focus on the patient's respiratory status, prevention of indirect complications (such as pressure ulcers), maintaining range of motion, and keeping available musculature active.

For people whose injuries are high enough to interfere with breathing, there is great emphasis on airway clearance during this stage of recovery. Weakness of respiratory muscles impairs the ability to cough effectively, allowing secretions to accumulate within the lungs. As SCI patients suffer from reduced total lung capacity and tidal volume, physical therapists teach them accessory breathing techniques (e.g. apical breathing, glossopharyngeal breathing) that typically are not taught to healthy individuals. Physical therapy treatment for airway clearance may include manual percussions and vibrations, postural drainage, respiratory muscle training, and assisted cough techniques. Patients are taught to increase their intra-abdominal pressure by leaning forward to induce cough and clear mild secretions. The quad cough technique is done lying on the back with the therapist applying pressure on the abdomen in the rhythm of the cough to maximize expiratory flow and mobilize secretions. Manual abdominal compression is another technique used to increase expiratory flow which later improves coughing. Other techniques used to manage respiratory dysfunction include respiratory muscle pacing, use of a constricting abdominal binder, ventilator-assisted speech, and mechanical ventilation.

The amount of functional recovery and independence achieved in terms of activities of daily living, recreational activities, and employment is affected by the level and severity of injury. The Functional Independence Measure (FIM) is an assessment tool that aims to evaluate the function of patients throughout the rehabilitation process following a spinal cord injury or other serious illness or injury. It can track a patient's progress and degree of independence during rehabilitation. People with SCI may need to use specialized devices and to make modifications to their environment in order to handle activities of daily living and to function independently. Weak joints can be stabilized with devices such as ankle-foot orthoses (AFOs) and knee-AFOs, but walking may still require a lot of effort. Increasing activity will increase chances of recovery.

Prognosis

Spinal cord injuries generally result in at least some incurable impairment even with the best possible treatment. The best predictor of prognosis is the level and completeness of injury, as measured by the ASIA impairment scale.The neurological score at the initial evaluation done 72 hours after injury is the best predictor of how much function will return. Most people with ASIA scores of A (complete injuries) do not have functional motor recovery, but improvement can occur. Most patients with incomplete injuries recover at least some function. Chances of recovering the ability to walk improve with each AIS grade found at the initial examination; e.g. an ASIA D score confers a better chance of walking than a score of C. The symptoms of incomplete injuries can vary and it is difficult to make an accurate prediction of the outcome. A person with a mild, incomplete injury at the T5 vertebra will have a much better chance of using his or her legs than a person with a severe, complete injury at exactly the same place. Of the incomplete SCI syndromes, Brown-Séquard and central cord syndromes have the best prognosis for recovery and anterior cord syndrome has the worst. People with nontraumatic causes of SCI have been found to be less likely to suffer complete injuries and some complications such as pressure sores and deep vein thrombosis, and to have shorter hospital stays. Their scores on functional tests were better than those of people with traumatic SCI upon hospital admission, but when they were tested upon discharge, those with traumatic SCI had improved such that both groups' results were the same. In addition to the completeness and level of the injury, age and concurrent health problems affect the extent to which a person with SCI will be able to live independently and to walk. However, in general people with injuries to L3 or below will likely be able to walk functionally, T10 and below to walk around the house with bracing, and C7 and below to live independently.

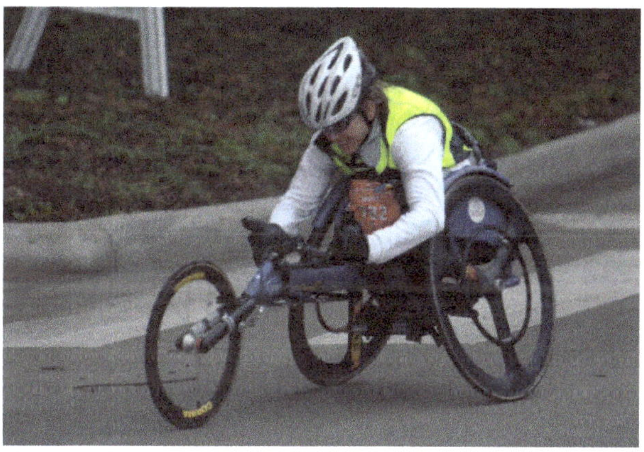

Holly Koester incurred a spinal injury as a result of a motor vehicle collision and is now a wheelchair racer.

One important predictor of motor recovery in an area is presence of sensation there, particularly pain perception. Most motor recovery occurs in the first year post-injury, but modest improvements can continue for years; sensory recovery is more limited. Recovery is typically quickest during the first six months. Spinal shock, in which reflexes are suppressed, occurs immediately after the injury and resolves largely within three months but continues resolving gradually for another 15.

Sexual dysfunction after spinal injury is common. Problems that can occur include erectile dysfunction, loss of ability to ejaculate, insufficient lubrication of the vagina, and reduced sensation and impaired ability to orgasm. Despite this, many people learn ways to adapt their sexual practices so they can lead satisfying sex lives.

Although life expectancy has improved with better care options, it is still not as good as the uninjured population. The higher the level of injury, and the more complete the injury, the greater the reduction in life expectancy. Mortality is very elevated within a year of injury.

Complications

Complications of spinal cord injuries include pulmonary edema, respiratory failure, neurogenic shock, and paralysis below the injury site. In the long term, the loss of muscle function can have additional effects from disuse, including atrophy of the muscle. Immobility can lead to pressure sores, particularly in bony areas, requiring precautions such as extra cushioning and turning in bed every two hours (in the acute setting) to relieve pressure. In the long term, people in wheelchairs must shift periodically to relieve pressure. Another complication is pain, including nociceptive pain (indication of potential or actual tissue damage) and neuropathic pain, when nerves affected by damage convey erroneous pain signals in the absence of noxious stimuli. Spasticity, the uncontrollable tensing of muscles below the level of injury, occurs in 65–78% of chronic SCI. It results from lack of input from the brain that quells muscle responses to stretch reflexes. It can be treated with drugs and physical therapy. Spasticity increases the risk of contractures (shortening of muscles, tendons, or ligaments that result from lack of use of a limb); this problem can be prevented by moving the limb through its full range of motion multiple times a day. Another problem lack of mobility can cause is loss of bone density and changes in bone structure. Loss of bone density (bone demineralization), thought to be due to lack of input from weakened or paralysed muscles, can increase the risk of fractures. Conversely, a poorly understood phenomenon is the overgrowth of bone tissue in soft tissue areas, called heterotopic ossification. It occurs below the level of injury, possibly as a result of inflammation, and happens to a clinically significant extent in 27% of people.

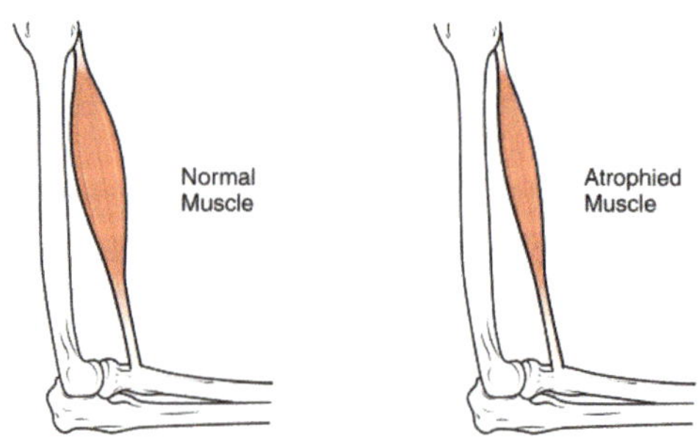

Muscle mass is reduced as muscles atrophy with disuse.

People with SCI are at especially high risk for respiratory and cardiovascular problems, so hospital staff must be watchful to avoid them. Respiratory problems (especially pneumonia) are the leading cause of death in people with SCI, followed by infections, usually of pressure sores, urinary tract infections and respiratory infections. Pneumonia can be accompanied by shortness of breath, fever, and anxiety.

Another potentially deadly threat to respiration is deep venous thrombosis (DVT), in which blood forms a clot in immobile limbs; the clot can break off and form a pulmonary embolism, lodging in the lung and cutting off blood supply to it. DVT is an especially high risk in SCI, particularly within 10 days of injury, occurring in over 13% in the acute care setting. Preventative measures include anticoagulants, pressure hose, and moving the patient's limbs. The usual signs and symptoms of DVT and pulmonary embolism may be masked in SCI cases due to effects such as alterations in pain perception and nervous system functioning.

Urinary tract infection (UTI) is another risk that may not display the usual symptoms (pain, urgency and frequency); it may instead be associated with worsened spasticity. The risk of UTI, likely the most common complication in the long term, is heightened by use of indwelling urinary catheters. Catheterization may be necessary because SCI interferes with the bladder's ability to empty when it gets too full, which could trigger autonomic dysreflexia or damage the bladder permanently. The use of intermittent catheterization to empty the bladder at regular intervals throughout the day has decreased the mortality due to kidney failure from UTI in the first world, but it is still a serious problem in developing countries.

An estimated 24–45% of people with SCI suffer disorders of depression, and the suicide rate is as much as six times that of the rest of the population. The risk of suicide is worst in the first five years after injury. In young people with SCI, suicide is the leading cause of death. Depression is associated with an increased risk of other complications such as UTI and pressure ulcers that occur more when self-care is neglected.

Epidemiology

Worldwide, the incidence (number of new cases) since 1995 of SCI ranges from 10.4 to 83 people per million per year. This wide range of numbers is probably partly due to differences among regions in whether and how injuries are reported. In North America, about 39 people per every million incur SCI traumatically each year, and in Western Europe the incidence is 16 per million. In the United States, the incidence of spinal cord injury has been estimated to be about 40 cases per 1 million people per year or around 12,000 cases per year. In China, the incidence is approximately 60,000 per year. The estimated prevalence (number of people living with SCI) in the world ranges from 236 to 4187 per million. Estimates vary widely due to differences in how data are collected and what techniques are used to extrapolate the figures. Little information is available from Asia, and even less from Africa and South America. In Western Europe the estimated prevalence is 300 per million people and in North America it is 853 per million. It is estimated at 440 per million in Iran, 526 per million in Iceland, and 681 per million in Australia. In the United States there are between 225,000 and 296,000 individuals living with spinal cord injuries, and different studies have estimated prevalences from 525 to 906 per million.

SCI is present in about 2% of all cases of blunt force trauma. Anyone who has undergone force sufficient to cause a thoracic spinal injury is at high risk for other injuries also. In 44% of SCI cases, other serious injuries are sustained at the same time; 14% of SCI patients also suffer head trauma or facial trauma. Other commonly associated injuries include chest trauma, abdominal trauma, pelvic fractures, and long bone fractures.

Males account for four out of five traumatic spinal cord injuries. Most of these injuries occur in men under 30 years of age. The average age at the time of injury has slowly increased from about 29 years in the 1970s to 41. Rates of injury are at their lowest in children, at their highest in the late teens to early twenties, then get progressively lower in older age groups; however rates may rise in the elderly. In Sweden between 50 and 70% of all cases of SCI occur in people under 30, and 25% occur in those over 50. While SCI rates are highest among people age 15–20, fewer than 3% of SCIs occur in people under 15. Neonatal SCI occurs in one in 60,000 births, e.g. from breech births or injuries by forceps. The difference in rates between the sexes diminishes in injuries at age 3 and younger; the same number of girls are injured as boys, or possibly more. Another cause of pediatric injury is child abuse such as shaken baby syndrome. For children, the most common cause of SCI (56%) is vehicle crashes. High numbers of adolescent injuries are attributable in a large part to traffic accidents and sports injuries. For people over 65, falls are the most common cause of traumatic SCI. The elderly and people with severe arthritis are at high risk for SCI because of defects in the spinal column. In nontraumatic SCI, the gender difference is smaller, the average age of occurrence is greater, and incomplete lesions are more common.

History

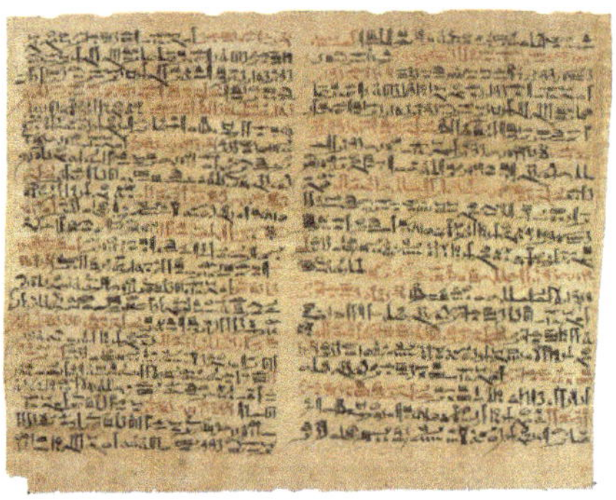

The ancient Egyptian Edwin Smith Papyrus is the earliest known description of SCI.

SCI has been known to be devastating for millennia; the ancient Egyptian Edwin Smith Papyrus from 2500 BC, the first known description of the injury, says it is "not to be treated". Hindu texts dating back to 1800 BC also mention SCI and describe traction techniques to straighten the spine. The Greek physician Hippocrates, born in the fifth century BC, described SCI in his Hippocratic Corpus and invented traction devices to straighten dislocated vertebrae. But it was not until Aulus Cornelius Celsus, born 30 BC, noted that a cervical injury resulted in rapid death that the spinal cord itself was implicated in the condition. In the second century AD the Greek physician Galen experimented on monkeys and reported that a horizontal cut through the spinal cord caused them to lose all sensation and motion below the level of the cut. The seventh-century Greek physician Paul of Aegina described surgical techniques for treatment of broken vertebrae by removing bone fragments, as well as surgery to relieve pressure on the spine. Little medical progress was made during the Middle Ages in Europe; it was not until the Renaissance that the spine and nerves were accurately depicted in human anatomy drawings by Leonardo da Vinci and Andreas Vesalius.

In 1762 a surgeon named Andre Louis removed a bullet from the lumbar spine of a patient, who regained motion in the legs. In 1829 the surgeon Gilpin Smith performed a successful laminectomy that improved the patient's sensation. However, the idea that SCI was untreatable remained predominant until the early 20th century. In 1934, the mortality rate in the first two years after injury was over 80%, mostly due to infections of the urinary tract and pressure sores. It was not until the latter half of the century that breakthroughs in imaging, surgery, medical care, and rehabilitation medicine contributed to a substantial improvement in SCI care. The relative incidence of incomplete compared to complete injuries has improved since the mid-20th century, due mainly to the emphasis on faster and better initial care and stabilization of spinal cord injury patients. The creation of emergency medical services to professionally transport people to the hospital is given partial credit for an improvement in outcomes since the 1970s. Improvements in care have been accompanied by increased life expectancy of people with SCI; survival times have improved by about 2000% since 1940.

Research Directions

Scientists are investigating various avenues for treatment of spinal cord injury. Therapeutic research is focused on two main areas: neuroprotection and neuroregeneration. The former seeks to prevent the harm that occurs from secondary injury in the minutes to weeks following the insult, and the latter aims to reconnect the broken circuits in the spinal cord to allow function to return. Neuroprotective drugs target secondary injury effects including inflammation, damage by free radicals, excitotoxicity (neuronal damage by excessive glutamate signaling), and apoptosis (cell suicide). Several potentially neuroprotective agents that target pathways like these are under investigation in human clinical trials.

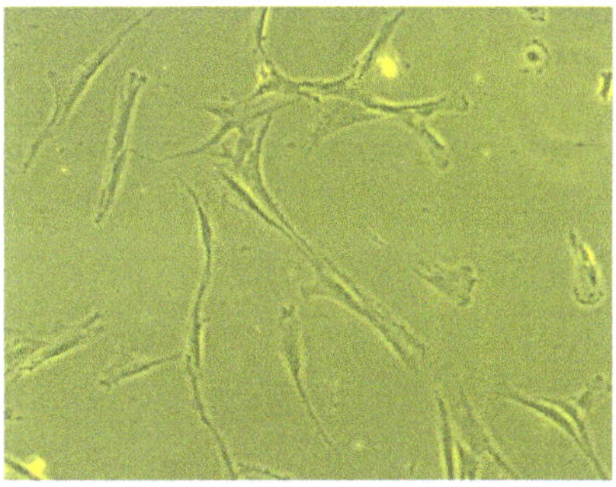

Human bone marrow derived mesenchymal stem cells seen under phase contrast microscope (63 x magnification)

Cell transplantation is an important avenue for SCI research: the goal is to replace lost spinal cord cells, allow reconnection in broken neural circuits by regrowing axons, and to create an environment in the tissues that is favorable to growth. A key avenue of SCI research is research on stem cells, which can differentiate into other types of cells—including those lost after SCI. Types of cells being researched for use in SCI include embryonic stem cells, neural stem cells, mesenchymal stem cells, olfactory ensheathing cells, Schwann cells, activated macrophages, and induced pluripotent stem cells. Hundreds of stem cell studies have been done in humans, with promising but inconclusive results. An ongoing Phase 2 trial in 2016 presented data showing that after 90 days, 2 out of 4 subjects had already improved two motor levels and had thus already achieved its endpoint of 2/5 patients improving two levels within 6–12 months. Six-month data is expected in January 2017.

Another type of approach is tissue engineering, using biomaterials to help scaffold and rebuild damaged tissues. Biomaterials being investigated include natural substances such as collagen or agarose and synthetic ones like polymers and nitrocellulose. They fall into two categories: hydrogels and nanofibers. These materials can also be used as a vehicle for delivering gene therapy to tissues.

One avenue being explored to allow paralyzed people to walk and to aid in rehabilitation of those with some walking ability is the use of wearable powered robotic exoskeletons. The devices, which have motorized joints, are put on over the legs and supply a source of power to move and walk. Several such devices are already available for sale, but investigation is still underway as to how they can be made more useful.

Electromyography

Electromyography (EMG) is an electrodiagnostic medicine technique for evaluating and recording the electrical activity produced by skeletal muscles. EMG is performed using an instrument called an electromyograph to produce a record called an electromyogram. An electromyograph detects the electric potential generated by muscle cells when these cells are electrically or neurologically activated. The signals can be analyzed to detect medical abnormalities, activation level, or recruitment order, or to analyze the biomechanics of human or animal movement.

Medical Uses

EMG testing has a variety of clinical and biomedical applications. EMG is used as a diagnostics tool for identifying neuromuscular diseases, or as a research tool for studying kinesiology, and disorders of motor control. EMG signals are sometimes used to guide botulinum toxin or phenol injections into muscles. EMG signals are also used as a control signal for prosthetic devices such as prosthetic hands, arms, and lower limbs.

EMG then an acceleromyograph may be used for neuromuscular monitoring in general anesthesia with neuromuscular-blocking drugs, in order to avoid postoperative residual curarization (PORC).

Except in the case of some purely primary myopathic conditions EMG is usually performed with another electrodiagnostic medicine test that measures the conducting function of nerves. This is called a nerve conduction studies (NCS). Needle EMG and NCSs are typically indicated when there is pain in the limbs, weakness from spinal nerve compression, or concern about some other neurologic injury or disorder. Spinal nerve injury does not cause neck, mid back pain or low back pain, and for this reason, evidence has not shown EMG or NCS to be helpful in diagnosing causes of axial lumbar pain, thoracic pain, or cervical spine pain. Needle EMG may aid with the diagnosis of nerve compression or injury (such as carpal tunnel syndrome), nerve root injury (such as sciatica), and with other problems of the muscles or nerves. Less common medical conditions include amyotrophic lateral sclerosis, myasthenia gravis, and muscular dystrophy.

Technique

Skin Preparation and Risks

The first step before insertion of the needle electrode is skin preparation. This typically involves simply cleaning the skin with an alcohol pad.

The actual placement of the needle electrode can be difficult and depends on a number of factors, such as specific muscle selection and the size of that muscle. Proper needle EMG placement is very important for accurate representation of the muscle of interest, although EMG is more effective on superficial muscles as it is unable to bypass the action potentials of superficial muscles and detect deeper muscles. Also, the more body fat an individual has, the weaker the EMG signal. When placing the EMG sensor, the ideal location is at the belly of the muscle: the longitudinal midline. The belly of the muscle can also be thought of as in-between the motor point (middle) of the muscle and the tendonus insertion point.

Cardiac pacemakers and implanted cardiac defibrillators (ICDs) are used increasingly in clinical practice, and no evidence exists indicating that performing routine electrodiagnostic studies on patients with these devices pose a safety hazard. However, there are theoretical concerns that electrical impulses of nerve conduction studies (NCS) could be erroneously sensed by devices and result in unintended inhibition or triggering of output or reprogramming of the device. In general, the closer the stimulation site is to the pacemaker and pacing leads, the greater the chance for inducing a voltage of sufficient amplitude to inhibit the pacemaker. Despite such concerns, no immediate or delayed adverse effects have been reported with routine NCS.

No known contraindications exist from performing needle EMG or NCS on pregnant patients. In addition, no complications from these procedures have been reported in the literature. Evoked potential testing, likewise, has not been reported to cause any problems when it is performed during pregnancy.

Patients with lymphedema or patients at risk for lymphedema are routinely cautioned to avoid percutaneous procedures in the affected extremity, namely venipuncture, to prevent development or worsening of lymphedema or cellulitis. Despite the potential risk, the evidence for such complications subsequent to venipuncture is limited. No published reports exist of cellulitis, infection, or other complications related to EMG performed in the setting of lymphedema or prior lymph node dissection. However, given the unknown risk of cellulitis in patients with lymphedema, reasonable caution should be exercised in performing needle examinations in lymphedematous regions to avoid complications. In patients with gross edema and taut skin, skin puncture by needle electrodes may result in chronic weeping of serous fluid. The potential bacterial media of such serous fluid and the violation of skin integrity may increase the risk of cellulitis. Prior to proceeding, the physician should weigh the potential risks of performing the study with the need to obtain the information gained.

Surface and Intramuscular EMG Recording Electrodes

There are two kinds of EMG: surface EMG and intramuscular EMG. Surface EMG assesses muscle function by recording muscle activity from the surface above the muscle on the skin. Surface electrodes are able to provide only a limited assessment of the muscle activity. Surface EMG can be recorded by a pair of electrodes or by a more complex array of multiple electrodes. More than one electrode is needed because EMG recordings display the potential difference (voltage difference) between two separate electrodes. Limitations of this approach are the fact that surface electrode recordings are restricted to superficial muscles, are influenced by the depth of the subcutaneous tissue at the site of the recording which can be highly variable depending of the weight of a patient, and cannot reliably discriminate between the discharges of adjacent muscles.

Intramuscular EMG can be performed using a variety of different types of recording electrodes. The simplest approach is a monopolar needle electrode. This can be a fine wire inserted into a muscle with a surface electrode as a reference; or two fine wires inserted into muscle referenced to each other. Most commonly fine wire recordings are for research or kinesiology studies. Diagnostic monopolar EMG electrodes are typically stiff enough to penetrate skin and insulated, with only the tip exposed using a surface electrode for reference. Needles for injecting therapeutic botulinum toxin or phenol are typically monopolar electrodes that use a surface reference, in this case, however, the metal shaft of a hypodermic needle, insulated so that only the tip is exposed, is used both to record signals and to inject. Slightly more complex in design is the concentric needle electrode. These needles have a fine wire, embedded in a layer of insulation that fills the barrel of a hypodermic needle, that has an exposed shaft, and the shaft serves as the reference electrode. The exposed tip of the fine wire serves as the active electrode. As a result of this configuration, signals tend to be smaller when recorded from a concentric electrode than when recorded from a monopolar electrode and they are more resistant to electrical artifacts from tissue and measurements tend to be somewhat more reliable. However, because the shaft is exposed throughout its length, superficial muscle activity can contaminate the recording of deeper muscles. Single fiber EMG needle electrodes are designed to have very tiny recording areas, and allow for the discharges of individual muscle fibers to be discriminated.

To perform intramuscular EMG, typically either a monopolar or concentric needle electrode is inserted through the skin into the muscle tissue. The needle is then moved to multiple spots within a relaxed muscle to evaluate both insertional activity and resting activity in the muscle. Normal muscles exhibit a brief burst of muscle fiber activation when stimulated by needle movement, but this rarely lasts more than 100ms. The two most common pathologic types of resting activity in muscle are fasciculation and fibrillation potentials. A fasciculation potential is an involuntary activation of a motor unit within the muscle, sometimes visible with the naked eye as a muscle twitch or by surface electrodes. Fibrillations, however, are only detected by needle EMG, and represent the isolated activation of individual muscle fibers, usually as the result of nerve or muscle disease. Often, fibrillations are triggered by needle movement (insertional activity) and persist for several seconds or more after the movement ceases.

After assessing resting and insertional activity, the electromyographer assess the activity of muscle during voluntary contraction. The shape, size, and frequency of the resulting electrical signals are judged. Then the electrode is retracted a few millimetres, and again the activity is analyzed. This is repeated, sometimes until data on 10–20 motor units have been collected in order to draw conclusions about motor unit function. Each electrode track gives only a very local picture of the activity of the whole muscle. Because skeletal muscles differ in the inner structure, the electrode has to be placed at various locations to obtain an accurate study.

Single fiber electromyography assessed the delay between the contractions of individual muscle fibers within a motor unit and is a sensitive test for dysfunction of the neuromuscular junction caused by drugs, poisons, or diseases such as myasthenia gravis. The technique is complicated and typically only performed by individuals with special advanced training. Surface EMG is used in a number of settings; for example, in the physiotherapy clinic, muscle activation is monitored using surface EMG and patients have an auditory or visual stimulus to help them know when they are activating the muscle (biofeedback). A review of the literature on surface EMG published in 2008 concluded that surface EMG may be useful to detect the presence of neuromuscular disease (level C rating, class III data), but there are insufficient data to support its utility for distinguishing between neuropathic and myopathic conditions or for the diagnosis of specific neuromuscular diseases. EMGs may be useful for additional study of fatigue associated with post-poliomyelitis syndrome and electromechanical function in myotonic dystrophy (level C rating, class III data).

Certain US states limit the performance of needle EMG by nonphysicians. New Jersey declared that it cannot be delegated to a physician's assistant. Michigan has passed legislation saying needle EMG is the practice of medicine. Special training in diagnosing medical diseases with EMG is required only in residency and fellowship programs in neurology, clinical neurophysiology, neuromuscular medicine, and physical medicine and rehabilitation. There are certain subspecialists in otolaryngology who have had selective training in performing EMG of the laryngeal muscles, and subspecialists in urology, obstetrics and gynecology who have had selective training in performing EMG of muscles controlling bowel and bladder function.

Maximal Voluntary Contraction

One basic function of EMG is to see how well a muscle can be activated. The most common way that can be determined is by performing a maximal voluntary contraction (MVC) of the muscle that is being tested.

Muscle force, which is measured mechanically, typically correlates highly with measures of EMG activation of muscle. Most commonly this is assessed with surface electrodes, but it should be recognized that these typically only record from muscle fibers in close approximation to the surface.

Several analytical methods for determining muscle activation are commonly used depending on the application. The use of mean EMG activation or the peak contraction value is a debated topic. Most studies commonly use the maximal voluntary contraction as a means of analyzing peak force and force generated by target muscles. According to the article, Peak and average rectified EMG measures: Which method of data reduction should be used for assessing core training exercises?, concluded that the "average rectified EMG data (ARV) is significantly less variable when measuring the muscle activity of the core musculature compared to the peak EMG variable." Therefore, these researchers would suggest that "ARV EMG data should be recorded alongside the peak EMG measure when assessing core exercises." Providing the reader with both sets of data would result in enhanced validity of the study and potentially eradicate the contradictions within the research.

Other Measurements

EMG can also be used for indicating the amount of fatigue in a muscle. The following changes in the EMG signal can signify muscle fatigue: an increase in the mean absolute value of the signal, increase in the amplitude and duration of the muscle action potential and an overall shift to lower frequencies. Monitoring the changes of different frequency changes the most common way of using EMG to determine levels of fatigue. The lower conduction velocities enable the slower motor neurons to remain active.

A motor unit is defined as one motor neuron and all of the muscle fibers it innervates. When a motor unit fires, the impulse (called an action potential) is carried down the motor neuron to the muscle. The area where the nerve contacts the muscle is called the neuromuscular junction, or the motor end plate. After the action potential is transmitted across the neuromuscular junction, an action potential is elicited in all of the innervated muscle fibers of that particular motor unit. The sum of all this electrical activity is known as a motor unit action potential (MUAP). This electrophysiologic activity from multiple motor units is the signal typically evaluated during an EMG. The composition of the motor unit, the number of muscle fibres per motor unit, the metabolic type of muscle fibres and many other factors affect the shape of the motor unit potentials in the myogram.

Nerve conduction testing is also often done at the same time as an EMG to diagnose neurological diseases.

Some patients can find the procedure somewhat painful, whereas others experience only a small amount of discomfort when the needle is inserted. The muscle or muscles being tested may be slightly sore for a day or two after the procedure.

EMG Signal Decomposition

EMG signals are essentially made up of superimposed motor unit action potentials (MUAPs) from several motor units. For a thorough analysis, the measured EMG signals can be decomposed into their constituent MUAPs. MUAPs from different motor units tend to have different characteristic shapes, while MUAPs recorded by the same electrode from the same motor unit are typically similar. Notably MUAP size and shape depend on where the electrode is located with respect to the fibers and so can appear to be different if the electrode moves position. EMG decomposition is non-trivial, although many methods have been proposed.

EMG Signal Processing

Rectification is the translation of the raw EMG signal to a single polarity frequency (usually positive). The purpose of rectifying a signal is to ensure the raw signal does not average zero, due to the raw EMG signal having positive and negative components. It facilitates the signals and process and calculates the mean, integration and the fast fourier transform (FFT). The two types of rectification of signals refer to what happens to the EMG wave when it is processed. These types include full length frequency and half length. Full length frequency adds the EMG signal below the baseline (usually negative polarity) to the signal above the baseline making a conditioned signal that is all positive. This is the preferred method of rectification because it conserves all signal energy for analysis, usually in the positive polarity. Half length rectification deletes the EMG signal below the baseline. In doing so, the average of the data is no longer zero therefore it can be used in statistical analyses. The only difference between the two types of rectification is that full-wave rectification takes the absolute value of the signal array of data points.

Limitations

Needle EMG use in clinical settings has practical applications such as helping to discover disease. Needle EMG has limitations, however, in that it does involve voluntary activation of muscle, and as such is less informative in patients unwilling or unable to cooperate, children and infants, and in individuals with paralysis., Surface EMG can have limited applications due to inherent problems associated with surface EMG. Adipose tissue (fat) can affect EMG recordings. Studies show that as adipose tissue increased the active muscle directly below the surface decreased. As adipose tissue increased, the amplitude of the surface EMG signal directly above the center of the active muscle decreased. EMG signal recordings are typically more accurate with individuals who have lower body fat, and more compliant skin, such as young people when compared to old. Muscle cross talk occurs when the EMG signal from one muscle interferes with that of another limiting reliability of the signal of the muscle being tested. Surface EMG is limited due to lack of deep muscles reliability. Deep muscles require intramuscular wires that are intrusive and painful in order to achieve an EMG signal. Surface EMG can only measure superficial muscles and even then it is hard to narrow down the signal to a single muscle.

Electrical Characteristics

The electrical source is the muscle membrane potential of about –90 mV. Measured EMG potentials range between less than 50 μV and up to 20 to 30 mV, depending on the muscle under observation.

Typical repetition rate of muscle motor unit firing is about 7–20 Hz, depending on the size of the muscle (eye muscles versus seat (gluteal) muscles), previous axonal damage and other factors. Damage to motor units can be expected at ranges between 450 and 780 mV.

Procedure Outcomes

Normal Results

Muscle tissue at rest is normally electrically inactive. After the electrical activity caused by the irritation of needle insertion subsides, the electromyograph should detect no abnormal spontaneous activity (i.e., a muscle at rest should be electrically silent, with the exception of the area of the neuromuscular junction, which is, under normal circumstances, very spontaneously active). When the muscle is voluntarily contracted, action potentials begin to appear. As the strength of the muscle contraction is increased, more and more muscle fibers produce action potentials. When the muscle is fully contracted, there should appear a disorderly group of action potentials of varying rates and amplitudes (a complete recruitment and interference pattern).

Abnormal Results

EMG findings vary with the type of disorder, the duration of the problem, the age of the patient, the degree to which the patient can be cooperative, the type of needle electrode used to study the patient, and sampling error in terms of the number of areas studied within a single muscle and the number of muscles studied overall. Interpreting EMG findings is usually best done by an individual informed by a focused history and physical examination of the patient, and in conjunction with the results of other relevant diagnostic studies performed including most importantly, nerve conduction studies, but also, where appropriate, imaging studies such as MRI and ultrasound, muscle and nerve biopsy, muscle enzymes, and serologic studies.

Abnormal results may be caused by the following medical conditions (please note this is not an exhaustive list of conditions that can result in abnormal EMG studies):

Disorders of Muscle:	Disorders of Nerves:	Plexus disorders:
• Inflammatory myopathies • Polymyositis • Dermatomyositis • Inclusion body myopathy • Myotonia Congenita • Muscular dystrophies: • Duchenne Muscular Dystrophy • Becker muscular dystrophy • Facioscapulohumeral dystrophy • Limb girdle muscular dystrophy • Centronuclear myopathy • Myotonic dystrophy • Mitochondrial myopathies Disorders of the neuromuscular junction: • Myasthenia Gravis • Lambert–Eaton myasthenic syndrome • Botulism poisoning • Organophosphate poisoning • Hypermagnesemia • Hypocalcemia	• Carpal tunnel syndrome • Ulnar neuropathy at the elbow • Radial nerve palsy (Saturday night palsy) • Peroneal (fibular) nerve palsy • Diabetic neuropathy • Alcohol related neuropathy • Nutritional neuropathy • Amyloid neuropathy • AIDP • CIDP • Bell's palsy • Laryngeal neuropathy • Pudendal neuropathy • Femoral neuropathy • Sciatic Neuropathy • Tibial neuropathy • Tarsal tunnel syndrome • Charcot-Marie-Tooth syndrome • Zoster neuropathy • Oculomotor, Facial, vagal, trigeminal, glossopharyngeal, spinal accessory neuropathies • Hemifacial spasm • Multifocal motor neuropathy • Axillary neuropathy • Long thoracic neuropathy • Suprascapular neuropathy • Toxic neuropathies • Drug-induced neuropathies	• Neuralgic Amyotrophy (idiopathic brachial plexitis) • Traumatic brachial plexopathy • Lumbosacral radiculopathy • Hirayama disease Root disorders: • Cervical, thoracic, lumbar, sacral radiculopathy • Spinal stenosis • Arachnoiditis • Leptomeningeal disorders Motor neuron disease • Amyotrophic lateral sclerosis • West Nile virus • Poliomyelitis • Kennedy's syndrome (Spinobulbar muscular atrophy).

History

The first documented experiments dealing with EMG started with Francesco Redi's works in 1666. Redi discovered a highly specialized muscle of the electric ray fish (Electric Eel) generated electricity. By 1773, Walsh had been able to demonstrate that the eel fish's muscle tissue could generate a spark of electricity. In 1792, a publication entitled *De Viribus Electricitatis in Motu Musculari Commentarius* appeared, written by Luigi Galvani, in which the author demonstrated that electricity could initiate muscle contraction. Six decades later, in 1849, Emil du Bois-Reymond discovered that it was also possible to record electrical activity during a voluntary muscle contraction. The first actual recording of this activity was made by Marey in 1890, who also introduced the term electromyography. In 1922, Gasser and Erlanger used an oscilloscope to show the electrical signals from muscles. Because of the stochastic nature of the myoelectric signal, only rough information could be obtained from its observation. The capability of detecting electromyographic signals improved steadily from the 1930s through the 1950s, and researchers began to use improved electrodes more widely for the study of muscles. The AANEM was formed in 1953 as one of several currently active medical societies with a special interest in advancing the science and clinical use of the technique. Clinical use of surface EMG (sEMG) for the treatment of more specific disorders began in the 1960s. Hardyck and his researchers were the first (1966) practitioners to use sEMG. In the early 1980s, Cram and Steger introduced a clinical method for scanning a variety of muscles using an EMG sensing device.

It was not until the middle of the 1980s that integration techniques in electrodes had sufficiently advanced to allow batch production of the required small and lightweight instrumentation and amplifiers. At present, a number of suitable amplifiers are commercially available. In the early 1980s, cables that produced signals in the desired microvolt range became available. Recent research has resulted in a better understanding of the properties of surface EMG recording. Surface electromyography is increasingly used for recording from superficial muscles in clinical or kinesiological protocols, where intramuscular electrodes are used for investigating deep muscles or localized muscle activity.

There are many applications for the use of EMG. EMG is used clinically for the diagnosis of neurological and neuromuscular problems. It is used diagnostically by gait laboratories and by clinicians trained in the use of biofeedback or ergonomic assessment. EMG is also used in many types of research laboratories, including those involved in biomechanics, motor control, neuromuscular physiology, movement disorders, postural control, and physical therapy.

Research

EMG can be used to sense isometric muscular activity where no movement is produced. This enables definition of a class of subtle motionless gestures to control interfaces without being noticed and without disrupting the surrounding environment. These signals can be used to control a prosthesis or as a control signal for an electronic device such as a mobile phone or PDA.

EMG signals have been targeted as control for flight systems. The Human Senses Group at the NASA Ames Research Center at Moffett Field, CA seeks to advance man-machine interfaces by directly connecting a person to a computer. In this project, an EMG signal is used to substitute for mechanical joysticks and keyboards. EMG has also been used in research towards a "wearable cockpit," which employs EMG-based gestures to manipulate switches and control sticks necessary for flight in conjunction with a goggle-based display.

Unvoiced speech recognition recognizes speech by observing the EMG activity of muscles associated with speech. It is targeted for use in noisy environments, and may be helpful for people without vocal cords and people with aphasia.

EMG has also been used as a control signal for computers and other devices. An interface device based on EMG could be used to control moving objects, such as mobile robots or an electric wheelchair. This may be helpful for individuals that cannot operate a joystick-controlled wheelchair. Surface EMG recordings may also be a suitable control signal for some interactive video games.

A joint project involving Microsoft, the University of Washington in Seattle, and the University of Toronto in Canada has explored using muscle signals from hand gestures as an interface device. A patent based on this research was submitted on June 26, 2008.

Postural Restoration

Postural restoration is a posture based integrative treatment approach to physical medicine. It includes the science of postural adaptations, the influence of the respiratory system and polyarticular chains of muscle, and asymmetrical patterns. Treatment aims to maximize neutrality in the body through manual and non-manual exercise techniques designed to reposition, retrain, and restore these asymmetrical patterned positions. It is used by some physical therapy and athletic trainers. There is little quality evidence on its usefulness in any health condition.

Effectiveness

Although there is no research based evidence on its effectiveness. Postural restoration has been used with people who have sciatica and low back pain, anterior knee pain, temporomandibular disorders (TMD) and orofacial pain.

Mechanism

The Zone of Apposition (ZOA) is a term for the area of the diaphragm that directly opposes the rib cage. The diaphragm's mechanical action and respiratory advantage depends on its relationship and anatomical arrangement with the rib cage. Respiratory function, proper diaphragmatic breathing and acquiring a zone of apposition are common principles utilized with Postural Restoration.

Evidence Base

Hruska 1997, reviewed the influence of faulty breathing patterns and overactive cervical musculature on normal resting position of the mandible and cervical cranial alignment. Clinical recommendations were offered regarding the importance of balancing the respiratory system through diaphragmatic breathing, along with strengthening the internal oblique and gluteal muscles when treating orofacial pain and TMD.

Hruska 2002, discussed temporomandibular dysfunction (TMD) and its relationship to thoracopelvic position. In addition to discussing proper respiratory mechanics and rib positioning, Postural Restoration non-manual technique recommendations were provided to improve abdominal oblique strength with concomitant latissimus dorsi and pectoralis major stretching.

Boyle et al. 2010, authored a journal article discussing the clinical use of a Postural Restoration non-manual technique (90-90 Hip Lift with Balloon). They review effectiveness of a balloon blowing exercise (BBE) technique to restore the zone of apposition and spinal position, allowing the diaphragm to optimally perform its respiratory and postural roles.

History

Physical therapist Ron Hruska developed the science of Postural Restoration in the early 1990s as a result of his clinical experience and dedication to the study of the asymmetrical human body. In 1999, he founded the Postural Restoration Institute, located in Lincoln, Nebraska, as a way to educate healthcare professionals across the world in postural restoration.

References

- Hardy, Paul A. J. (1997). Chronic pain management: the essentials. U.K.: Greenwich Medical Media. ISBN 1-900151-85-5.
- Main, Chris J.; Spanswick, Chris C. (2000). Pain management: an interdisciplinary approach. Churchill Livingstone. ISBN 0-443-05683-8.
- Thienhaus, Ole; Cole, B. Eliot (2002). "The classification of pain". In Weiner, Richard S,. Pain management: A practical guide for clinicians. CRC Press. p. 29. ISBN 0-8493-0926-3.
- Marijuana and Medicine: Assessing the Science Base. Institute of Medicine. 1999. ISBN 0-309-07155-0. Retrieved 3 May 2013.
- McKenzie, R A (1998). The Cervical and Thoracic Spine: Mechanical Diagnosis and Therapy. New Zealand: Spinal Publications Ltd. pp. 16–20. ISBN 978-0-9597746-7-2.

- Cameron, Michelle H. (2003). Physical agents in rehabilitation: from research to practice. Philadelphia: W. B. Saunders. ISBN 0-7216-9378-4.
- Human Rights Watch (2 June 2011), Global State of Pain Treatment: Access to Medicines and Palliative Care, Human Rights Watch, retrieved 28 July 2016.
- "Asterias Biotherapeutics Announces Positive Efficacy Data in Patients with Complete Cervical Spinal Cord Injuries Treated with AST-OPC1". asteriasbiotherapeutics.com. Retrieved 2016-09-15.
- Chris, Collora,. "Master's of Physical Therapy (MPT) vs. Doctor of Physical Therapy (DPT) Degree". Exercise Science Guide. Retrieved 2016-02-15.
- "Enhance your Athleticism with Sports massage therapy". Archived from the original on March 17, 2016. Retrieved March 17, 2016.
- Consumer Reports (April 28, 2016). "Pain Relief: What You Need to Know". Consumer Reports. Retrieved 26 May 2016.
- "ACGME Sports, ACGME Pain, or Non-ACGME Sports and Spine: Which Is the Ideal Fellowship Training for PM&R Physicians Interested in Musculoskeletal Medicine?". ResearchGate. Retrieved 2015-09-19.

4

Various Types of Rehabilitation Medicine

Orthopedic surgery is the surgery that is performed or is concerned with the conditions involving the musculoskeletal system. The alternative types of rehabilitation medicine are aquatic therapy, hydrotherapy, medicine ball, stroke recovery, vocational rehabilitation and barthel scale. This section provides a plethora of the categories related to the subject matter for better comprehension of rehabilitation medicine.

Infinity Walk

Infinity Walk is a therapeutic method for progressively developing coordination and certain areas of cognitive functioning. It is typically used with compromised individuals such as those with brain injuries or learning disabilities. Teachers and therapists use it to improve some of the essential foundation skills that must be mastered before learning can occur.

A beginning student or patient learns to walk smoothly in a figure-eight pattern while looking at an object or person across the room. As they become able to do that consistently, other physical and mental activities are added to the coordinated walking. An advanced walker can maintain a smooth figure-eight walk while doing several other activities, *e.g.*, simultaneously gesturing and doing mental arithmetic as they converse with their teacher or therapist.

Infinity Walking can be done under a variety of conditions: indoors or outdoors, on foot or when riding a wheelchair, therapeutic riding horse, or other means of seated ambulation. There are systems of curved handrails that facilitate Infinity Walking by those unable to stand or walk on their own.

Developed in the 1980s by clinical psychologist Deborah Sunbeck, the Infinity Walk is based on studies of cognitive science, neuropsychology, and practical applications of EEG research on lateralized readiness potential. It strives to improve the sensorimotor functioning of those who practice it. In developing the method, Dr. Sunbeck also applied knowledge of social facilitation and intrinsic motivation to the task of creating a self-motivating method of physical and mental skill-building that would help the user develop resilient self-regulated learning strategies for future challenges.

Uses

The Infinity Walk is used in fields including elementary education, special education, physical therapy and occupational therapy.

- It has been used by U.S. physical and occupational therapists in the rehabilitation of persons with brain injuries.
- It has been recognized as a particularly effective activity in developing multi-sensory integration in occupational therapy, including some clients with learning disabilities.
- In a 1993 study, learning disabled elementary school students who completed an Infinity Walk program showed significant improvement in reading readiness, word identification, word comprehension, and reading passage comprehension.

Orthopedic Surgery

Orthopedic surgery or orthopedics (alternatively spelled orthopaedic surgery and orthopaedics) is the branch of surgery concerned with conditions involving the musculoskeletal system. Orthopedic surgeons use both surgical and nonsurgical means to treat musculoskeletal trauma, spine diseases, sports injuries, degenerative diseases, infections, tumors, and congenital disorders.

Etymology

As with many words derived with the "æ" ligature, simplification to either "ae" or just "e" is common. In the US the majority of college, university and residency programs, and even the American Academy of Orthopaedic Surgeons, still use the spelling with the Latinate digraph ae. Elsewhere, usage is not uniform; in Canada, both spellings are acceptable; *orthopaedics* usually prevails in the rest of the British Commonwealth, especially in the UK.

History

Early Orthopedics

Many developments in orthopedic surgery have resulted from experiences during wartime. On the battlefields of the Middle Ages the injured were treated with bandages soaked in horses' blood which dried to form a stiff, but unsanitary, splint.

Originally, the term orthopedics meant the correcting of musculoskeletal deformities in children. Nicolas Andry, a French professor at the University of Paris coined the term in the first textbook written on the subject in 1741. He advocated the use of exercise, manipulation and splinting to treat deformities in children. His book was directed towards parents, and while some topics would be familiar to orthopedists today, it also included 'excessive sweating of the palms' and freckles.

Jean-André Venel established the first orthopedic institute in 1780, which was the first hospital dedicated to the treatment of children's skeletal deformities. He developed the club-foot shoe for children born with foot deformities and various methods to treat curvature of the spine.

Advances made in surgical technique during the 18th century, such as John Hunter's research on tendon healing and Percival Pott's work on spinal deformity steadily increased the range of new methods available for effective treatment. Antonius Mathijsen, a Dutch military surgeon, invented the plaster of Paris cast in 1851. However, up until the 1890s, orthopedics was still a study limited to the correction of deformity in children. One of the first surgical procedures developed was percutaneous tenotomy. This involved cutting a tendon, originally the Achilles tendon, to help treat deformities alongside bracing and exercises. In the late 1800s and first decades of the 1900s, there was significant controversy about whether orthopedics should include surgical procedures at all.

Modern Orthopedics

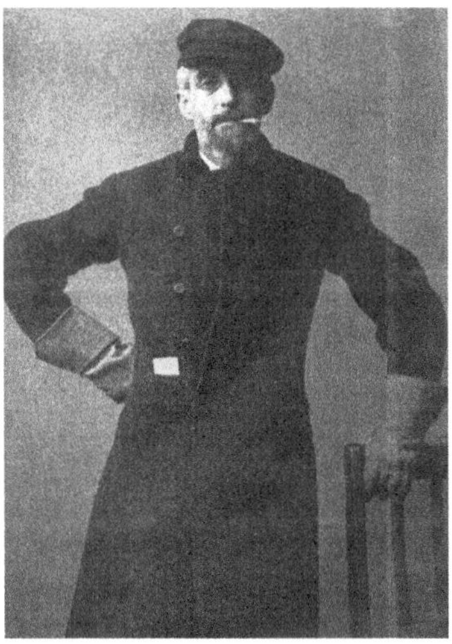

Hugh Owen Thomas, a pioneer of modern orthopedic surgery.

Examples of people who aided the development of modern orthopedic surgery were Hugh Owen Thomas, a surgeon from Wales, and his nephew, Robert Jones. Thomas became interested in orthopedics and bone-setting at a young age and, after establishing his own practice, went on to expand the field into general treatment of fracture and other musculoskeletal problems. He advocated enforced rest as the best remedy for fractures and tuberculosis and created the so-called 'Thomas Splint', to stabilize a fractured femur and prevent infection. He is also responsible for numerous other medical innovations that all carry his name: 'Thomas's collar' to treat tuberculosis of the cervical spine, 'Thomas's manoeuvre', an orthopedic investigation for fracture of the hip joint, Thomas test, a method of detecting hip deformity by having the patient lying flat in bed, 'Thomas's wrench' for reducing fractures, as well as an osteoclast to break and reset bones.

Thomas's work was not fully appreciated in his own lifetime. It was only during the First World War that his techniques came to be used for injured soldiers on the battlefield. His nephew, Sir Robert Jones, had already made great advances in orthopedics in his position as Surgeon-Superintendent for the construction of the Manchester Ship Canal in 1888. He was responsible for the injured among the 20,000 workers, and he organized the first comprehensive accident service in the world, dividing the 36 mile site into 3 sections, and establishing a hospital and a string of first aid posts in each section. He had the medical personnel trained in fracture management. He personally managed 3,000 cases and performed 300 operations in his own hospital. This position enabled him to learn new techniques and improve the standard of fracture management. Physicians from around the world came to Jones' clinic to learn his techniques. Along with Alfred Tubby, Jones founded the British Orthopaedic Society in 1894.

During the First World War, Jones served as a Territorial Army surgeon. He observed that treatment of fractures both at the front and in hospitals at home was inadequate, and his efforts led to the introduction of military orthopedic hospitals. He was appointed Inspector of Military Orthopaedics, with responsibility over 30,000 beds. The hospital in Ducane Road, Hammersmith became the model for both British and American military orthopedic hospitals. His advocacy of the use of Thomas splint for the initial treatment of femoral fractures reduced mortality of compound fractures of the femur from 87% to less than 8% in the period from 1916 to 1918.

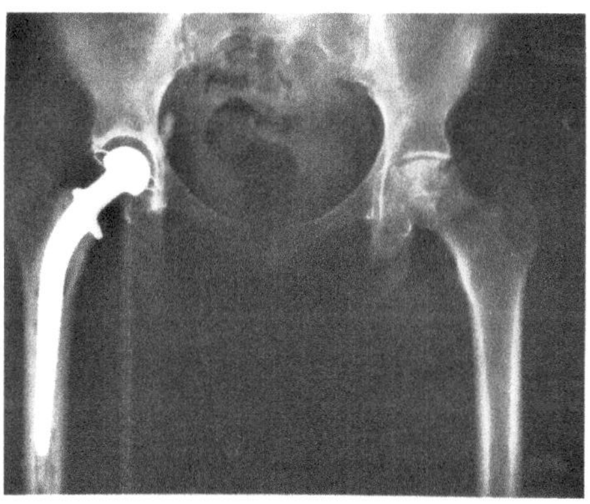

X-ray of a hip replacement.

The use of intramedullary rods to treat fractures of the femur and tibia was pioneered by Gerhard Küntscher of Germany. This made a noticeable difference to the speed of recovery of injured German soldiers during World War II and led to more widespread adoption of intramedullary fixation of fractures in the rest of the world. However, traction was the standard method of treating thigh bone fractures until the late 1970s when the Harborview Medical Center in Seattle group popularized intramedullary fixation without opening up the fracture.

The modern total hip replacement was pioneered by Sir John Charnley, expert in tribology at Wrightington Hospital, England in the 1960s. He found that joint surfaces could be replaced by implants cemented to the bone. His design consisted of a stainless steel one-piece femoral stem and head and a polyethylene, acetabular component, both of which were fixed to the bone using PMMA (acrylic) bone cement. For over two decades, the Charnley Low Friction Arthroplasty and its derivative designs were the most-used systems in the world. This formed the basis for all modern hip implants.

The Exeter hip replacement system (with a slightly different stem geometry) was developed at the same time.Since Charnley, there have been continuous improvements in the design and technique of joint replacement (arthroplasty) with many contributors, including W. H. Harris, the son of R. I. Harris, whose team at Harvard pioneered uncemented arthroplasty techniques with the bone bonding directly to the implant.

Knee replacements using similar technology were started by McIntosh in rheumatoid arthritis patients and later by Gunston and Marmor for osteoarthritis in the 1970s developed by Dr. John Insall in New York utilizing a fixed bearing system, and by Dr. Frederick Buechel and Dr. Michael Pappas utilizing a mobile bearing system.

External fixation of fractures was refined by American surgeons during the Vietnam War but a major contribution was made by Gavril Abramovich Ilizarov in the USSR. He was sent, without much orthopedic training, to look after injured Russian soldiers in Siberia in the 1950s. With no equipment he was confronted with crippling conditions of unhealed, infected, and malaligned fractures. With the help of the local bicycle shop he devised ring external fixators tensioned like the spokes of a bicycle. With this equipment he achieved healing, realignment and lengthening to a degree unheard of elsewhere. His Ilizarov apparatus is still used today as one of the distraction osteogenesis methods.

Modern orthopedic surgery and musculoskeletal research has sought to make surgery less invasive and to make implanted components better and more durable.

Training

In the United States, orthopedic surgeons have typically completed four years of undergraduate education and four years of medical school. Subsequently, these medical school graduates undergo residency training in orthopedic surgery. The five-year residency is a categorical orthopedic surgery training.

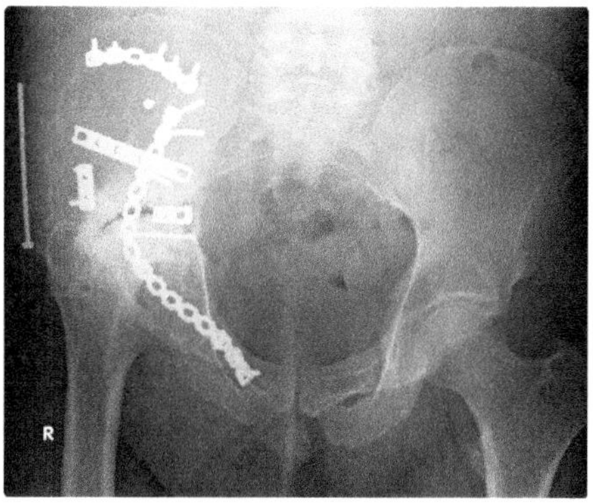

This image, taken in September 2006, shows extensive repair work to the right acetabulum 6 years after it was carried out (2000). Further damage to the joint is visible due to the onset of arthritis - a bone/joint disease.

Selection for residency training in orthopedic surgery is very competitive. Approximately 700 physicians complete orthopedic residency training per year in the United States. About 10 percent of current orthopedic surgery residents are women; about 20 percent are members of minority groups. There are approximately 20,400 actively practicing orthopedic surgeons and residents in the United States. According to the latest Occupational Outlook Handbook (2011–2012) published by the United States Department of Labor, between 3–4% of all practicing physicians are orthopedic surgeons.

Many orthopedic surgeons elect to do further training, or fellowships, after completing their residency training. Fellowship training in an orthopedic sub-specialty is typically one year in duration (sometimes two) and sometimes has a research component involved with the clinical and operative training. Examples of orthopedic sub-specialty training in the United States are:

- Hand surgery
- Shoulder and elbow surgery
- Total joint reconstruction (arthroplasty)
- Pediatric orthopedics
- Foot and ankle surgery
- Spine surgery
- Musculoskeletal oncology
- Surgical sports medicine
- Orthopedic trauma

These specialty areas of medicine are not exclusive to orthopedic surgery. For example, hand surgery is practiced by some plastic surgeons and spine surgery is practiced by most neurosurgeons. Additionally, foot and ankle surgery is practiced by board-certified Doctors of Podiatric Medicine (D.P.M.) in the United States. Some family practice physicians practice sports medicine; however, their scope of practice is non-operative.

After completion of specialty residency/registrar training, an orthopedic surgeon is then eligible for board certification by the American Board of Medical Specialties or the American Osteopathic Association Bureau of Osteopathic Specialists. Certification by the American Board of Orthopaedic Surgery or the American Osteopathic Board of Orthopedic Surgery means that the orthopedic surgeon has met the specified educational, evaluation, and examination requirements of the Board. The process requires successful completion of a standardized written exam followed by an oral exam focused on the surgeon's clinical and surgical performance over a 6-month period. In Canada, the certifying organization is the Royal College of Physicians and Surgeons of Canada; in Australia and New Zealand it is the Royal Australasian College of Surgeons.

In the United States, specialists in hand surgery and orthopedic sports medicine may obtain a Certificate of Added Qualifications (CAQ) in addition to their board primary certification by successfully completing a separate standardized examination. There is no additional certification process for the other sub-specialties.

Practice

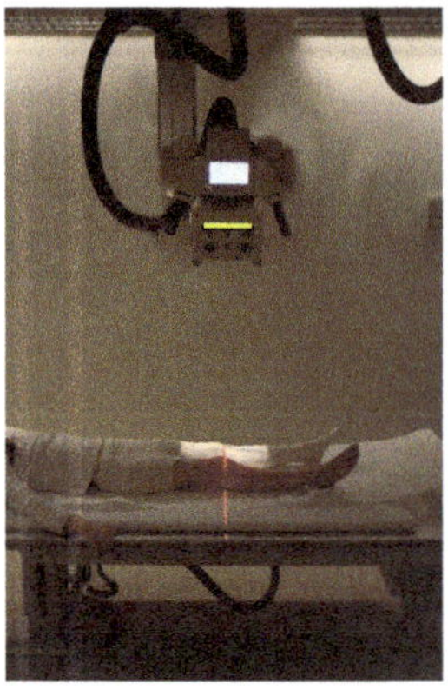

Radiography to identify eventual bone fractures after a knee injury.

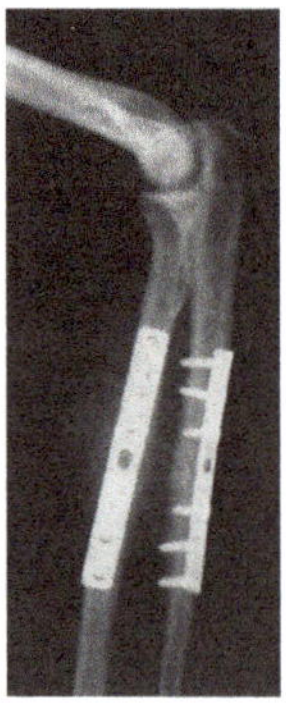

Orthopedic implants to repair fractures to the radius and ulna. Note the visible break in the ulna. (right forearm)

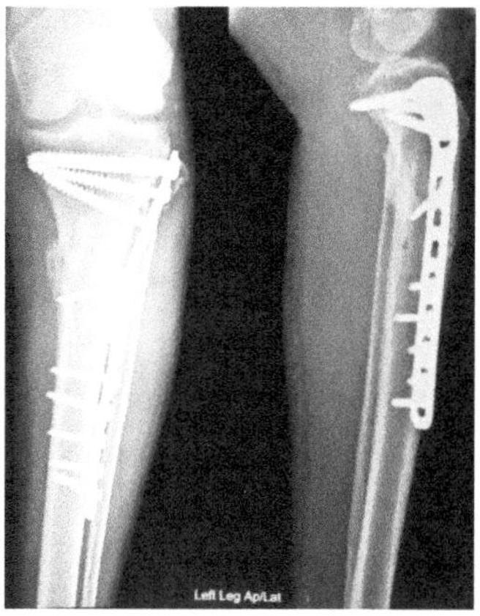

Anterior and lateral view x-rays of fractured left leg with internal fixation after surgery

According to applications for board certification from 1999 to 2003, the top 25 most common procedures (in order) performed by orthopedic surgeons are as follows:

1. Knee arthroscopy and meniscectomy
2. Shoulder arthroscopy and decompression
3. Carpal tunnel release
4. Knee arthroscopy and chondroplasty
5. Removal of support implant
6. Knee arthroscopy and anterior cruciate ligament reconstruction
7. Knee replacement
8. Repair of femoral neck fracture
9. Repair of trochanteric fracture
10. Debridement of skin/muscle/bone/fracture
11. Knee arthroscopy repair of both menisci
12. Hip replacement
13. Shoulder arthroscopy/distal clavicle excision
14. Repair of rotator cuff tendon
15. Repair fracture of radius (bone)/ulna
16. Laminectomy
17. Repair of ankle fracture (bimalleolar type)

18. Shoulder arthroscopy and debridement
19. Lumbar spinal fusion
20. Repair fracture of the distal part of radius
21. Low back intervertebral disc surgery
22. Incise finger tendon sheath
23. Repair of ankle fracture (fibula)
24. Repair of femoral shaft fracture
25. Repair of trochanteric fracture

A typical schedule for a practicing orthopedic surgeon involves 50–55 hours of work per week divided among clinic, surgery, various administrative duties and possibly teaching and/or research if in an academic setting.

Arthroscopy

The use of arthroscopic techniques has been particularly important for injured patients. Arthroscopy was pioneered in the early 1950s by Dr. Masaki Watanabe of Japan to perform minimally invasive cartilage surgery and reconstructions of torn ligaments. Arthroscopy helped patients recover from the surgery in a matter of days, rather than the weeks to months required by conventional, 'open' surgery. It is a very popular technique. Knee arthroscopy is one of the most common operations performed by orthopedic surgeons today and is often combined with meniscectomy or chondroplasty. The majority of orthopedic procedures are now performed arthroscopically.

Arthroplasty

Arthroplasty is an orthopedic surgery where the articular surface of a musculoskeletal joint is replaced, remodeled, or realigned by osteotomy or some other procedure. It is an elective procedure that is done to relieve pain and restore function to the joint after damage by arthritis (rheumasurgery) or some other type of trauma. As well as the standard total knee replacement surgery, the uni-compartmental knee replacement, in which only one weight-bearing surface of an arthritic knee is replaced, is a popular alternative.

Joint replacements are available for other joints on a limited basis, most notably the knee, shoulder, elbow, wrist, ankle, spine, and finger joints.

In recent years, surface replacement of joints, in particular the hip joint, have become more popular amongst younger and more active patients. This type of operation delays the need for the more traditional and less bone-conserving total hip replacement, but carries significant risks of early failure from fracture and bone death.

One of the main problems with joint replacements is wear of the bearing surfaces of components. This can lead to damage to surrounding bone and contribute to eventual failure of the implant. Use of alternative bearing surfaces has increased in recent years, particularly in younger patients, in an attempt to improve the wear characteristics of joint replacement components. These include ceramics and all-metal implants (as opposed to the original metal-on-plastic). The plastic (actually ultra high-molecular-weight polyethylene) can also be altered in ways that may improve wear characteristics.

Epidemiology

Between 2001 and 2016, the prevalence of musculoskeletal procedures drastically increased in the U.S, from 17.9% to 24.2% of all operating room procedures performed during hospital stays.

In a study of hospitalizations in the United States in 2012, spine and joint procedures were common among all age groups except infants. Spinal fusion was one of the five most common OR procedures performed in every age group except infants younger than 1 year and adults 85 years and older. Laminectomy was common among adults aged 18–84 years. Knee arthroplasty and hip replacement were in the top five OR procedures for adults aged 45 years and older.

Aquatic Therapy

Aquatic therapy refers to treatments and exercises performed in water for relaxation, fitness, physical rehabilitation, and other therapeutic benefit. Typically a qualified aquatic therapist gives constant attendance to a person receiving treatment in a heated therapy pool. Aquatic therapy techniques include Ai Chi, Aqua Running, Bad Ragaz Ring Method, Burdenko Method, Halliwick, Watsu, and other aquatic bodywork forms. Therapeutic applications include neurological disorders, spine pain, musculoskeletal pain, postoperative orthopedic rehabilitation, pediatric disabilities, and pressure ulcers.

Overview

Aquatic therapy refers to water-based treatments or exercises of therapeutic intent, in particular for relaxation, fitness, and physical rehabilitation. Treatments and exercises are performed while floating, partially submerged, or fully submerged in water. Many aquatic therapy procedures require constant attendance by a trained therapist, and are performed in a specialized temperature-controlled pool. Rehabilitation commonly focuses on improving the physical function associated with illness, injury, or disability.

Aquatic therapy encompasses a broad set of approaches and techniques, including aquatic exercise, physical therapy, aquatic bodywork, and other movement-based therapy in water (hydrokinesiotherapy). Treatment may be passive, involving a therapist or giver and a patient or receiver, or active, involving self-generated body positions, movement, or exercise. Examples include Halliwick Aquatic Therapy, Bad Ragaz Ring Method, Watsu, and Ai chi.

For orthopedic rehabilitation, aquatic therapy is considered to be synonymous with therapeutic aquatic exercise, aqua therapy, aquatic rehabilitation, water therapy, and pool therapy. Aquatic therapy can support restoration of function for many areas of orthopedics, including sports medicine, work conditioning, joint arthroplasty, and back rehabilitation programs. A strong aquatic component is especially beneficial for therapy programs where limited or non-weight bearing is desirable and where normal functioning is limited by inflammation, pain, guarding, muscle spasm, and limited range of motion (ROM). Water provides a controllable environment for reeducation of weak muscles and skill development for neurological and neuromuscular impairment, acute orthopedic or neuromuscular injury, rheumatological disease, or recovery from recent surgery.

Various properties of water contribute to therapeutic effects, including the ability to use water for resistance in place of gravity or weights; thermal stability that permits maintenance of near-constant temperature; hydrostatic pressure that supports and stabilizes, and that influences heart and lung function; buoyancy that permits floatation and reduces the effects of gravity; and turbulence and wave propagation that allow gentle manipulation and movement.

Techniques

Techniques for aquatic therapy include the following:

- Ai Chi: Ai Chi, developed in 1993 by Jun Konno, uses diaphragmatic breathing and active progressive resistance training in water to relax and strengthen the body, based on elements of qigong and Tai chi chuan.
- Aqua running: Aqua running (Deep Water Running or Aquajogging) is a form of cardiovascular conditioning, involving running or jogging in water, useful for injured athletes and those who desire a low-impact aerobic workout. Aqua running is performed in deep water using a floatation device (vest or belt) to support the head above water.
- Bad Ragaz Ring Method: The Bad Ragaz Ring Method (BRRM) focuses on rehabilitation of neuromuscular function using patterns of therapist-assisted exercise performed while the patient lies horizontal in water, with support provided by rings or floats around the neck, arms, pelvis, and knees. BRRM is an aquatic version of Proprioceptive Neuromuscular Facilitation (PNF) developed by

physiotherapists at Bad Ragaz, Switzerland, as a synthesis of aquatic exercises designed by a German physician in the 1930s and land-based PNF developed by American physiotherapists in the 1950s and 1960s.

- Burdenko Method: The Burdenko Method, originally developed by Soviet professor of sports medicine Igor Burdenko, is an integrated land-water therapy approach that develops balance, coordination, flexibility, endurance, speed, and strength using the same methods as professional athletes. The water-based therapy uses buoyant equipment to challenge the center of buoyancy in vertical positions, exercising with movement in multiple directions, and at multiple speeds ranging from slow to fast.
- Halliwick Concept: The Halliwick Concept, originally developed by fluid mechanics engineer James McMillan in the late 1940s and 1950s at the Halliwick School for Girls with Disabilities in London, focuses on biophysical principles of motor control in water, in particular developing sense of balance (equilibrioception) and core stability. The Halliwick Ten-Point-Program implements the concept in a progressive program of mental adjustment, disengagement, and development of motor control, with an emphasis on rotational control, and applies the program to teach physically disabled people balance control, swimming, and independence. Halliwick Aquatic Therapy (also known as Water Specific Therapy, WST), implements the concept in patient-specific aquatic therapy.
- Watsu: Watsu is a form of aquatic bodywork, originally developed in the early 1980s by Harold Dull at Harbin Hot Springs, California, in which an aquatic therapist continuously supports and guides the person receiving treatment through a series of flowing movements and stretches that induce deep relaxation and provide therapeutic benefit. In the late 1980s and early 1990s physiotherapists began to use Watsu for a wide range of orthopedic and neurologic conditions, and to adapt the techniques for use with injury and disability.

Applications and Effectiveness

Applications of aquatic therapy include neurological disorders, spine pain, musculoskeletal pain, postoperative orthopedic rehabilitation, pediatric disabilities, and pressure ulcers.

A 2006 systematic review of effects of aquatic interventions in children with neuromotor impairments found "substantial lack of evidence-based research evaluating the specific effects of aquatic interventions in this population".

Professional Training and Certification

Aquatic therapy is performed by diverse professionals with specific training and certification requirements.

For medical purposes, aquatic therapy, as defined by the American Medical Association (AMA), can be performed by various legally-regulated healthcare professionals who have scopes of practice that permit them to offer such services and who are permitted to use AMA Current Procedural Terminology (CPT) codes.

Hydrotherapy

Hydrotherapy, formerly called hydropathy, is a part of medicine and alternative medicine, in particular of naturopathy, occupational therapy and physiotherapy, that involves the use of water for pain relief and treatment. The term encompasses a broad range of approaches and therapeutic methods that take advantage of the physical properties of water, such as temperature and pressure, for therapeutic purposes, to stimulate blood circulation and treat the symptoms of certain diseases.

Various therapies used in the present-day hydrotherapy employ water jets, underwater massage and mineral baths (e.g. balneotherapy, Iodine-Grine therapy, Kneipp treatments, Scotch hose, Swiss shower, thalassotherapy) and/or whirlpool bath, hot Roman bath, hot tub, Jacuzzi, cold plunge and mineral bath.

Uses

Water therapy may be restricted to use in physical therapy, and as a cleansing agent. However, it is also used as a medium for delivery of heat and cold to the body, which has long been the basis for its application. Hydrotherapy involves a range of methods and techniques, many of which use water as a medium to facilitate thermoregulatory reactions for therapeutic benefit.

Practitioners of hydrotherapy may seek use it to produce vasodilation and vasoconstriction. These cause changes in blood flow and associated metabolic functions, via physiological mechanisms, including those of thermoregulation, that are these days fairly well understood, and which underpin the contemporary use of hydrotherapy.

When removal of tissue is necessary for the treatment of wounds, hydrotherapy which performs selective mechanical debridement can be used. Examples of this include directed wound irrigation and therapeutic irrigation with suction.

It continues to be used as an adjunct to therapy, including in nursing, where its use is now long established. It continues to be widely used for burn treatment, although shower-based hydrotherapy techniques have been increasingly used in preference to full-immersion methods, partly for the ease of cleaning the equipment and reducing infections due to contamination.

Hydrotherapy is used today in alternative medicine.

Technique

The appliances and arrangements by means of which heat and cold are brought to bear are (a) packings, hot and cold, general and local, sweating and cooling; (b) hot air and steam baths; (c) general baths, of hot water and cold; (d) sitz (sitting), spinal, head and foot baths; (e) bandages (or compresses), wet and dry; also (f) fomentations and poultices, hot and cold, sinapisms, stupes, rubbings and water potations, hot and cold.

Hydrotherapy which involves submerging all or part of the body in water can involve several types of equipment:

- Full body immersion tanks (a "Hubbard tank" is a large size)
- Arm, hip, and leg whirlpool

Whirling water movement, provided by mechanical pumps, has been used in water tanks since at least the 1940s. Similar technologies have been marketed for recreational use under the terms "hot tub" or "spa".

In some cases Baths with whirlpool water flow aren't used to manage wounds because a whirlpool will not selectively target the tissue to be removed and can damage all tissue. Whirlpools also create an unwanted risk of bacterial infection, can damage fragile body tissue, and in the case of treating arms and legs, bring risk of complications from edema.

Society and Culture

Modern medicine's successes, particularly with drug therapy, removed or replaced many water-related therapies during the mid-20th century.

While the physiological mechanisms were initially poorly understood, the therapeutic benefits have long been recognised, even if the reason for the therapeutic benefit was in dispute. For example, in November 1881, the *British Medical Journal* noted that hydropathy was a specific instance, or "particular case", of general principles of thermodynamics. That is, "the application of heat and cold in general", as it applies to physiology, mediated by hydropathy. In 1883, another writer stated "Not, be it observed, that hydropathy is a water treatment after all, but that water is the medium for the application of heat and cold to the body". Thus, the "active agents in the treatment (are) heat and cold", of which water is little more than the vehicle, and not the only one".

Although standard anatomy and physiology textbooks make only passing reference, if any, to hydrotherapy, some of the best descriptions of the underlying physiology upon which hydrotherapy relies, are to be found in such textbooks. For example, one of the best succinct descriptions of blood redistribution (which is fundamental to the above-mentioned reflex reaction), quoted below, is from a standard textbook.

By constricting or dilating arterioles in specific areas of the body, such as skeletal muscles, the skin, and the abdominal region, it is possible not only to regulate the blood pressure but also to alter the distribution of blood in various parts of the body.

British and other hydrotherapy establishments are discussed from another standpoint in a recent history of psychiatry.

Before World War II, various forms of hydrotherapy were used to treat alcoholism. The basic text of the Alcoholics Anonymous fellowship, *Alcoholics Anonymous*, reports that A.A. co-founder Bill Wilson was treated by hydrotherapy for his alcoholism in the early 1930s.

The use of water to treat rheumatic diseases has a long history.

The growth of hydrotherapy, and various forms of hydropathic establishments, resulted in a form of tourism, both in the UK, and in Europe. At least one book listed English, Scottish, Irish and European establishments suitable for each specific malady, while another focused primarily on German spas and hydropathic establishments, but including other areas. While many bathing establishments were open all year round, doctors advised patients not to go before May, "nor to remain after October. English visitors rather prefer cold weather, and they often arrive for the baths in May, and return again in September. Americans come during the whole season, but prefer summer. The most fashionable and crowded time is during July and August". In Europe, interest in various forms of hydrotherapy and spa tourism continued unabated through the 19th century and into the 20th century, where "in France, Italy and Germany, several million people spend time each year at a spa." In 1891, when Mark Twain toured Europe and discovered that a bath of spring water at Aix-les-Bains soothed his rheumatism, he described the experience as "so enjoyable that if I hadn't had a disease I would have borrowed one just to have a pretext for going on".

This was not the first time such forms of spa tourism had been popular in Europe and the U.K. Indeed,

in Europe, the application of water in the treatment of fevers and other maladies had, since the seventeenth century, been consistently promoted by a number of medical writers. In the eighteenth century, taking to the waters became a fashionable pastime for the wealthy classes who decamped to resorts around Britain and Europe to cure the ills of over-consumption. In the main, treatment in the heyday of the British spa consisted of sense and sociability: promenading, bathing, and the repetitive quaffing of foul-tasting mineral waters.

A hydropathic establishment is a place where people receive hydropathic treatment. They are commonly built in spa towns, where mineral-rich or hot water occurs naturally.

Several hydropathic institutions wholly transferred their operations away from therapeutic purposes to become tourist hotels in the late 20th century whilst retaining the name 'Hydro'. There are several prominent examples in Scotland at Crieff, Peebles and Seamill amongst others.

History

Various forms of hydrotherapy have been recorded in ancient Egyptian, Persian, Greek and Roman civilizations. Egyptian royalty bathed with essential oils and flowers, while Romans had communal public baths for their citizens. Hippocrates prescribed bathing in spring water for sickness. Other cultures noted for a long history of hydrotherapy include China and Japan, this latter being centred primarily around Japanese hot springs, or (onsen). Many such histories predate the Roman thermae.

Modern Revival of Hydrotherapy

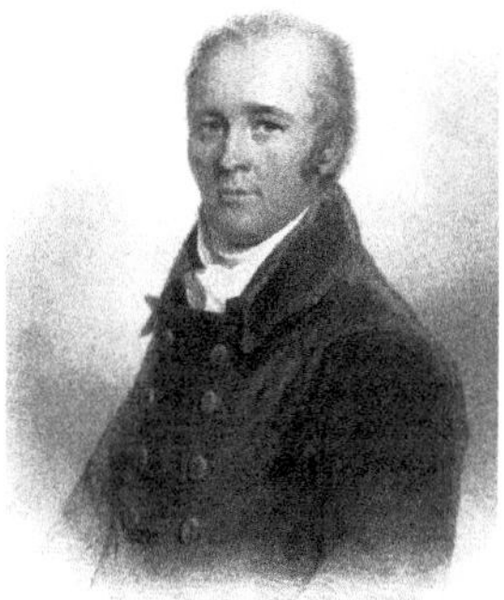

James Currie, who, according to Captain R. T. Claridge discovered "...the merit of settling the use of cold water...[and who established] the scientific base of Hydropathy"

Two English works on the medical uses of water were published in the 18th century that inaugurated the new fashion for hydrotherapy. One of these was by Sir John Floyer, a physician of Lichfield, who, struck by the remedial use of certain springs by the neighbouring peasantry, investigated the history of cold bathing and published a book on the subject in 1702. The book ran through six editions within a few years and the translation of this book into German was largely drawn upon by Dr J. S. Hahn of Silesia as the basis for his book called *On the Healing Virtues of Cold Water, Inwardly and Outwardly Applied, as Proved by Experience*, published in 1738.

The other work was a 1797 publication by Dr James Currie of Liverpool on the use of hot and cold water in the treatment of fever and other illness, with a fourth edition published in 1805, not long before his death. It was also translated into German by Michaelis (1801) and Hegewisch (1807). It was highly popular and first placed the subject on a scientific basis. Hahn's writings had meanwhile created much enthusiasm among his countrymen, societies having been formed everywhere to promote the medicinal and dietetic use of water; and in 1804 Professor E.F.C. Oertel of Anspach republished them and quickened the popular movement by unqualified commendation of water drinking as a remedy for all diseases.

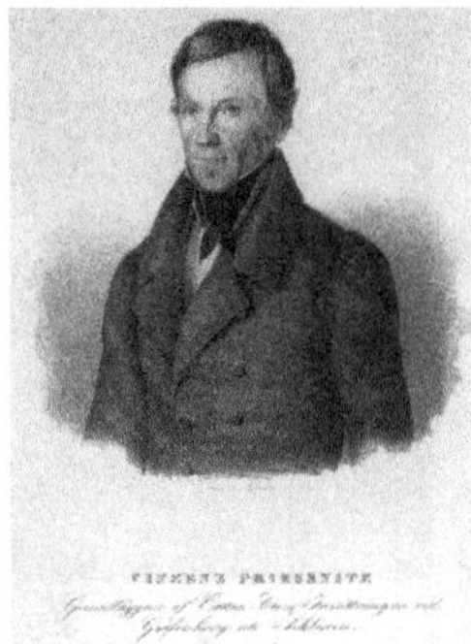

Vincenz Priessnitz, who initiated the popular revival of hydrotherapy at Gräfenberg

In the 19th century, a popular revival followed the application of hydrotherapy around 1829, by Vincenz Priessnitz, a peasant farmer in Gräfenberg, then part of the Austrian Empire. This revival was continued by a Bavarian priest, Sebastian Kneipp (1821–1897), "an able and enthusiastic follower" of Priessnitz, "whose work he took up where Priessnitz left it", after he read a treatise on the cold water cure. In Wörishofen (south Germany), Kneipp developed the systematic and controlled application of hydrotherapy for the support of medical treatment that was delivered only by doctors at that time. Kneipp's own book *My Water Cure* was published in 1886 with many subsequent editions, and translated into many languages.

A significant factor in the popular revival of hydrotherapy was that it could be practised relatively cheaply at home. The growth of hydrotherapy (or 'hydropathy' to use the name of the time), was thus partly derived from two interacting spheres: "the hydro and the home".

Hydrotherapy as a formal medical tool dates from about 1829 when Vincenz Priessnitz (1799–1851), a farmer of Gräfenberg in Silesia, then part of the Austrian Empire, began his public career in the paternal homestead, extended so as to accommodate the increasing numbers attracted by the fame of his cures.

At Gräfenberg, to which the fame of Priessnitz drew people of every rank and many countries, medical men were conspicuous by their numbers, some being attracted by curiosity, others by the desire of knowledge, but the majority by the hope of cure for ailments which had as yet proved incurable. Many records of experiences at Gräfenberg were published, all more or less favorable to the claims of Priessnitz, and some enthusiastic in their estimate of his genius and penetration.

Spread of Hydrotherapy

Captain R. T. Claridge was responsible for introducing and promoting hydropathy in Britain, first in London in 1842, then with lecture tours in Ireland and Scotland in 1843.

His 10-week tour in Ireland included Limerick, Cork, Wexford, Dublin and Belfast, over June, July and August 1843, with two subsequent lectures in Glasgow.

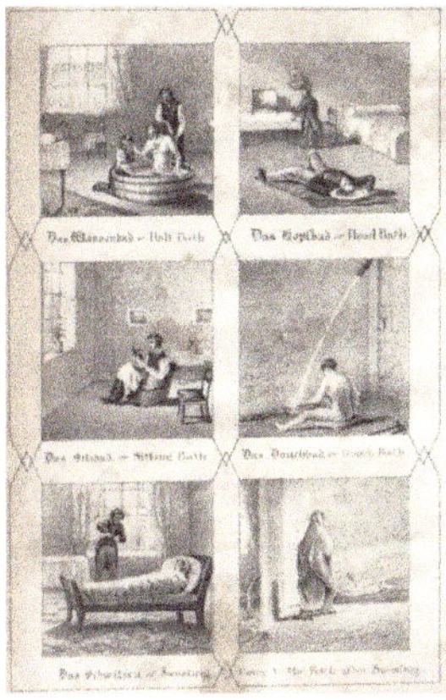

Hydropathic applications according to Claridge's Hydropathy book.

Some other Englishmen preceded Claridge to Graefenberg, although not many. One of these was Dr. James Wilson, who himself, along with Dr James Manby Gully, established and operated a water cure establishment at Malvern in 1842. In 1843, Wilson and Gully published a comparison of the efficacy of the water-cure with drug treatments, including accounts of some cases treated at Malvern, combined with a prospectus of their Water Cure Establishment. Then in 1846 Gully published *The Water Cure in Chronic Disease*, further describing the treatments available at the clinic.

The fame of the water-cure establishment grew, and Gully and Wilson became well-known national figures. Two more clinics were opened at Malvern. Famous patients included Charles Darwin, Charles Dickens, Thomas Carlyle, Florence Nightingale, Lord Tennyson and Samuel Wilberforce. With his fame he also attracted criticism: Sir Charles Hastings, a physician and founder of the British Medical Association, was a forthright critic of hydropathy, and Dr Gully in particular.

From the 1840s, hydropathics were established across Britain. Initially, many of these were small institutions, catering to at most dozens of patients. By the later nineteenth century the typical hydropathic establishment had evolved into a more substantial undertaking, with thousands of patients treated annually for weeks at a time in a large purpose-built building with lavish facilities – baths, recreation rooms and the like – under the supervision of fully trained and qualified medical practitioners and staff.

In Germany, France and America, and in Malvern, England, hydropathic establishments multiplied with great rapidity. Antagonism ran high between the old practice and the new. Unsparing condemnation was heaped by each on the other; and a legal prosecution, leading to a royal commission of inquiry, served but to make Priessnitz and his system stand higher in public estimation.

Increasing popularity soon diminished caution whether the new method would help minor ailments and be of benefit to the more seriously injured. Hydropathists occupied themselves mainly with studying chronic invalids well able to bear a rigorous regimen and the severities of unrestricted crisis. The need of a radical adaptation to the former class was first adequately recognized by John Smedley, a manufacturer of Derbyshire, who, impressed in his own person with the severities as well as the benefits of the cold water cure, practised among his workpeople a milder form of hydropathy, and began about 1852 a new era in its history, founding at Matlock a counterpart of the establishment at Gräfenberg.

Ernst Brand (1827–1897) of Berlin, Raljen and Theodor von Jürgensen of Kiel, and Karl Liebermeister of Basel, between 1860 and 1870, employed the cooling bath in abdominal typhus with striking results, and led to its introduction to England by Dr Wilson Fox. In the Franco-German War the cooling bath was largely employed, in conjunction frequently with quinine; and it was used in the treatment of hyperpyrexia.

Hot Baths

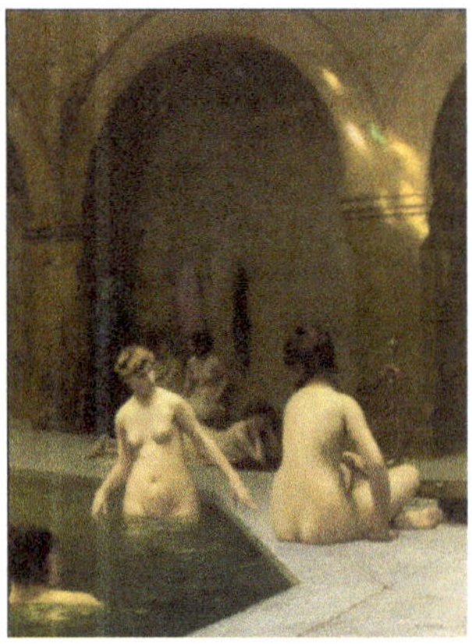

Baigneuses, oil on canvas, Jean-Léon Gérôme (1824-1904)

Hydrotherapy, especially as promoted during the height of its Victorian revival, has often been associated with the use of cold water, as evidenced by many titles from that era. However, not all therapists limited their practice of hydrotherapy to cold water, even during the height of this popular revival.

The specific use of heat was however often associated with the Turkish bath. This was introduced by David Urquhart into England on his return from the East in the 1850s, and ardently adopted by Richard Barter. The Turkish bath became a public institution, and, with the morning tub and the general practice of water drinking, is the most noteworthy of the many contributions by hydropathy to public health.

Spread to the United States

The first U.S. hydropathic facilities were established by Joel Shew and R. T. Trall in the 1840s. Dr Charles Munde also established early hydrotherapy facilities in the 1850s. Trall also co-edited the *Water Cure Journal*.

By 1850, it was said that "there are probably more than one hundred" facilities, along with numerous books and periodicals, including the New York *Water Cure Journal*, which had "attained an extent of circulation equalled by few monthlies in the world". By 1855, there were attempts by some to weigh the evidence of treatments in vogue at that time.

Following the introduction of hydrotherapy to the U.S., John Harvey Kellogg employed it at Battle Creek Sanitarium, which opened in 1866, where he strove to improve the scientific foundation for hydrotherapy. Other notable hydropathic centers of the era included the Cleveland Water Cure Establishment, founded in 1848, which operated successfully for two decades, before being sold to an organization which transformed it into an orphanage.

At its height, there were over 200 water-cure establishments in the United States, most located in the northeast. Few of these lasted into the postbellum years, although some survived into the 20th century including institutions in Scott (Cortland County), Elmira, Clifton Springs and Dansville. While none were located in Jefferson County, the Oswego Water Cure operated in the city of Oswego.

The technique is also mentioned in the 1951 film *A Streetcar Named Desire*.

Recent Techniques

Cryotherapy, cold water immersion or ice bath is a new form of hydrotherapy used by physical therapists, sports medicine facilities and rehab clinics. Proponents claim improved return of blood flow and byproducts of cellular breakdown to the lymphatic system and more efficient recycling.

Alternating the temperatures, either in a shower or complementary tanks, combines the use of hot and cold in the same session. Proponents claim improvement in circulatory system and lymphatic drainage. Experimental evidence suggests that contrast hydrotherapy helps to reduce injury in the acute stages by stimulating blood flow and reducing swelling.

For Animals

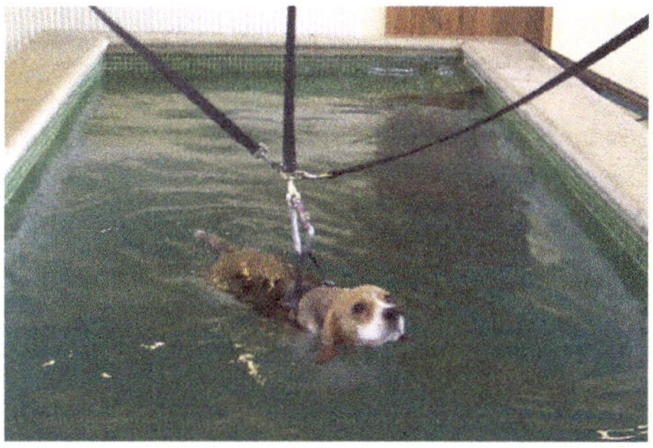

A Beagle swimming in a harness in a hydrotherapy pool

Canine hydrotherapy is a form of hydrotherapy directed at the treatment of chronic conditions, post-operative recovery, and pre-operative or general fitness in dogs.

Rehabilitation in Spinal Cord Injury

When treating a person with a spinal cord injury, repairing the damage created by injury is the ultimate goal. By using a variety of treatments, greater improvements are achieved, and, therefore, treatment should not be limited to one method. Furthermore, increasing activity will increase his/her chances of recovery.

Acute Recovery

The rehabilitation process following a spinal cord injury typically begins in the acute care setting. Occupational therapy plays an important role in the management of SCI. Recent studies emphasize the importance of early occupational therapy, started immediately after the client is stable. This process includes teaching of coping skills, and physical therapy. Physical therapists, occupational therapists, social workers, psychologists and other health care professionals typically work as a team under the coordination of a physiatrist to decide on goals with the patient and develop a plan of discharge that is appropriate for the patient's condition. In the first step, the focus is on support and prevention. Interventions aim to give the individual a sense of control over a situation in which the patient likely feels little independence.

As the patient becomes more stable, they may move to a rehabilitation facility or remain in the acute care setting. The patient begins to take more of an active role in their rehabilitation at this stage and works with the team to develop reasonable functional goals.

Respiration

In the acute phase physical and occupational therapists focus on the patient's respiratory status, prevention of indirect complications (such as pressure sores), maintaining range of motion, and keeping available musculature active.

Depending on the Neurological Level of Impairment (NLI), the muscles responsible for expanding the thorax, which facilitate inhalation, may be affected. If the NLI is such that it affects some of the ventilatory muscles, more emphasis will then be placed on the muscles with intact function. For example, the intercostal muscles receive their innervation from T1–T11, and if any are damaged, more emphasis will need to be placed on the unaffected muscles which are innervated from higher levels of the CNS. As SCI patients suffer from reduced total lung capacity and tidal volume it is pertinent that physical therapists teach SCI patients accessory breathing techniques (e.g. apical breathing, glossopharyngeal breathing, etc.) that typically are not taught to healthy individuals.

Functional Electrical Stimulation

Physical therapists can assist immobilized patients with effective cough techniques, secretion clearance, stretching of the thoracic wall, and suggest abdominal support belts when necessary. The amount of time a patient is immobilized may depend on the level of the spinal cord injury. Physical therapists work with the patient to prevent any complications that may arise due to this immobilization. Other complications that arise from immobilization include muscle atrophy and osteoporosis, especially to the lower limbs, increasing the risk of fractures to the femur and tibia. While passive weight bearing of paralyzed lower extremities appears to be ineffective, stressing the bones through muscular contractions initiated by functional electrical stimulation (FES) has yielded positive results in some cases. The intensity, frequency, and duration of stress to the bones appear to be important determinants of improved bone parameters. Generally, the frequency is effective with three or more weekly exercise sessions. Studies of duration suggest that several months to one or more years of FES are necessary.

Improving Locomotor Function

Improvement of locomotor function is one of the primary goals for people with a spinal cord injury. SCI treatments may focus on specific goals such as to restore walking or locomotion to an optimal level for the individual. The most effective way to restore locomotion is by complete repair, but techniques are not yet developed for regeneration. Treadmill training, over groundtraining, and functional electrical stimulation can all be used to improve walking or locomotor activity. These activities work if neurons of the central pattern generator (CPG) circuits, which generate rhythmic movements of the body, are still functioning. With inactivity, the neurons of CPG degenerate. Therefore, the above activities are important for keeping neurons active until regeneration activities are developed. A 2012 systematic review found insufficient evidence to conclude *which* locomotor training strategy improves walking function most for people with spinal cord injury. This suggests that it is not the type of training used, but the goals and the routines that have the biggest impact. Applying spinal cord stimulation (transcutaneous or epidurally) during weight supported walking have been shown to improve locomotor output.

Post-discharge Rehabilitation Therapy

Though rehabilitation interventions are performed during the acute phase, recent literature suggests that 44% of the total hours spent on rehabilitation during the first year after spinal cord injury, occur after discharge from inpatient rehabilitation. Participants in this study received 56% of their total physical therapy hours and 52% of their total occupational therapy hours after discharge. This suggests that inpatient rehabilitation lengths of stay are reduced and that post-discharge therapy may replace some of the inpatient treatment.

Functional Independence

Whether patients are placed in inpatient rehabilitation or discharged, occupational therapists attempt to maximize functional independence at this stage. Depending on the level of the spinal cord injury, whatever sparing the patient has is optimized. Bed mobility, transfers, wheelchair mobility skills, and performing other activities of daily living (ADLs) are just a few of the interventions that occupational therapists can help the patient with. A major problem for spinal cord injury patients is restricted range of motion. Massage therapy has been used to aid in range of motion rehabilitation. Literature has shown that participants with spinal cord injuries that had massage therapy added into their rehabilitation had significant improvement observed by physical therapist in functional living activities and limb range of motion. This could be due to the decrease in H-Reflex amplitudes measured by EMG that is critical for the comfort of spinal cord injury patients for reducing cramps and spasms.

ADLs can be difficult for an individual with a spinal cord injury; however, through the rehabilitation process, individuals with SCI may be able to live independently in the community with or without full-time attendant care, depending on the level of their injury.

Further interventions focus on support and education for the individual and caregivers. This includes an evaluation of limb function to determine what the patient is capable of doing independently, and teaching the patient self-care skills. Independence in daily activities like eating, bowel and bladder management, and mobility is the goal, as obtaining competency in self-care tasks contributes significantly to an individual's sense of self-confidence and reduces the burden on caregivers. Quality of life issues such as sexual health and function after spinal cord injury are also addressed.

Assistive Devices

Assistive devices such as wheelchairs have a substantial effect on the quality of life of the patient, and careful selection is important. Teaching the patient how to transfer from different positions, such as from a wheelchair into bed, is an important part of therapy, and devices such as sliding transfer boards and grab bars can assist in these tasks. Individuals who are able to transfer independently from their wheelchair to the driver's seat using a sliding transfer board may be able to return to driving in an adapted vehicle. Complete independence with driving also requires the ability to load and unload one's wheelchair from the vehicle. In addition to acquiring skills such as wheelchair transfers, individuals with a spinal cord injury can greatly benefit from exercise reconditioning. In the majority of cases, spinal cord injury leaves the lower limbs either entirely paralyzed, or with insufficient strength, endurance, or motor control to support safe and effective physical training. Therefore, most exercise training employs the use of arm crank ergometry, wheelchair ergometry, and swimming. In one study, subjects with traumatic spinal cord injury participated in a progressive exercise training program, which involved arm ergometry and resistance training. Subjects in the exercise group experienced significant increases in strength for almost all muscle groups when compared to the control group. Exercisers also reported less stress, fewer depressive symptoms, greater satisfaction with physical functioning, less pain, and better quality of life. Physical therapists are able to provide a variety of exercise interventions, including, passive range of motion exercises, upper body wheeling (arm crank ergometry), functional electrical stimulation, and electrically stimulated resistance exercises all of which can improve arterial function in those living with SCI. Physical therapists can improve the quality of life of individuals with spinal cord injury by developing exercise programs that are tailored to meet individual patient needs. Adapted physical activity equipment can also be used to allow for sport participation: for example, sit-skiis can be used by individuals with a spinal cord injury for cross-country or downhill skiing.

The patient's living environment can also be modified to improve independence. For example, ramps or lifts can be added to a patient's home, and part of rehabilitation involves investigating options for returning to previous interests as well as developing new pursuits. Community participation is an important aspect in maintaining quality of life.

Gait Training

Body weight supported treadmill training is another intervention that physiotherapists may assist with. Body weight supported treadmill training has been researched in an attempt to prevent bone loss in the lower extremities in individuals with spinal cord injury. Research has shown that early weight-bearing after acute spinal cord injury by standing or treadmill walking (5 times weekly for 25 weeks) resulted in no loss or only moderate loss in trabecular bone compared with immobilized subjects who lost 7-9% of trabecular bone at the tibia. Gait training with body weight support, among patients with incomplete spinal cord injuries, has also recently been shown to be more effective than conventional physiotherapy for improving the spatial-temporal and kinematic gait parameters.

A combination of Body weight supported treadmill training (BWSTT) and robotic-assisted BWSTT is being implemented into some training programs. The benefits include: (1) assist in reproducing leg movements and optimizing gait pattern (speed, step length, amplitude); (2) training sessions can be prolonged and walking speed can be adjusted, increasing motor outcome; (3) provides consistency of movement, where manual interventions/cues by a trainer may be variable (although a trainer should analyze the gait pattern and outcome measures of the training and supervise training). It is important to note that the patient must be an active participant during the robotic movements and try to move with the robot. This type of training would be implemented during the beginning of rehabilitation and progressed to independent locomotion as improvements are made. However, robotic-assisted BWSTT is expensive and often not affordable by physiotherapy clinics. As an alternative, the development of non-motorized exoskeletons are currently being investigated for patients with incomplete SCI. The development of the exoskeleton locomotor device would provide an inexpensive alternative to the robotic devices. The exoskeleton may be used in areas that can not afford robotic devices, or, in areas that can not provide adequate physiotherapy care.

Restorative neurology offers a different paradigm of treating spinal cord injury by focusing on the residual remaining motor control and on the intrinsic function of the sub-lesional spinal cord segments.

Medicine Ball

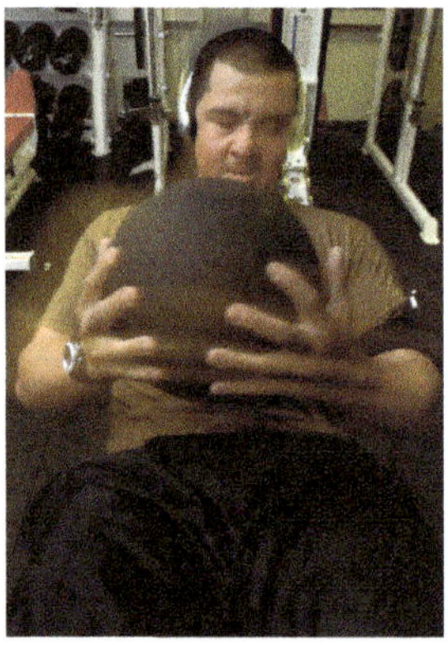

Exercising with a medicine ball

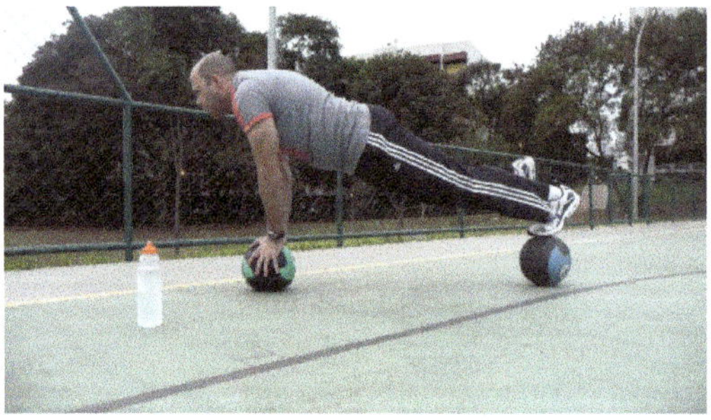

Medicine Ball Plank

A medicine ball (also known as an exercise ball, a med ball, or a fitness ball) is a weighted ball roughly the diameter of the shoulders (approx. 13.7 inches), often used for rehabilitation and strength training. The medicine ball also serves an important role in the field of sports medicine. However, it should not be confused with the larger, inflated exercise ball.

Medicine balls are usually sold as 2–25 lb (1–11 kg) balls and are used effectively in plyometric weight training to increase explosive power in athletes in all sports. Some medicine balls are up to 14” wide and up to 14 lbs weight, or in the form of weighted basketballs. Modern exercise balls are larger, up to 36” diameter.

A med ball is used for children training as the best way to overcome fear of free weights exercises. It is also one of the favorite equipment in gyms because if a med ball falls down it doesn't damage the floor.

Hippocrates is said to have stuffed animal skins for patients to toss for "medicinal" purposes. Persia in 1705 used similar large balls. The term "medicine ball" dates back to at least 1876, in *American Gymnasia and Academic Record,* by Robert Jenkins Roberts, JR. Mr. Roberts also invented the Indian Club and the sand pile as a play scape. Mr. Roberts through the Boston YMCA started the Boston Marathon. The name "medicine ball" is a play on the American Indian device, the "medicine bag" which the medicine ball resembles. Native American culture was experiencing a rebirth of appreciation in the minds of European Americans as witnessed by the creation of the American Boy Scouts movement at the same time as the invention of these exercise tools by Mr. Roberts.

Stroke Recovery

The primary goals of stroke management are to reduce brain injury and promote maximum patient recovery. Rapid detection and appropriate emergency medical care are essential for optimizing health outcomes. When available, patients are admitted to an acute stroke unit for treatment. These units specialize in providing medical and surgical care aimed at stabilizing the patient's medical status. Standardized assessments are also performed to aid in the development of an appropriate care plan. Current research suggests that stroke units may be effective in reducing in-hospital fatality rates and the length of hospital stays.

Once a patient is medically stable, the focus of their recovery shifts to rehabilitation. Some patients are transferred to in-patient rehabilitation programs, while others may be referred to out-patient services or home-based care. In-patient programs are usually facilitated by an interdisciplinary team that may include a physician, nurse, pharmacist, physical therapist, occupational therapist, speech and language pathologist, psychologist, and recreation therapist. The patient and their family/caregivers also play an integral role on this team. The primary goals of this sub-acute phase of recovery include preventing secondary health complications, minimizing impairments, and achieving functional goals that promote independence in activities of daily living.

In the later phases of stroke recovery, patients are encouraged to participate in secondary prevention programs for stroke. Follow-up is usually facilitated by the patient's primary care provider.

The initial severity of impairments and individual characteristics, such as motivation, social support, and learning ability, are key predictors of stroke recovery outcomes.

Responses to treatment and overall recovery of function are highly dependent on the individual. Current evidence indicates that most significant recovery gains will occur within the first 12 weeks following a stroke.

History of Stroke Neuro-rehabilitation

In 1620, Johann Jakob Wepfer, by studying the brain of a pig, developed the theory that stroke was caused by an interruption of the flow of blood to the brain. After that, the focus became how to treat patients with stroke.

For most of the last century, people were discouraged from being active after a stroke. Around the 1950s, this attitude changed, and health professionals began prescription of therapeutic exercises for stroke patient with good results. At that point, a good outcome was considered to be achieving a level of independence in which patients are able to transfer from the bed to the wheelchair without assistance.

In the early 1950s, Twitchell began studying the pattern of recovery in stroke patients. He reported on 121 patients whom he had observed. He found that by four weeks, if there is some recovery of hand function, there is a 70% chance of making a full or good recovery. He reported that most recovery happens in the first three months, and only minor recovery occurs after six months. More recent research has demonstrated that significant improvement can be made years after the stroke.

Around the same time, Brunnstrom also described the process of recovery, and divided the process into seven stages. As knowledge of the science of brain recovery improved, intervention strategies have evolved. Knowledge of strokes and the process of recovery after strokes has developed significantly in the late 20th century and early 21st century.

Current Perspectives and Therapeutic Avenues

Motor Re-learning

"Neurocognitive Rehabilitation by Carlo Perfetti concept", widespread in many countries, is an original motor re-learning theories application.

Constraint-induced Movement Therapy

The idea for constraint-induced therapy is at least 100 years old. Significant research was carried out by Robert Oden. He was able to simulate a stroke in a monkey's brain, causing hemiplegia. He then bound up the monkey's good arm, and forced the monkey to use his bad arm, and observed what happened. After two weeks of this therapy, the monkeys were able to use their once hemiplegic arms again. This is due to neuroplasticity. He did the same experiment without binding the arms, and waited six months past their injury. The monkeys without the intervention were not able to use the affected arm even six months later. In 1918, this study was published, but it received little attention.

Eventually, researchers began to apply his technique to stroke patients, and it came to be called constraint-induced movement therapy. Notably, the initial studies focused on chronic stroke patients who were more than 12 months past their stroke. This challenged the belief held at that time that no recovery would occur after one year. The therapy entails wearing a soft mitt on the good hand for 90% of the waking hours, forcing use of the affected hand. The patients undergo intense one-on-one therapy for six to eight hours per day for two weeks.

Evidence that supports the use of constraint induced movement therapy has been growing since its introduction as an alternative treatment method for upper limb motor deficits found in stroke populations. Recently, constraint induced movement therapy has been shown to be an effective rehabilitation technique at varying stages of stroke recovery to improve upper limb motor function and use during daily activities of living. The greatest gains are seen among persons with stroke who exhibit some wrist and finger extension in the effected limb. Transcranial magnetic stimulation and brain imaging studies have demonstrated that the brain undergoes plastic changes in function and structure in patients that perform constraint induced movement therapy. These changes accompany the gains in motor function of the paretic upper limb. However, there is no established causal link between observed changes in brain function/structure and the motor gains due to constraint induced movement therapy.

Constraint induced movement therapy has recently been modified to treat aphasia in patients post CVA as well. This treatment intervention is known as Constraint Induced Aphasia Therapy (CIAT). The same general principals apply, however in this case, the client is constricted from using compensatory strategies to communicate such as gestures, writing, drawing, and pointing, and are encouraged to use verbal communication. Therapy is typically carried out in groups and barriers are used so hands, and any compensatory strategies are not seen. <Cohen, A. (2014). Constraint Induced Aphasia Therapy. Retrieved from http://researchandhope.com/constraint-induced-aphasia-therapy>

Mental Practice/Mental Imagery

Mental practice of movements, has been shown in many studies to be effective in promoting recovery of both arm and leg function after a stroke. It is often used by physical or occupational therapists in the rehab or homehealth setting, but can also be used as part of a patient's independent home exercise program. Mental Movement Therapy is one product available for assisting patients with guided mental imagery.

Brain Repair

Electrical Stimulation

Such work represents a paradigm shift in the approach towards rehabilitation of the stroke-injured brain away from pharmacologic flooding of neuronal receptors and instead, towards targeted physiologic stimulation. In layman's terms, this electrical stimulation mimics the action of healthy muscle to improve function and aid in retraining weak muscles and normal movement. Functional Electrical Stimulation (FES) is commonly used in 'foot-drop' following stroke, but it can be used to help retrain movement in the arms or legs.

Bobath (NDT)

In patients undergoing rehabilitation with a stroke population or other central nervous system disorders (cerebral palsy,etc.), Bobath, also known as Neurodevelopmental Treatment (NDT), is often the treatment of choice in North America. The Bobath concept is best viewed as a framework for interpretation and problem solving of the individual patient's presentation, along with their potential for improvement. Components of motor control that are specifically emphasized, are the integration of postural control and task performance, the control of selective movement for the production of coordinated sequences of movement and the contribution of sensory inputs to motor control and motor learning. Task practice is a component of a broad approach to treatment that includes in-depth assessment of the movement strategies utilized by the patient to perform tasks, and identification of specific deficits of neurological and neuromuscular functions. Many studies have been conducted comparing NDT with other treatment techniques such as proprioceptive neuromuscular facilitation (PNF stretching), as well as conventional treatment approaches (utilizing traditional exercises and functional activities), etc. Despite being widely used, based on the literature, NDT has failed to demonstrate any superiority over other treatment techniques available. In fact, the techniques compared with NDT in these studies often produce similar results in terms of treatment effectiveness. Research has demonstrated significant findings for all these treatment approaches when compared with control subjects and indicate that overall, rehabilitation is effective. It is important to note, however, that the NDT philosophy of "do what works best" has led to heterogeneity in the literature in terms of what constitutes an NDT technique, thus making it difficult to directly compare to other techniques.

Mirror Therapy

Mirror therapy (MT) has been employed with some success in treating stroke patients. Clinical studies that have combined mirror therapy with conventional rehabilitation have achieved the most positive outcomes. However, there is no clear consensus as to its effectiveness. In a recent survey of the published research, Rothgangel concluded that

In stroke patients, we found a moderate quality of evidence that MT as an additional therapy improves recovery of arm function after stroke. The quality of evidence regarding the effects of MT on the recovery of lower limb functions is still low, with only one study reporting effects. In patients with CRPS and PLP, the quality of evidence is also low.

Stem Cells Therapies (In Research)

Use of Bone-marrow Derived Mesenchymal Stem Cells (MSCs) in the treatment of Ischemic Stroke

The terminal differentiation of some somatic stem cells has recently been called into question after studies of transplanted haematopoietic stem cells showed the development of myoblasts, endothelium, epithelium and neuroectodermal cells, suggesting pluripotency. These findings have led to MSCs being considered for treatment of ischemic stroke, specifically in directly enhancing neuroprotection and the neurorestorative processes of neurogenesis, angiogenesis and synaptic plasticity.

Possible Mechanisms of Neurorestoration and Neuroprotection by MSCs After Stroke

Transdifferentiation of MSCs into excitable neuron-like cells has been shown to be possible in vitro and these cells respond to common central nervous system neurotransmitters. However, it is unlikely that this degree of transdifferentiation occurs in vivo and that <1% of injected MSCs become truly differentiated and integrate in the damaged area. This suggests that transdifferentiation of MSCs into neurons or neuron-like cells is not a major mechanism by which MSCs cause neurorestoration.

Induction of neurogenesis (development of new neurons) is another possible mechanism of neurorestoration; however its correlation with functional improvement after stroke is not well established. The inducted cells likely originate from the ventricular zone, subventricular zone and choroid plexus, and migrate to the areas in their respective hemispheres which are damaged. Unlike the induction of neurogenesis, the induction of angiogenesis (development of new blood vessels) by MSCs has been associated with improvements in brain function after ischemic strokes and is linked to improved neuronal recruitment. In addition, synaptogenesis (formation of new synapses between neurons) has been shown to increase after MSC treatment; this combination of improved neurogenesis, angiogenesis and synaptogenesis may lead to a more significant functional improvement in damaged areas as a result of MSC treatment.

MSC treatment also has shown to have various neuroprotective effects, including reductions in apoptosis, inflammation and demyelination, as well as increased astrocyte survival rates. MSC treatment also appears to improve the control of cerebral blood flow and blood–brain barrier permeability, as well as what is currently thought to be the most important mechanism of MSC treatment after stroke, the activation of endogenous neuroprotection and neurorestoration pathways by the release of cytokines and trophic factors.

Although activation of endogenous neuroprotection and neurorestoration probably has a major part in the improvement of brain function after stroke, it is likely that the functional improvements as a result of MSC treatment are due to combined action via multiple cellular and molecular mechanisms to affect neurorestoration and neuroprotection, rather than just a single mechanism. These effects are also modulated by key variables, including the number of and type of MSCs used, timing of treatment relative to when the patient's stroke occurred, route of delivery of the MSCs, as well as patient variables (e.g. age, underlying conditions).

What this Means for Stroke Patients and the Limitations or concerns With MSCs as a Potential Treatment

If MSC treatment becomes available for stroke patients, it is possible that current mortality and morbidity rates could substantially improve due to the direct enhancement of neuroprotection and neurorestoration mechanisms rather than only indirect facilitation or prevention of further damage, e.g. decompressive surgery. However, for MSC treatment to be used effectively and safely in a clinical setting, more research needs to be conducted, specifically in the areas of determining the relative influences of key variables (especially patient variables) on patient outcomes as well quantifying potential risks, e.g. tumour formation. Although ethical concerns are mostly limited to the use of embryonic stem cells, it may also be important to address any possible ethical concerns (however unlikely) over the use of somatic stem cells.

Training of Muscles Affected by the Upper Motor Neuron Syndrome

Muscles affected by the Upper Motor Neuron Syndrome have many potential features of altered performance including: weakness, decreased motor control, clonus (a series of involuntary rapid muscle contractions), exaggerated deep tendon reflexes, spasticity and decreased endurance. The term "spasticity" is often erroneously used interchangeably with Upper Motor Neuron Syndrome, and it is not unusual to see patients labeled as spastic who demonstrate an array of UMN findings.

It has been estimated that approximately 65% of individuals develop spasticity following stroke, and studies have revealed that approximately 40% of stroke victims may still have spasticity at 12 months post-stroke. The changes in muscle tone probably result from alterations in the balance of inputs from reticulospinal and other descending pathways to the motor and interneuronal circuits of the spinal cord, and the absence of an intact corticospinal system. In other words, there is damage to the part of the brain or spinal cord that controls voluntary movement.

Various means are available for the treatment of the effects of the Upper Motor Neuron Syndrome. These include: exercises to improve strength, control and endurance, non-pharmacologic therapies, oral drug therapy, intrathecal drug therapy, injections, and surgery. While Landau suggests that researchers do not believe that treating spasticity is worthwhile, many scholars and clinicians continue to attempt to manage/treat it.

Another group of researchers concluded that while spasticity may contribute to significant motor and activity impairments post-stroke, the role of spasticity has been overemphasized in stroke rehabilitation. In a survey done by the National Stroke Association, while 58 percent of survivors in the survey experienced spasticity, only 51 percent of those had received treatment for the condition.

Nonpharmacologic Therapies

Treatment should be based on assessment by the relevant health professionals. For muscles with mild-to-moderate impairment, exercise should be the mainstay of management, and is likely to need to be prescribed by a physiotherapist.

Muscles with severe impairment are likely to be more limited in their ability to exercise and may require help to do this. They may require additional interventions, to manage the greater neurological impairment and also the greater secondary complications. These interventions may include serial casting, flexibility exercise such as sustained positioning programs, and patients may require equipment, such as using a standing frame to sustain a standing position. Applying specially made Lycra garments may also be beneficial.

Physiotherapy

Physiotherapy is beneficial in this area as it helps post-stroke individuals to progress through the stages of motor recovery. These stages were originally described by Twitchell and Brunnstrom, and may be known as the Brunnstrom Approach. Initially, post-stroke individuals suffer from flaccid paralysis. As recovery begins, and progresses, basic movement synergies will develop into more complex and difficult movement combinations. Concurrently, spasticity may develop and become quite severe before it begins to decline (if it does at all). Although an overall pattern of motor recovery exists, there is much variability between each individual's recovery. As previously described, the role of spasticity in stroke rehabilitation is controversial. However, physiotherapy can help to improve motor performance, in part, through the management of spasticity.

Unaddressed spasticity will result in the maintenance of abnormal resting limb postures which can lead to contracture formation. In the arm, this may interfere with hand hygiene and dressing, whereas in the leg, abnormal resting postures may result in difficulty transferring. In order to help manage spasticity, physiotherapy interventions should focus on modifying or reducing muscle tone. Strategies include mobilizations of the affected limbs early in rehabilitation, along with elongation of the spastic muscle and sustained stretching. In addition, the passive manual technique of rhythmic rotation can help to increase initial range. Activating the antagonist (muscle) in a slow and controlled movement is a beneficial training strategy that can be used by post-stroke individuals. Splinting, to maintain muscle stretch and provide tone inhibition, and cold (i.e. in the form of ice packs), to decrease neural firing, are other strategies that can be used to temporarily decrease the extent of spasticity. The focus of physiotherapy for post-stroke individuals is to improve motor performance, in part, through the manipulation of muscle tone.

Oral Drug Therapies

Oral medications used for the treatment of spasticity include: diazepam (Valium), dantrolene sodium, baclofen, tizanidine, clonidine, gabapentin, and even cannabinoid-like compounds.[3] The exact mechanism of these medications is not fully understood, but they are thought to act on neurotransmitters or neuromodulators within the central nervous system (CNS) or muscle itself, or to decrease the stretch reflexes. The problem with these medications is their potential side effects and the fact that, other than lessening painful or disruptive spasms and dystonic postures, drugs in general have not been shown to decrease impairments or lessen disabilities.

Intrathecal Drug Therapy

Intrathecal administration of drugs involves the implantation of a pump that delivers medication directly to the CNS. The benefit of this is that the drug remains in the spinal cord, without traveling in the bloodstream, and there are often fewer side effects. The most commonly used medication for this is baclofen but morphine sulfate and Fentanyl have been used as well, mainly for severe pain as a result of the spasticity.

Injections

Injections are focal treatments administered directly into the spastic muscle. Drugs used include: Botulinum toxin (BTX), phenol, alcohol, and lidocaine. Phenol and alcohol cause local muscle damage by denaturing protein, and thus relaxing the muscle. Botulinum toxin is a neurotoxin and it relaxes the muscle by preventing the release of a neurotransmitter (acetylcholine). Many studies have shown the benefits of BTX and it has also been demonstrated that repeat injections of BTX show unchanged effectiveness.

Surgery

Surgical treatment for spasticity includes lengthening or releasing of muscle and tendons, procedures involving bones, and also selective dorsal rhizotomy. Rhizotomy, usually reserved for severe spasticity, involves cutting selective sensory nerve roots, as they probably play a role in generating spasticity.

Shoulder Subluxation Following Stroke

Glenohumeral (or shoulder) subluxation is defined as a partial or incomplete dislocation of the shoulder joint that typically results from changes in the mechanical integrity of the joint. Subluxation is a common problem with hemiplegia, or weakness of the musculature of the upper limb. Traditionally this has been thought to be a significant cause of post-stroke shoulder pain, although a few recent studies have failed to show a direct correlation between shoulder subluxation and pain.

The exact etiology of subluxation in post-stroke patients is unclear but appears to be caused by weakness of the musculature supporting the shoulder joint. The shoulder is one of the most mobile joints in the body. To provide a high level of mobility the shoulder sacrifices ligamentous stability and as a result relies on the surrounding musculature (i.e., rotator cuff muscles, latissimus dorsi, and deltoid) for much of its support. This is in contrast to other less mobile joints such as the knee and hip, which have a significant amount of support from the joint capsule and surrounding ligaments. If a stroke damages the upper motor neurons controlling muscles of the upper limb, weakness and paralysis, followed by spasticity occurs in a somewhat predictable pattern. The muscles supporting the shoulder joint, particularly the supraspinatus and posterior deltoid become flaccid and can no longer offer adequate support leading to a downward and outward movement of arm at the shoulder joint causing tension on the relatively weak joint capsule. Other factors have also been cited as contributing to subluxation such as pulling on the hemiplegic arm and improper positioning.

Diagnosis can usually be made by palpation or by feeling the joint and surrounding tissues, although there is controversy as to whether or not the degree of subluxation can be measured clinically. If shoulder subluxation occurs, it can become a barrier to the rehabilitation process. Treatment involves measures to support the subluxed joint such as taping the joint, using a lapboard or armboard. A shoulder sling may be used, but is controversial and a few studies have shown no appreciable difference in range-of-motion, degree of subluxation, or pain when using a sling. A sling may also contribute to contractures and increased flexor tone if used for extended periods of time as it places the arm close to the body in adduction, internal rotation and elbow flexion. Use of a sling can also contribute to learned nonuse by preventing the functional and spontaneous use of the affected upper extremity. That said, a sling may be necessary for some therapy activities. Slings may be considered appropriate during therapy for initial transfer and gait training, but overall use should be limited. As the patient begins to recover, spasticity and voluntary movement of the shoulder will occur as well as reduction in the shoulder subluxation. Slings are of no value at this point.

Functional electrical stimulation (FES) has also shown promising results in treatment of subluxation, and reduction of pain, although some studies have shown a return of pain after discontinuation of FES. More recent research has failed to show any reduction of pain with the use of FES.

Logical treatment consists of preventive measures such as early range of motion, proper positioning, passive support of soft tissue structures and possibly early re-activation of shoulder musculature using functional electrical stimulation. Aggressive exercises such as overhead pulleys should be avoided with this population.

Post-stroke Pain Syndromes

Central Post-stroke Pain (CPSP) is neuropathic pain which is caused by damage to the neurons in the brain (central nervous system), as the result of a vascular injury. One study found that up to 8% of people who have had a stroke will develop Central Post-stroke Pain, and that the pain will be moderate to severe in 5% of those affected. The condition was formerly called "thalamic pain", because of the high incidence among those with damage to the thalamus or thalamic nuclei. Now known as CPSP, it is characterized by perceived pain from non-painful stimuli, such as temperature and light touch. This altered perception of stimuli, or allodynia, can be difficult to assess due to the fact that the pain can change daily in description and location, and can appear anywhere from months to years after the stroke. CPSP can also lead to a heightened central response to painful sensations, or hyperpathia. Affected persons may describe the pain as cramping, burning, crushing, shooting, pins and needles, and even bloating or urinary urgency. Both the variation and mechanism of pain in CPSP have made it difficult to treat. Several strategies have been employed by physicians, including intravenous lidocaine, opioids/narcotics, anti-depressants, anti-epileptic medications and neurosurgical procedures with varying success. Higher rates of successful pain control in persons with CPSP can be achieved by treating other sequelae of stroke, such as depression and spasticity. As the age of the population increases, the diagnosis and management of CPSP will become increasingly important to improve the quality of life of an increasing number of stroke survivors.

Apraxia

An uncommon, less understood result of stroke is a condition called apraxia. This condition was initially recognized as: 'Disorders of the execution of learned movements which cannot be accounted for by either weakness, incoordination, or sensory loss, nor by incomprehension of, or inattention to commands.' Several forms of apraxia are recognized. Limb-kinetic apraxia is the inability to make precise or exact movements with a finger, an arm or a leg. idiomotor apraxia is the inability to carry out a command from the brain to mimic limb or head movements performed or suggested by others. Conceptual apraxia is similar to idiomotor apraxia, but infers a more profound malfunctioning in which the function of tools or objects is no longer understood. Ideational apraxia is the inability to create a plan for a specific movement. Buccofacial apraxia, or facial-oral apraxia, is the inability to coordinate and carry out facial and lip movements such as whistling, winking, coughing, etc. on command. Constructional apraxia affects the person's ability to draw or copy simple diagrams, or to construct simple figures. Oculomotor apraxia is a condition in which the patient finds it difficult to move his/her eyes. Many believe that the most common form of apraxia is ideamotor apraxia, in which a disconnection between the area of the brain containing plans for a movement and the area of the brain that is responsible for executing that movement occurs.

Unlike many effects of stroke, where the clinician is able to judge the particular area of the brain that a stroke has injured by certain signs or symptoms, the causation of apraxia is less clear. A common theory is that the part of the brain that contains information for previously learned skilled motor activities has been either lost or cannot be accessed. The condition is usually due to an insult to the dominant hemisphere of the brain. More often this is located in the frontal lobe of the left hemisphere of the brain. Treatment of acquired apraxia due to stroke usually consists of physical, occupational, and speech therapy. The Copenhagen Stroke Study, which is a large important study published in 2001, showed that out of 618 stroke patients, manual apraxia was found in 7% and oral apraxia was found in 6%. Both manual and oral apraxia were related to increasing severity of stroke. Oral apraxia was related with an increase in age at the time of the stroke. There was no difference in incidence among gender. It was also found that the finding of apraxia has no negative influence on ability to function after rehabilitation is completed. The National Institute of Neurological Disorders and Stroke (NINDS) is currently sponsoring a clinical trial to gain an understanding of how the brain operates while carrying out and controlling voluntary motor movements in normal subjects. The objective is to determine what goes wrong with these processes in the course of acquired apraxia due to stroke or brain injury.

Lateral Medullary Syndrome

Lateral medullary syndrome, also known as Wallenberg's Syndrome, is caused by blockage of the posterior inferior cerebellar artery (PICA) or the vertebral arteries. Signs and symptoms include decreased pain and temperature on the same side of the face and opposite side of the body compared to the lesion, ataxia on the same side of the lesion, and Horner's syndrome on the same side of the face.

Treatment in the acute setting is mostly focused on symptomatic management. After initial treatment in the hospital, some patients will need short-term placement in a nursing home or rehabilitation facility before going home. In hospital settings the doctors work with speech pathologists in issues like these. Typically, a commonly used tool to assess the degree of severity of dysphagia and speech issues is the Barnes Jewish Hospital Stroke Dysphagia Screen, which offers a validated guide to assessing plan of action (solid food diet, all liquid diet, IV hydration, etc.) for the patient while in the hospital and the proper course of action in the outpatient setting. Rehabilitation in Wallenberg's Syndrome focuses on improving balance, coordination, working on activities of daily living, and improving speech and swallowing function. Severe nausea and vertigo can be present and limit progress in rehabilitation and recovery. Symptomatic treatment with anti-emetics and medications for the hiccups are important. Commonly used anti-emetics include ondansetron, metoclopramide, prochlorperazine, and promethazine. These medications are also used to treat hiccups, along with chlorpromazine. There are case reports of other medications useful in treating hiccups in Wallenberg's Syndrome including baclofen and anti-epileptic medications. The prognosis for someone with lateral medullary syndrome depends upon the size and location of damaged area of the brain stem. Some individuals recover quickly while others may have significant neurological disabilities for months to years after the initial injury.

Post-stroke Depression

Depression is a commonly reported consequence of stroke and is seen in anywhere from 25-50% of patients. The Diagnostic and Statistical Manual (DSM-IV-TR) defines post-stroke depression as "a mood disorder due to a general medical condition (i.e. stroke) that is judged to be due to the direct physiological effects of [that] condition." Post-stroke depression may involve depressed mood and decreased interest and pleasure that impairs social and occupational functioning, but does not necessarily need to meet the full criteria of a major depressive disorder.

The first studies to look for an association between specific stroke lesions and the occurrence of depression reported a correlation between left frontal lesions and major depression. Damage to the frontal noradrenergic, dopaminergic, and serotonergic projections were thought to cause a depletion of catecholamines, leading to depression. However, more recent studies have demonstrated that the anatomic aspects of a lesion do not necessarily correlate with the occurrence of depression. Other psychological factors can lead to the development of depression including personal and social losses related to the physical disabilities often caused by a stroke.

The incidence of post-stroke depression peaks at 3–6 months and usually resolves within 1–2 years after the stroke, although a minority of patients can go on to develop chronic depression. The diagnosis of post-stroke depression is complicated by other consequences of stroke such as fatigue and psychomotor retardation – which do not necessarily indicate the presence of depression. Loss of interest in activities and relationships should prompt an evaluation for depression.

Traditionally, tricyclic antidepressants (TCAs), such as nortriptyline, have been used in the treatment of post-stroke depression. More recently, the selective serotonin reuptake inhibitors (SSRIs), such as fluoxetine and citalopram, have become the pharmacologic therapy of choice due to the lower incidence of side effects. Also, psychologic treatment such as cognitive behavioral therapy, group therapy, and family therapy are reported to be useful adjuncts to treatment.

Overall, the development of post-stroke depression can play a significant role in a patient's recovery from a stroke. For instance, the severity of post-stroke depression has been associated with severity of impairment in activities of daily living (ADLs). By effectively treating depression, patients experience a greater recovery of basic ADLs such as dressing, eating and ambulating, as well as instrumental ADLs, such as the ability to take care of financial and household matters. In essence, recognition and treatment of post-stroke depression leads to greater functional ability for the patient over time.

Horticultural Therapy

Horticultural therapy (also known as social and therapeutic horticulture or STH) is defined by the American Horticultural Therapy Association (AHTA) as the engagement of a person in gardening and plant-based activities, facilitated by a trained therapist, to achieve specific therapeutic treatment goals. The visual aesthetics of plants are known to elicit feelings of inner peace, which generates positive emotions toward a meaningful appreciation of life. Direct contact with plants guides the individual's focus away from stress enhancing their overall quality of life. The AHTA believes that horticultural therapy is an active process which occurs in the context of an established treatment plan. Horticultural therapists are specially educated and trained members of rehabilitation teams (with doctors, psychiatrists, psychologists, occupational therapists and other) who involve the client in all phases of gardening, from propagation to selling products, as a means of bringing about improvement in their life.

History

The first modern documentation of horticulture being used as a treatment for mental health purposes was in the 1800s. Dr. Benjamin Rush discovered that field labor in a farm setting helped attain positive outcomes for clients with mental illness (Simson & Straus, 2003). This discovery lead many hospitals in the western world to begin using horticulture as a means to start therapeutically treating patients with mental health and developmental disabilities. In 1817, the Asylum for Persons Deprived of Their Reason, now known as Friends Hospital, constructed an environment with landscaping, paths and a park atmosphere in effort to assist patients in their recovery. In 1879 Friends Hospital built the first greenhouse that was used for therapy (Simson & Straus, 2003). "During World War I and II, servicemen worked in gardens to improve functioning of injured limbs and increase mental function, but also to learn new skills and to provide food" (http://tiadjones.tripod.com/horttherapy.htm#d). Plants and gardening also came to be used as a diversion for those who were hospitalized long-term.

The 1950s and 1960s brought the first degree in horticultural therapy at Michigan State University. In 1972, Kansas State University created the first curriculum that provided students with dual training in both psychology and horticulture (Simson & Straus, 2003). The first graduate degree program was offered by Clemson University in 1973 (Simson & Straus, 2003). In 1973 the Council for Therapy and Rehabilitation though Horticulture (NCTRH) was established by a group of horticulture therapy professionals. In 1988, they changed their name to the American Horticulture Therapy Association (AHTA) which they are still called today. AHTA is a non-profit organization with about 25% off their members being professionally registered

Credentials

American Horticulture Therapy Association (AHTA) offers the opportunity for professionals interested in practicing horticultural therapy to register as Horticultural Therapists (Horticulture Therapy Registered, HTR). Some colleges and universities have academic programs in horticulture therapy that are accredited through AHTA. AHTA has a set core curriculum for accredited programs to follow. Along with specific classes to take, internships are a very critical component. AHTA requires that to be Horticultural Therapist Registered, 480 hours of field experience are to be completed.

Programs

Horticultural Therapy can be used with a variety of populations and settings. Simson and Straus (2003) have categorized Horticultural Therapy services into three main types of programming; vocational, social, and therapeutic. Clients benefiting from the therapeutic arm of Horticultural Therapy typically include those individuals with psychiatric challenges, substance abuse issues, and those who are in recovery from a physical injury. Clients served under the vocational arm of Horticultural Therapy may include individuals who are incarcerated, have a developmental or psychiatric disability, or people who have experienced socioeconomic disadvantages. Clients typically served under the social arm of Horticultural Therapy might include the elderly, and community-based programs.

Electrodiagnostic Medicine

Electrodiagnosis (EDX) is a method of medical diagnosis that obtains information about diseases by passively recording the electrical activity of body parts (that is, their natural electrophysiology) or by measuring their response to external electrical stimuli (evoked potentials). The most widely used methods of recording spontaneous electrical activity are various forms of electrodiagnostic testing (electrography) such as electrocardiography (ECG), electroencephalography (EEG), and electromyography (EMG). Electrodiagnostic medicine (also EDX) is a medical subspecialty of neurology, clinical neurophysiology, cardiology, and physical medicine and rehabilitation. Electrodiagnostic physicians apply electrophysiologic techniques, including needle electromyography and nerve conduction studies to diagnose, evaluate, and treat people with impairments of the neurologic, neuromuscular, and/or muscular systems. The provision of a quality electrodiagnostic medical evaluation requires extensive scientific knowledge that includes anatomy and physiology of the peripheral nerves and muscles, the physics and biology of the electrical signals generated by muscle and nerve, the instrumentation used to process these signals, and techniques for clinical evaluation of diseases of the peripheral nerves and sensory pathways

Training

In the United States, neurologists receive training in performing needle electromyography and nerve conduction studies during a fellowship in clinical neurophysiology or neuromuscular medicine. Physical medicine and rehabilitation physicians receive this training during their residency. and can get further training in a neuromuscular fellowship. The American Board of Electrodiagnostic Medicine certifies US physicians in electrodiagnostic medicine. In Europe, nerve conduction studies and electromyography training may be part of neurology, physical medicine and rehabilitation, or clinical neurophysiology training. In the United States, there is also a certification in neuromuscular medicine. This certification is open only to neurologists and physical medicine and rehabilitation specialists that have completed a fellowship in neuromuscular medicine. The neuromuscular medicine examination includes electrodiagnostic testing as part of the certification examination but also includes broader topics such as genetics, biopsy, and rehabilitation. Technologists sometimes assist in the performance of the NCSs but do not the interpretation. In the United States, the Current Procedural Terminology code of the American Medical Association, states ""Waveforms must be reviewed on site in real time..." In addition, it states that the "Reports must be prepared on site by the examiner, and consists of the work product of the interpretation of numerous test results...along with summarization of clinical and electrodiagnostic data, and physician or other qualified health care professional interpretation.

Patients will typically be referred to a specialist in electrodiagnostic medicine if they have numbness, tingling, pain, weakness or spasms. Common muscle and nerve disorders seen by these type of specialists include pinched nerves in the neck or back (radiculopathy), carpal tunnel syndrome, and neuropathies. More uncommon diseases include ALS, myasthenia gravis, and chronic inflammatory demyelinating polyneuropathy. Using their broader training, physicians in electrodiagnostic medicine, often perform more detailed evaluations which may include laboratory tests, CT or MRI scans, genetic evaluation, biopsy of nerve, skin, or muscle, or perform neuromuscular ultrasound. A more complete listing of disorders and testing can be found under neuromuscular medicine.

Relationship to Neurophysiology

Clinical neurophysiology, is a broader field that includes EEG, intraoperative monitoring, nerve conduction studies, EMG and evoked potentials. The American Board of Psychiatry and Neurology provides certification examination in clinical neurophysiology. The American Board of Electrodiagnostic Medicine provides certification in EDX medicines. The American Board of Clinical Neurophysiology certifies in electroencephalography (EEG), Evoked Potentials (EP), Polysomnography (PSG), Epilepsy Monitoring, and Neurologic Intraoperative Monitoring (NIOM). In the US physicians typically specialize in EEG or EDX medicine but not both.

History

Electrodiagnostic medicine traces its origin back to a 1791 experiment by Luigi Galvani. Galvani depolarized frog leg muscles by using metal rods to make contact with the leg muscles. The development of the oscilloscope in 1897 significantly enhanced the ability of scientists to record signals from nerve and muscle. However, it was the needs of those with severe injuries during World War II that created the field of modern electrodiagnostic medicine. In the early 1950s, the first society dedicated to the development of this field, the AAEE, was founded in Chicago by a group of interested specialists in neurology and physical medicine and rehabilitation. James Golseth was instrumental in creating this organization. Over time, newer techniques, such as somatosensory evoked potentials, single fiber electromyography, autonomic testing, and neuromuscular ultrasound have evolved as useful complementary techniques to nerve conduction studies and elecytromyography, which remain the core of electrodiagnostic medicine.

Telerehabilitation

Telerehabilitation (or e-rehabilitation) is the delivery of rehabilitation services over telecommunication networks and the internet. Most types of services fall into two categories: clinical assessment (the patient's functional abilities in his or her environment), and clinical therapy. Some fields of rehabilitation practice that have explored telerehabilitation are: neuropsychology, speech-language pathology, audiology, occupational therapy, and physical therapy. Telerehabilitation can deliver therapy to people who cannot travel to a clinic because the patient has a disability or because of travel time. Telerehabilitation also allows experts in rehabilitation to engage in a clinical consultation at a distance.

Most telerehabilitation is highly visual. As of 2006 the most commonly used modalities are via webcams, videoconferencing, phone lines, videophones and webpages containing rich Internet applications. The visual nature of telerehabilitation technology limits the types of rehabilitation services that can be provided. It is most widely used for neuropsychological rehabilitation; fitting of rehabilitation equipment such as wheelchairs, braces or artificial limbs; and in speech-language pathology. Rich internet applications for neuropsychological rehabilitation (aka cognitive rehabilitation) of cognitive impairment (from many etiologies) was first introduced in 2001. This endeavor has recently (2006) expanded as a teletherapy application for cognitive skills enhancement programs for school children. Tele-audiology (hearing assessments) is a growing application. As of 2006, telerehabilitation in the practice of occupational therapy and physical therapy are very limited, perhaps because these two disciplines are more "hands on".

Two important areas of telerehabilitation research are (1) demonstrating equivalence of assessment and therapy to in-person assessment and therapy, and (2) building new data collection systems to digitize information that a therapist can use in practice. Ground-breaking research in telehaptics (the sense of touch) and virtual reality may broaden the scope of telerehabilitation practice, in the future.

In the United States, the National Institute on Disability and Rehabilitation Research's (NIDRR) supports research and the development of telerehabilitation. NIDRR's grantees include the "Rehabilitation Engineering and Research Center" (RERC) at the University of Pittsburgh, the Rehabilitation Institute of Chicago, the State University of New York at Buffalo, and the National Rehabilitation Hospital in Washington DC. Other federal funders of research are the Veterans Administration, the Health Services Research Administration in the US Department of Health and Human Services, and the Department of Defense. Outside the United States, excellent research is conducted in Australia and Europe.

As of 2006, only a few health insurers in the United States will reimburse for telerehabilitation services. If the research shows that tele-assessments and tele-therapy are equivalent to clinical encounters, it is more likely that insurers and Medicare will cover telerehabilitation services.

History

In 1999, D.M. Angaran published "Telemedicine and Telepharmacy: Current Status and Future Implications" in the American Journal of Health-System Pharmacy. He provided a comprehensive history of telecommunications, the internet and telemedicine since the 1950s. The Department of Defense (DoD) and the National Aeronautics and Space Administration (NASA) spearheaded the technology in the United States during the Vietnam War and the space program; both agencies continue to fund advances in telemedicine.

Three early adopters of telemedicine were state penitentiary systems, rural health care systems, and the radiology profession. Telemedicine makes business sense for the states because they do not have to pay for security escorts to have a prisoner receive care outside the prison.

Rural telemedicine in the United States is heavily subsidized through federal agency grants for telecommunications operations. Most of this funding comes through the Health Services Research Administration and the Department of Commerce. Some state universities have obtained state funding to operate tele-clinics in rural areas. As of 2006, few (if any) of these programs are known to financially break-even, mostly because the Medicare program for people over age 65 (the largest payer) is very restrictive about paying for telehealth.

In contrast, the Veterans Administration is relatively active in using telemedicine for people with disabilities. There are several programs that provide annual physical exams or monitoring and consultation for veterans with spinal cord injuries. Similarly, some state Medicaid programs (for poor people and people with disabilities) have pilot programs using telecommunications to connect rural practitioners with subspecialty therapists. A few school districts in Oklahoma and Hawaii offer school-based rehabilitation therapy using therapy assistants who are directed by a remote therapist. The National Rehabilitation Hospital in Washington DC and Sister Kenny Rehabilitation Institute in Minneapolis provided assessment and evaluations to patients living in Guam and American Samoa. Cases included post-stroke, post-polio, autism, and wheel-chair fitting.

An argument can be made that "telerehabilitation" began in 1998 when NIDRR funded the first RERC on tele-rehabilitation. It was awarded to a consortium of biomedical engineering departments at the National Rehabilitation Hospital and The Catholic University of America, both located in Washington, DC; the Sister Kenny Rehabilitation Institute in Minnesota; and the East Carolina University in North Carolina. Some of this early research work, and its motivation, is reviewed in Winters (2002). The State of Science Conference held in 2002 convened most of military and civilian clinicians, engineers, and government officials interested in using telecommunications as a modality for rehabilitation assessment and therapy; a summary is provided in Rosen, Winters & Lauderdale (2002). The conference was attended by the incoming president of the American Telemedicine Association (ATA). This led to an invitation by ATA to the conference attendees to form a special interest group on telerehabilitation. NIDRR funded the second 5-year RERC on telerehabilitation in 2004, awarding it to the University of Pittsburgh. This RERC was renewed in 2010.

In 2001, O. Bracy, a neuropsychologist, introduced the first web based, rich internet application, for the telerehabilitation presentation of cognitive rehabilitation therapy. This system first provides the subscriber clinician with an economical means of treating their own patients over the internet. Secondly, the system then provides, directly to the patient, the therapy prescription set up and controlled by the member clinician. All applications and response data are transported via the internet in real time. The patient can login to do their therapy from home, the library or anywhere they have access to an internet computer. In 2006, this system formed the basis of a new system designed as a cognitive skills enhancement program for school children. Individual children or whole classrooms can participate in this program over the internet.

In 2006, M.J. McCue and S.E. Palsbo published an article in the Journal of Telemedicine and Telecare that explored how telemedicine can become a profitable business for hospitals. They argue that telerehabilitation should be expanded so that people with disabilities and people in pain (perhaps after hip-replacement surgery or people with arthritis) can get the rehabilitative therapy they need. It is unethical to limit paymente for telerehabilitation services only to patients in rural areas.

Research in telerehabilitation is in its infancy, with only a handful of equivalence trials. As of 2006, most peer-reviewed research in telemedicine are case reports of pilot programs or new equipment. Rehabilitation researchers need to conduct many more controlled experiments and present the evidence to clinicians (and payers) that telerehabilitation is clinically effective. The discipline of speech-language pathology is far head of occupational therapy and physical therapy in demonstrating equivalence over various types of telecommunications equipment.

Technologies

1. Plain old telephone service (POTS) with videophones/phones in telerehabilitation

   There are several types of connections used with real time exchanges. Plain old telephone service (POTS) uses standard analog telephone lines. Videophones are used with POTS lines and include a camera, display screen, and telephone. Videophones use telephone lines that are available in most homes, so are easy to set up; however small display screens make them problematic for individuals with vision problems. This can be solved by using a large screen or television as a screen.

2. Videotelephony/Videotelephony in telerehabilitation

   The use of improved quality video-assisted telecommunication devices, such as videoconferencing, webcams and telepresence to assist in treatments.

3. Virtual reality/Virtual reality in telerehabilitation

   Virtual reality in telerehabilitation is one of the newest tools available in that area. This computer technology allows the development of three-dimensional virtual environments.

4. Motion technology/Motion technology in telerehabilitation
5. Web-based approaches/Web-based approaches in telerehabilitation

   Applications that run over the internet, just as if they were installed in your computer (called Rich Internet Applications), represent a new direction in software development. A person subscribes to the website rather than purchase the software. Any updates or changes to the software system are instantly available to all subscribers. The applications can be accessed from any location where one has access to an internet connected computer. Likewise, a patient's data is accessible from where ever the therapist is located. Neither the application nor the patient's data is tied to one computer.

6. Sensors and body monitoring/Sensors and body monitoring in telerehabilitation
7. Haptic technology/Haptic technology in telerehabilitation
8. Artificial intelligence/Artificial intelligence in telerehabilitation

9. Wireless technology/Wireless technology in telerehabilitation
10. PDAs/PDA in telerehabilitation
11. Mobile telephony/Mobile telephony in telerehabilitation
12. Electronic medical records/Electronic medical record telerehabilitation
13. Mobile apps/Mobile apps telerehabilitation

Clinical Applications

1. Review of telerehabilitation research on clinical populations
2. Professional to professional (clinic to clinic applications)
3. Telehealth – Information access
4. Clinical approaches
    1. Assessment
    2. Monitoring
    3. Intervention
    4. Telesupervision (of licensed assistants)
    5. Telementoring
    6. Tele-education
    7. Telementoring

Speech-language Pathology

The clinical services provided by speech-language pathology readily lend themselves to telerehabilitation applications due to the emphasis on auditory and visual communicative interaction between the client and the clinician. As a result, the number of telerehabilitation applications in speech-language pathology tend to outnumber those in other allied health professions. To date, applications have been developed to assess and/or treat acquired adult speech and language disorders, stuttering, voice disorders, speech disorders in children, and swallowing dysfunction. The technology involved in these applications has ranged from the simple telephone (Plain Old Telephone System – POTS) to the use of dedicated Internet-based videoconferencing systems.

Early applications to assess and treat acquired adult speech and language disorders involved the use of the telephone to treat patients with aphasia and motor speech disorders (Vaughan, 1976, Wertz, et al., 1987), a computer controlled video laserdisc over the telephone and a closed-circuit television system to assess speech and language disorders (Wertz et al., 1987), and a satellite-based videoconferencing system to assess patients in rural areas (Duffy, Werven & Aronson, 1997). More recent applications have involved the use of sophisticated Internet-based videoconferencing systems with dedicated software which enable the assessment of language disorders (Georgeadis, Brennan, Barker, & Baron, 2004, Brennan, Georgeadis, Baron & Barker, 2004) and the assessment and treatment of motor speech disorders (Hill, Theodoros, Russell, Cahill, Ward, Clark, 2006; Theodoros, Constantinescu, Russell, Ward, Wilson & Wootton, in press) following brain impairment and Parkinson's disease. Collectively, these studies have revealed positive treatment outcomes, while assessment and diagnoses have been found to be comparable to face-to-face evaluations.

The treatment of stuttering has been adapted to a telerehabilitation environment with notable success. Two Australian studies (Harrison, Wilson & Onslow, 1999; Wilson, Onslow & Lincoln, 2004) involving the distance delivery of the Lidcombe program to children who stutter have utilized the telephone in conjunction with offline video recordings to successfully treat several children. Overall, the parents and children responded positively to the program delivered at a distant. Using a high speed videoconferencing system link, Sicotte, Lehoux, Fortier-Blanc and Leblanc (2003) assessed and treated six children and adolescents with a positive reduction in the frequency of dysfluency that was maintained six months later. In addition, a videoconferencing platform has been used successfully to provide follow-up treatment to an adult who had previously received intensive therapy (Kully, 200).

Reports of telerehabilitation applications in paediatric speech and language disorders are sparse. A recent Australian pilot study has investigated the feasibility of an Internet-based assessment of speech disorder in six children (Waite, Cahill, Theodoros, Russell, Busuttin, in press). High levels of agreement between the online and face-to-face clinicians for single-word articulation, speech intelligibility, and oro-motor tasks were obtained suggesting that the Internet-based protocol had the potential to be a reliable method for assessing paediatric speech disorders.

Voice therapy across a variety of types of voice disorders has been shown to be effectively delivered via a telerehabilitation application. Mashima et al. (2003) using PC based videoconferencing and speech analysis software compared 23 patients treated online with 28 persons treated face-to-face. The authors reported positive post treatment results with no significant difference in measures between the traditional and videoconferencing group, suggesting that the majority of traditional voice therapy techniques can be applied to distance treatment.

Although obvious limitations exist, telerehabilitation applications for the assessment of swallowing function have also been used with success. Lalor, Brown and Cranfield (2000) were able to obtain an initial assessment of the nature and extent of swallowing dysfunction in an adult via a videoconferencing link although a more complete evaluation was restricted due to the inability to physically determine the degree of laryngeal movement. A more sophisticated telerehabilitation application for the assessment of swallowing was developed by Perlman and Witthawaskul (2002) who described the use of real-time videofluoroscopic examination via the Internet. This system enabled the capture and display of images in real-time with only a three to five second delay.

There continues to be a need for ongoing research to develop and validate the use of telerehabilitation applications in speech-language pathology in a greater number and variety of adult and paediatric communication and swallowing disorders.

Physical and Occupational Therapy

Disciplines and Therapies

1. Speech-language pathology
2. Audiology
3. Physical therapy
4. Occupational therapy
5. Psychology
6. Nursing
7. Social work
8. Rehabilitation counseling/Vocational rehabilitation

Standards and Training Requirements

1. Telerehabilitation standards
2. Reimbursement policies/Reimbursement in telerehabilitation
3. Legislative activities/Legislative activities in telerehabilitation
4. Ethics and privacy issues/Ethics and privacy issues in telerehabilitation
5. Clinical and technology training issues

Related Organizations

- American Telemedicine Association (ATA)
- American Speech-Language-Hearing Association (ASHA)
- Association of Telehealth Service Providers (ATSP)

- National Institute on Disability and Rehabilitation Research (NIDRR)
- Rehabilitation Engineering and Assistive Technology Society of North America (RESNA)
- Special Interest Group on Telerehabilitation (SIGOT)

Community-based Rehabilitation

The aim of **comm**unity-based rehabilitation (CBR) is to help people with disabilities, by establishing community-based programs for social integration, equalization of opportunities, and Physical therapy rehabilitation programs for the disabled. The strength of CBR programs is that they can be made available in rural areas, with limited infrastructure, as program leadership is not restricted to professionals in healthcare, educatiol, Occupational therapy vocational or social services. Rather, CBR programs involve the people with disabilities themselves, their families and communities, as well as appropriate professionals.

History

In the beginning of the 1960s, efforts to establish rehabilitation centers in developing countries had taken hold in urban centers, but failed to provide support and assistance to disabled people in rural areas throughout the world. The response of world aid organizations was to shift funding from city-based hospitals to rural community programs. The first CBR pilot projects were launched in the 1960s, and their continuing success has led to CBR programs being adopted throughout Africa, Asia and South America.

CBR Asia Pacific Network

A CBR Network is a formal or informal relationship among CBR implementers/ practitioners or their organizations to promote and strengthen CBR. The strength of the network depends on the strength of individual or organizational members and the co-ordination and collaboration between members. It is expected that the benefits from the network will be greater than any individual's effort. To enrich CBR further for the benefit of the people with disabilities, their family, community and the country, a network of CBR practitioners/implementers/promoters is required at least at a national level, regional level and global level.

These networks need to be democratic, national CBR network members need to select their national executive body; e.g., CBR Afghanistan Network, CBR India Network, CBR Indonesia Network. President or the secretary of the national networks should represent the general body of the Regional Network; e.g., CBR Asia Pacific Network. General body of the CBR AP Network to elect their Executive body and representatives for CBR Global Network. While electing the executive body one must ensure that committee represents with competent and committed people. CBR is for all, richness and success of CBR depends on diversity and respecting that diversity. An ideal CBR committee should be of people from various background; e.g., people with disabilities (different impairment groups), academicians, people with different socio economic background, people coming from rural areas or representing vulnerable groups policy makers, practitioners, promoters, representative from public and private sectors. Gender and disability balance are the key of the success of any CBR Networks.

Around the world there are existing networks: large and small, formal and informal, active and inactive, etc. For example the CBR Africa Network is a large network covering one continent.

In 2001 during the first Africa Regional Conference on CBR in Kampala, Uganda, the CBR Africa Network (CAN) was created. It started with four action points:

- Initiate the formation of National CBR Associations.
- Improve capacity for sharing information about good CBR practices.
- Review CBR training programmes in order to promote their synchronisation.
- Organize regular (every three years) CBR Conferences in Africa, starting with one in 2004.

There are other notable networks including the CBR South-Asia Network is a sub regional network and there exists across the world many National CBR Networks.

At present three larger continental (regional) networks are under development or expansion including the CBR Africa Network (CAN), CBR America Network (RED de RBC de las Américas y el Caribe) and the CBR Asia-Pacific Network. One of the main outcomes of the CBR Asia-Pacific Congress was to form the CBR Asia-Pacific Network.

The 1st CBR Asia Pacific Congress provided a great opportunity to form the general body of the CBR Asia-Pacific Network who eventually would meet and elect their executive body and take the CBR Asia-Pacific Network forward. The initial purpose of the CBR Asia-Pacific Network was to promote and strengthen CBR across the continent and in countries; mobilize resources, organize trainings and support information exchange.

Twenty-four country representatives have nominated and selected among CBR promoters/implementers/practitioners, including persons with disabilities, taking gender equity, organizational and regional diversity into consideration. The country representatives of the Network held their first meeting immediately after the Congress. Members present in the meeting have taken the responsibility to form the CBR Asia-Pacific Network, draft a constitution, draw a future plan of actions and take it forward (as a continuation of dialogue) with support from the Asia-Pacific Center on Disability (APCD) as the secretariat of the Network.

Vocational Rehabilitation

Vocational rehabilitation is a process which enables persons with functional, psychological, developmental, cognitive and emotional impairments or health disabilities to overcome barriers to accessing, maintaining or returning to employment or other useful occupation.

Vocational rehabilitation can require input from a range of health care professionals and other non-medical disciplines such as disability employment advisers and career counselors. Techniques used can include:

- assessment, appraisal, program evaluation and research.
- goal setting and intervention planning.
- provision of health advice and promotion, in support of returning to work.
- support for self-management of health conditions.
- making adjustments to the medical and psychological impact of a disability.
- case management, referral, and service co-ordination.
- psychosocial interventions.
- career counseling, job analysis, job development, and placement services.
- functional and work capacity evaluations.

Vocational rehabilitation practitioners are often governed by standards of practice. In the United Kingdom these are produced by the Vocational Rehabilitation Association.

Kinaesthetics

Kinaesthetics is the study of body motion, and of the perception (both conscious and unconscious) of one's own body motions. The perception of continuous movement (kinesthesia) is largely unconscious. A conscious proprioception is achieved through increased awareness. Kinaesthetics involves the teaching and personal development of such awareness.

Therapeutic Applications

Occupational therapy and physical therapy based on movement-associated awareness has been applied in the Western world since the mid-1980s, especially in Central European care facilities. It makes use of the psychophysiological finding that greater muscle tone reduces proprioceptive sensitivity.

Kinaesthetics may benefit patients who need:

- Assistance in activities of daily living (ADL)
- Somatic feedback
- To reduce the physical effort required to move

History

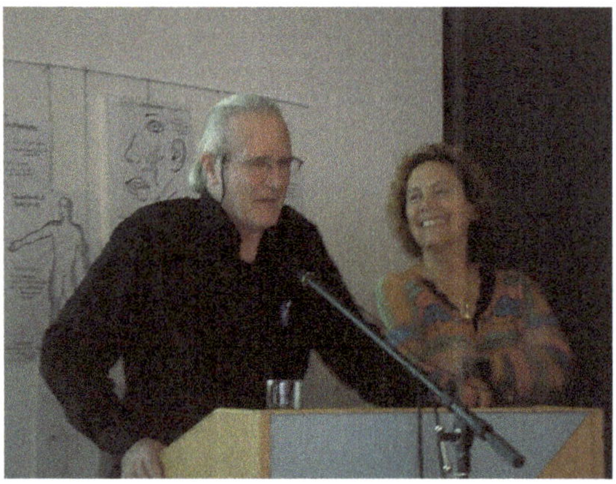

Kinaesthetics-founders Lenny Maietta and Frank Hatch (2011)

Kinaesthetics was developed in the early 1970s by Frank White Hatch, who was a choreographer and dancer. Hatch studied behavioral cybernetics at Madison/Wisconsin and developed academic programs for movement and dance called *Kinaesthetics* in three American universities. He then turned to working with disabled children as well as the field of rehabilitation. Psychologist Lenny Maietta developed a handling-training program for young parents that was also based on behavioral cybernetics. Hatch & Maietta taught and worked together in German-speaking countries beginning in 1974. With the dancer John Graham, they held workshops under the name of Gentle Dance.

Maietta & Hatch used Kinaesthetics-seminars the first time as therapy in the Ernest-Holmes Fachklinik in Germany 1974-77. Together with registered nurse Suzanne Bernard Schmidt, Maietta & Hatch developed a job-specific program "Kinaesthetics in Nursing." They were in dialogue and exchange with Gregory Bateson, Moshe Feldenkrais, Berta and Karel Bobath, Liliane Juchli, and Nancy Roper. In addition to behavioral cybernetics and dance, movement therapy and humanistic psychology were named as key sources of kinaesthetics.

Maietta & Hatch are still actively involved in the development of Kinaesthetics. In the last years, programs for caregivers, for workplace health and for older people especially were developed. Currently there are four organizations in which Kinaesthetics-programs are developed.

Literature

- Asmussen, M. (2010) (in German), *Praxisbuch Kinaesthetics. Erfahrungen zur individuellen Bewegungsunterstützung auf Basis der Kinästhetik* (2. ed.), München: Elsevier, ISBN 978-3-437-27570-8
- Bauder-Mißbach, H.; Eisenschink A. M.; Kirchner, E. (2009) (in German), *Kinästhetische Mobilisation. Wie Pflegekräfte die Genesung unterstützen können - eine Studie am Universitätsklinikum Ulm*, Hannover: Schlütersche, ISBN 3-87706-736-0
- Brandt, I., ed. (2008) (in German), *Pflegetechniken heute. Pflegehandeln Schritt für Schritt verstehen, S. 232-247* (2., vollst. überarb. ed.), München: Urban & Fischer, ISBN 978-3-437-27091-8
- Citron, I. (2004) (in German), *Kinästhetik - Kommunikatives Bewegungslernen*, Stuttgart: Thieme, ISBN 3-13-111862-8
- Hatch, F.; Maietta, L.; Schmidt, S. (1992) (in German), *Kinästhetik. Interaktion durch Berührung und Bewegung in der Pflege* (4., überarb. ed.), Eschborn: DBfK Verlag, ISBN 978-3927944022
- Hatch, F.; Maietta, L. (2003) (in German), *Kinästhetik. Gesundheitsentwicklung und menschliche Funktionen* (2. ed.), München: Urban & Fischer bei Elsevier, ISBN 3-437-26840-6
- Hatch, F.; Maietta, L. (2011) (in German), *Kinaesthetics. Infant Handling* (2., durchges. ed.), Bern: Huber, ISBN 978-3-456-84987-4

Films

- Asmussen-Clausen, M. / Knobel, S. (2006): *Fortbewegen statt heben - Kinästhetik in der Pflegepraxis* (DVD)
- Asmussen-Clausen, M. / Buschmann, U. (2004): *Kinästhetik Infant Handling - Bewegungsunterstützung in den ersten Lebensjahren* (DVD)
- Bauder-Mißbach, H. (2008): “Grundlagen der Bewegungsförderung “ (DVD)
- Marty-Teuber, M. (2000): *Ermöglichen statt Behindern - Kinaesthetics ein Lern- und Interaktionsmodell* (DVD)

Cognitive Rehabilitation Therapy

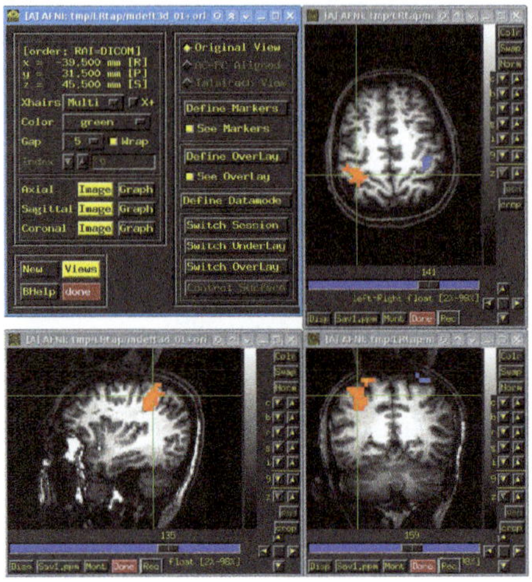

Effects of cognitive rehabilitation therapy, assessed using fMRI.

Cognitive rehabilitation is a program to help brain-injured or otherwise cognitively impaired individuals to restore normal functioning, or to compensate for cognitive deficits. It entails an individualized program of specific skills training and practice plus metacognitive strategies. Metacognitive strategies include helping the patient increase self-awareness regarding problem-solving skills by learning how to monitor the effectiveness of these skills and self-correct when necessary.

Cognitive rehabilitation therapy (offered by a trained therapist) is a subset of Cognitive Rehabilitation (community-based rehabilitation, often in traumatic brain injury; provided by rehabilitation professionals) and has been shown to be effective for individuals who suffered a stroke in the left or right hemisphere. or brain trauma. A computer-assisted type of cognitive rehabilitation therapy called cognitive remediation therapy has been used to treat schizophrenia, ADHD, and major depressive disorder.

Cognitive rehabilitation, in its narrow training of the client sense, builds upon brain injury strategies involving memory and in the community, Executive functions, activities planning and "follow through" (e.g., memory, task sequencing, lists).

It may also be recommended for traumatic brain injury, the primary population for which it was developed in the university medical and rehabiltation communities, such as that suffered by U.S. Representative Gabrielle Giffords, according to Dr. Gregory J. O'Shanick of the Brain Injury Association of America. Her new doctor has confirmed that it will be part of her rehabilitation. Cognitive rehabilitation may be part of a comprehensive community services program and integrated into residential services, such as supported living, supported employment, family support, professional education, home health (as personal assistance), recreation, or education programs in the community.

Assessments

According to the standard text by Sohlberg and Mateer:

Individuals and families respond differently to different interventions, in different ways, at different times after injury. Premorbid functioning, personality, social support, and environmental demands are but a few of the factors that can profoundly influence outcome. In this variable response to treatment, cognitive rehabilitation is no different from treatment for cancer, diabetes, heart disease, Parkinson's disease, spinal cord injury, psychiatric disorders, or any other injury or disease process for which variable response to different treatments is the norm.

Nevertheless, many different statistical analyses of the benefits of this therapy have been carried out. One study made in 2002 analyzed 47 treatment comparisons and reported "a differential benefit in favor of cognitive rehabilitation in 37 of 47 (78.7%) comparisons, with no comparison demonstrating a benefit in favor of the alternative treatment condition."

An internal study conducted by the Tricare Management Agency in 2009 is cited by the US Department of Defense as its reason for refusing to pay for this therapy for veterans who have suffered traumatic brain injury. According to Tricare, "There is insufficient, evidence-based research available to conclude that cognitive rehabilitation therapy is beneficial in treating traumatic brain injury." The ECRI Institute, whose report serves as the basis for this decision by the Department of Defense, has summed up their own findings this way:

In our report, we carried out several meta-analyses using data from 18 randomized controlled trials. Based on data from these studies, we were able to conclude the following:

- Adults with moderate to severe traumatic brain injury who receive social skills training perform significantly better on measures of social communication than patients who receive no treatment.
- Adults with traumatic brain injury who receive comprehensive cognitive rehabilitation therapy report significant improvement on measures of quality of life compared to patients who receive a less intense form of therapy.

The strength of the evidence supporting our conclusions was low due to the small number of studies that addressed the outcomes of interest. Further, the evidence was too weak to draw any definitive conclusions about the effectiveness of cognitive rehabilitation therapy for treating deficits related to the following cognitive areas: attention, memory, visuospacial skills, and executive function. The following factors contributed to the weakness of the evidence: differences in the outcomes assessed in the studies, differences in the types of cognitive rehabilitation therapy methods/strategies employed across studies, differences in the control conditions, and/or insufficient number of studies addressing an outcome.

Citing this 2009 assessment, US Department of Defense, one of the federal agencies not responsible for health care decisions in the US, has declared that cognitive rehabilitation therapy is scientifically unproved and should refer their concerns to the US Department of Health and Human Services, US Budget and Management, and/or the Government Accountability Office (GAO). As a result, it refuses to cover the cost of cognitive rehabilitation for brain-injured veterans. Cost-benefit and cost-effectiveness studies, together with an analysis of personnel and veterans' services for new our emerging groups in head and brain injuries, are recommended.

Barthel Scale

The Barthel scale or Barthel ADL index is an ordinal scale used to measure performance in activities of daily living (ADL). Each performance item is rated on this scale with a given number of points assigned to each level or ranking. It uses ten variables describing ADL and mobility. A higher number is associated with a greater likelihood of being able to live at home with a degree of independence following discharge from hospital. The amount of time and physical assistance required to perform each item are used in determining the assigned value of each item. External factors within the environment affect the score of each item. If adaptations outside the standard home environment are met during assessment, the participant's score will be lower if these conditions are not available. If adaptations to the environment are made, they should be described in detail and attached to the Barthel index.

The scale was introduced in 1965, and yielded a score of 0–20. Although this original version is still widely used, it was modified by Granger *et al.* in 1979, when it came to include 0–10 points for every variable, and further refinements were introduced in 1989. The modified Barthel index was designed as the original scale was insensitive to change and had arbitrary scores. The sensitized version sharply discriminates between good and better and poor and poorer performances. Its effectiveness is not just with in-patient rehabilitation but home care, nursing care, skilled nursing, and community. The Barthel index signifies one of the first contributions to the functional status literature and it represents occupational therapists' lengthy period of inclusion of functional mobility and ADL measurement within their scope of practice. The scale is regarded as reliable, although its use in clinical trials in stroke medicine is inconsistent. It has however, been used extensively to monitor functional changes in individuals receiving in-patient rehabilitation, mainly in predicting the functional outcomes related to stroke. The Barthel index has been shown to have portability and has been used in 16 major diagnostic conditions. The Barthel index has demonstrated high inter-rater reliability (0.95) and test–retest reliability (0.89) as well as high correlations (0.74–0.8) with other measures of physical disability.

Copyright Information: The Maryland State Medical Society holds the copyright for the Barthel Index. It may be used freely for noncommercial purposes with the following citation: Mahoney FI, Barthel D. "Functional evaluation: the Barthel Index." Maryland State Med Journal 1965;14:56-61. Used with permission. Permission is required to modify the Barthel Index or to use it for commercial purposes.

The ten variables addressed in the Barthel scale are:

- presence or absence of fecal incontinence
- presence or absence of urinary incontinence
- help needed with grooming
- help needed with toilet use
- help needed with feeding
- help needed with transfers (e.g. from chair to bed)
- help needed with walking
- help needed with dressing
- help needed with climbing stairs
- and help needed with bathing

Bobath Concept

The Bobath concept is an approach to neurological rehabilitation that is applied in patient assessment and treatment (such as with adults after stroke, or children with cerebral palsy). The goal of applying the Bobath concept is to promote motor learning for efficient motor control in various environments, thereby improving participation and function. This is done through specific patient handling skills to guide patients through initiation and completion of intended tasks. This approach to neurological rehabilitation is multidisciplinary, primarily involving physiotherapists, but may also include occupational therapists and speech and language therapists. In the United States, the Bobath concept is also known as 'neuro-developmental treatment' (NDT).

The concept and its international tutors / instructors, have embraced neuroscience and the developments in understanding motor control, motor learning, neuroplasticity and human movement science. They believe that this approach continues to develop.

Recent Criticism of the Bobath Approach

The concept that Bobath can "evolve" and still be called Bobath has been challenged by the president of the American Academy of Cerebral Palsy and Developmental

Medicine and the chair of the UK Association of Chartered Physiotherapists in Neurology (ACPIN). These eminent physiotherapists believe that several of the key original teachings of the founders have now been abandoned, whilst the ideas / concepts of others (non Bobath therapists & scientists) have unjustifiably been given the name of Bobath.

There is widespread use of the Bobath concept amongst therapists in stroke rehabilitation. Yet, a large review of randomized controlled trials (RCTs) of Bobath for stroke rehabilitation found only three instances of significant differences in favour of Bobath, yet 11 in favour of alternatives. The authors concluded:- "evidence-based guidelines, accepted rules of motor learning, and biological mechanisms of functional recovery, rather than therapist preference for any named therapy approach should serve as a framework from which therapists should derive the most effective treatment". This review pointed out that the approach is now regarded as "obsolete" in some European countries and it is therefore no longer taught.

National evidence based guidelines for stroke rehabilitation have been published for England, Netherlands, USA, Canada, Australia and New Zealand; yet in none of these is the Bobath approach recommended. However, in 2016 the American Stroke Association concluded that although the effectiveness of NDT/Bobath (compared with other treatment approaches) had not been established that it still "may be considered" as a treatment option for mobility. This however was their lowest classification of an acceptable treatment. Their two highest recommendation groups ("should be performed" and "reasonable to perform") contained a variety of treatments for which there was much better evidence. NDT/Bobath was not listed as an option for arm/hand rehabilitation.

In the UK, an NHS review of stroke rehabilitation by Professor Tyson concluded that "the strength of evidence that task specific functional training and strength training are effective, whilst Bobath is not, indicates that a paradigm shift is needed in UK stroke physiotherapy..... it is increasingly difficult to justify the continued use of the Bobath concept or its associated techniques".

The Bobath (NDT) approach is also widely used on children with cerebral palsy (CP). However, when the effectiveness of interventions for the treatment of CP was reviewed by Novak et al. they concluded "Consequently, there are no circumstances where any of the aims of NDT could not be achieved by a more effective treatment. Thus, on the grounds of wanting to do the best for children with CP, it is hard to rationalize a continued place for traditional NDT within clinical care". They consequently recommended "ceasing provision of the ever-popular NDT".

The dichotomy between the popularity and institutional funding of this approach versus the negative findings of most RCTs has been excused on the grounds that RCTs may not be suitable for neurorehabilitation. Yet, the British Bobath Tutors Association website does quote the minority of RCTs that support their approach.

More recently Professor Tyson has written a comprehensive and critical review of Bobath/NDT methods, theory and effectiveness.

History

The Bobath concept is named after its inventors: Berta Bobath (physiotherapist) and Karel Bobath (a psychiatrist/neurophysiologist). Their work focused mainly on patients with cerebral palsy and stroke. The main problems of these patient groups resulted in a loss of the normal postural reflex mechanism and normal movements. At its earliest inception, the Bobath concept was focused on regaining normal movements through re-education. Since then, it has evolved to incorporate new information on neuroplasticity, motor learning and motor control. Therapists that practice the Bobath concept today also embrace the goal of developing optimal movement patterns through the use of orthotics and appropriate compensations, instead of aiming for completely "normal" movement patterns.

Application in Stroke Rehabilitation

In the Bobath Concept, postural control is the foundation on which patients begin to develop their skills. Patients undergoing this treatment typically learn how to control postures and movements and then progress to more difficult ones. Therapists analyze postures and movements and look for any abnormalities that may be present when asked to perform them. Examples of common abnormal movement patterns include obligatory synergy patterns. These patterns can be described as the process of trying to perform isolated movement of a particular limb, but triggering the use of other typically uninvolved muscles (when compared to normal movement) in order to achieve movement. Obligatory synergy patterns can be further subdivided into flexion and extension synergy components for both the upper and lower extremities. This approach requires active participation from both the patient and the therapist. Depending on the patient, rehabilitation goals may work to improve any or all of the following: postural control, coordination of movement sequences, movement initiation, optimal body alignment, abnormal tone or muscle weakness. Treatment will therefore address both negative signs such as impaired postural control, and positive signs such as spasticity.

Intervention strategies and techniques for Bobath consist of therapeutic handling, facilitation, and activation of key points of control. Therapeutic handling is used in order to influence the quality of the patients' movements and incorporates both facilitation and inhibition. Facilitation is a key technique used by Bobath practitioners to promote motor learning. It is the use of sensory information (tactile cue through manual contacts, verbal directions) to reinforce weak movement patterns and to discourage overactive ones. The appropriate provision of facilitation during the motor task is regulated in time, modality, intensity and withdrawal, all of which affects the outcome of motor learning. Inhibition can be described as reducing parts of movement/posture that are abnormal and interfere with normal performance. Key points of control generally refers to parts of the body that are advantageous when facilitating or inhibiting movement/posture.

Activities assigned by a Physical Therapist or Occupational Therapist to an individual who has suffered from a stroke are selected based on functional relevance and are varied in terms of difficulty and the environment in which they are performed. The use of the individual's less involved segments, also known as compensatory training strategies, are avoided. Carryover of functional activities in the home and community setting is largely attributed to patient, family and caregiver education.

The Bobath Concepts theoretical underpinning and practice is clearly documented in a contemporary book published by Wiley Blackman in 2009: *Bobath Concept: Theory and Clinical Practice in Neurological Rehabilitation' written by the British Bobath Tutors Association (BBTA) and edited by Raine, Meadows and Lynch-Ellerington.* The chair of ACPIN (Association of Chartered Physiotherapists in Neurology) reviewed this book and concluded :- "I am not really sure that it is clear from the book what the Bobath approach actually is", "often the prose turns into jargon" and "this book will do little to quell the critics; in fact it will no doubt give them more fuel for the fire".

Research

Paci (2003) conducted an extensive critical appraisal of studies to determine the effectiveness of the Bobath concept for adults with hemiplegia following a stroke. Although selected trials showed no evidence proving the effectiveness of the Bobath Concept as the optimal type of treatment, neither did they show evidence of non-efficacy because of methodological limitations. Paci (2003) recommended that standardized guidelines for treatment be identified and described, and that further investigations are necessary to develop outcome measures concerning goals of the Bobath approach such as quality of motor performance.

Bobath therapy is nonstandardized as it responds, through clinical reasoning and the development of a clinical hypothesis, to the individual patient and their movement control problems. The decisions about specific treatment techniques are collaboratively made with the patient, and are guided by the therapist, through the use of goal setting and the development of close communication and interaction. Working to develop improved muscle tone, appropriate to the task, the individual and the environment, will enable better alignment and activation of movement, and allow for recruitment of, for example, arm activity in functional situations within various positions.

A study by Lennon et al. concluded that even under idealized conditions (patients with optimal rehabilitation potential, advanced trained therapists, unlimited therapy input and a movement analysis laboratory) the Bobath approach had no effect on the quality of gait for patients with a stroke.

References

- Sunbeck, Deborah (1996). Infinity Walk: Preparing your mind to learn!. Torrance, California: Jalmar Press. ISBN 1-880396-31-9.

- Sunbeck, Deborah (2002). The Complete Infinity Walk, Book 1: The Physical Self. The Leonardo Foundation Press. ISBN 0-9705164-6-0.
- Gundle KR. Rearticulations of Orthopaedic Surgery: The Process of Specialty Boundary Formation and the Provision of Fracture Care in the United States. Lulu: 2014. ISBN 1312540451.
- Gundle KR. "Rearticulations of Orthopaedic Surgery: The Process of Specialty Boundary Formation and the Provision of Fracture Care in the United States", Lulu: 2014. ISBN 1312540451.
- Becker, BE and Cole, AJ (eds). 2011. Comprehensive aquatic therapy, 3rd edition. Washington State University Press. ISBN 978-0615365671.
- Koury JM. 1996. Aquatic therapy programming: guidelines for orthopedic rehabilitation. Human Kinetics. ISBN 0-87322-971-1.
- Becker, BE. 2011. Biophysical aspects of hydrotherapy. pp 23-75. Chapter 2 In Becker, BE and Cole, AJ (eds). Comprehensive aquatic therapy, 3rd edition. Washington State University Press. ISBN 978-0615365671.
- Audette JF and Bailey A. 2008. Integrative pain medicine: the science and practice of complementary and alternative medicine in pain management. Humana Press. ISBN 978-1588297860.
- Wilder, RP and Brennan DK. 2011. Aqua running. pp 155-170, Chapter 6 In: Becker BE and Cole AJ (eds). Comprehensive aquatic therapy, 3rd edition. Washington State University Press. ISBN 978-0615365671.
- Dutton M. 2011. Orthopaedics for the physical therapist assistant. Jones & Bartlett Learning. ISBN 978-0763797553.
- Ainslie T. 2012. The concise guide to physiotherapy - 2-volume set: Assessment and Treatment. pp 1096-1106, Bad Ragaz Ring Method. Elsevier Health Sciences. ISBN 9780702053030.
- Gamper U and Lambeck J. 2011. The Bad Ragaz Ring Method. pp 109-136, Chapter 4 In: Becker BE and Cole AJ (eds). Comprehensive aquatic therapy, 3rd edition. Washington State University Press. ISBN 978-0615365671.

5

Rehabilitation Team: An Integrated Study

Audiology is a branch of science; it studies balance and also studies hearing. Those who practice audiology treat patients and prevent further damage related to hearing. Nursing, occupational therapist, orthotics, prosthetist and speech-language pathology are some of the topics discussed in the following chapter.

Athletic Training

Athletic Training has been recognized by the American Medical Association (AMA) as an allied health care profession since June 1991.

"Athletic training is practiced by athletic trainers, health care professionals who collaborate with physicians to optimize activity and participation of patients and clients. Athletic training encompasses the prevention, diagnosis, and intervention of emergency, acute and chronic medical conditions involving impairment, functional limitations and disabilities."

There are five domains of athletic training listed in the 7th edition (2015) of the Athletic Training Practice Analysis:

- Injury and Illness Prevention and Wellness Promotion
- Examination, Assessment and Diagnosis
- Immediate and Emergency Care
- Therapeutic Intervention
- Healthcare Administration and Professional Responsibility

An athletic trainer functions as an integral member of the health care team in clinics, secondary schools, colleges and universities, professional sports programs, and other athletic health care settings.

History

Athletic training in the United States began in October 1881 when Harvard University hired James Robinson to work conditioning their football team. At the time, the term "athletic trainer" meant one who worked with track and field athletes. Robinson had worked with track and field athletes and the name "athletic trainer" transferred to those working on conditioning these football players and later other athletes. Athletic trainers began to treat and rehabilitate injuries in order to keep the athletes participating. The first major text on athletic training and the care of athletic injuries was called Athletic Training (later changed to The Trainer's Bible) written in 1917 by Samuel E. Bilik. Early athletic trainers had "no technical knowledge, their athletic training techniques usually consisted of a rub, the application of some type of counterirritant, and occasionally the prescription of various home remedies and poultices". In 1918, Chuck Cramer started the Cramer Chemical Company (now Cramer Products) that produced a line of products used by athletic trainers and began publishing a newsletter in 1932 entitled The First Aider.

An organization named the National Athletic Trainers' Association (NATA) was founded in 1938 and folded in 1944. Another NATA was founded in 1950 and still exists. The first athletic training curriculum approved by NATA was in 1959 and the amount of athletic training programs began to grow throughout colleges and universities in the United States. In the early development of the major, athletic training was geared more towards prepping the student for teaching at the secondary level, emphasizing on health and physical education. This program was first introduced at an undergraduate level in 1969 to the schools of Mankato State University, Indiana State University, Lamar University, and the University of New Mexico.

Through the years athletic training has evolved to be defined as "health care professionals who specialize in preventing, recognizing, managing, and rehabilitating injures". During the 1970s the NATA Professional Education Committee formed a list of objectives to define athletic training as a major course of study and to eliminate it as a secondary-level teaching credential. By June 1982, there were nine NATA-approved graduate athletic training education programs. On July 1, 1986, this work was used to implement athletic training as a major course of study in at least 10 colleges and universities, and to only start the development of the major in a handful of others.

Once athletic training was recognized as an allied health profession the process of accrediting programs began. NATA's Professional Education Committee (PEC) was the first to take on this role of approving athletic training educational programs. The AMA's Committee on Allied Health Education and Accreditation (CAHEA) was given the responsibility in 1993 to develop requirements for the programs of entry-level athletic trainers. At this time all programs had to go through the CAHEA accreditation process. A year later CAHEA was broken up and replaced with the Commission on Accreditation of Allied Health Education Programs (CAAHEP), which then lead the accreditation process. In 2003 JRC-AT, Joint Review Committee on Athletic Training completely took over the process and became an independent accrediting agency like all other allied health professions had. Three years later JRC-AT officially became the Committee for Accreditation of Athletic Training Education (CAATE), which is fully in charge of accrediting athletic training programs in the United States. NATA produced the NATABOC in 1969 in order to implement a certification process for the profession for an entry-level athletic trainer. In 1989, became an independent non-profit corporation and soon later changed its name to the Board of Certification (BOC).

Roles and Responsibilities

Scope

The Board of Certification serves as the national certifying body for athletic trainers, and its Standards of Professional Practice outline the roles and responsibilities of certified athletic trainers. Such practice standards include practice expectations such as, "The Athletic Trainer renders service or treatment under the direction of a physician." Regardless of the setting, limitations and restrictions on what an athletic trainer can do and who can be treated are in large part determined by the regulatory statutes governing professional practice in individual states.

Referring

"In certain situations, an individual may require treatment from or consultation with a variety of both medical and nonmedical services and personnel other than the athletic trainer." It is the athletic trainer's responsibility to understand the limits of their scope of practice and recognize situations where a referral is necessary. "A number of support health services may be used including school health services, nurses, physicians, dentists, podiatrists, physician's assistants, physical therapists, strength and conditioning specialists, biomechanists, exercise physiologists, nutritionists, psychologists, massage therapists, occupational therapists, emergency medical technicians, paramedics, chiropractors, orthopedists, prosthesis, equipment personnel, referees, or social workers."

NATA Code of Ethics

"The National Athletic Trainers' Association Code of Ethics states the principles of ethical behavior that should be followed in the practice of athletic training. It is intended to establish and maintain high standards and professionalism for the athletic training profession."

Employment Settings

- Clinic
- Hospital
- Industrial/Occupational
- Corporate
- College/University

- Two-year Institution
- Secondary School
- Professional Sports
- Amateur/recreation/youth sports
- Performing Arts
- Military/Law Enforcement/Government
- Health/fitness/sports/performance enhancement clinics/clubs
- Independent Contractor

Education

Undergraduate Course Descriptions

All courses may have prerequisites to be completed before taking further coursework. Also, those prerequisites and content of the courses will vary upon the institute and professor. The courses listed below are commonly taken to increase knowledge regarding athletic training.

- Human Physiology- This course is designed to provide students with an understanding of the function and regulation of the human body and physiological integration of the organ systems to maintain homeostasis
- Human Anatomy- The anatomical structures of the body will be studied in this course. Including the muscular systems, organs, respiratory, bony anatomy, veins and arteries. This course will help you to learn all components of the body and is almost always accompanied with a lab section to reinforce the lectures.
- Exercise Physiology- This course investigates the acute responses and chronic adaptations of physiological functions to a wide range of physical exercise conditions, involving people of all ages and abilities.
- Kinesiology- Structural and applied musculoskeletal anatomy relative to human movement and sports skill. This course concentrates on muscles, their origins, insertions, and actions.
- Nutrition- This course emphasizes basic nutritional principles and concepts, their application to personal health and relationship between food and its use by the human body for energy, regulation, structure, and optimal health. Discussion of issues in nutrition during various stages of the life cycle and specific chronic diseases will be addressed.
- Therapeutic Modalities- This is a course looks into the background for clinical

application of therapeutic modalities in athletic training. Students will comprehend the underlying theories, physiological effects, indications, and contraindications of various therapeutic modalities utilized in the treatment of orthopedic injuries.

- Acute Care of Injury and Illness- This course focuses on the emergency management techniques that are commonly implemented when dealing with trauma and illnesses suffered during/through sport participation. Included will be field evaluation of medical emergencies, such as cessation of breathing or circulation, shock, concussion, and spinal injury to the athlete. Students will review policies and position statements issued by the NATA, NCAA, ACSM, AAP, and AMA regarding prevention, evaluation, and management of acute athletic injuries and illnesses.
- Physical Examination of the Lower Extremities- Intense in-depth study of the lower extremities including physical examinations, injury recognition, treatment, taping, bracing, and care. Laboratory experiences emphasize the methods and techniques in evaluating lower extremity injuries/conditions.

Undergraduate Athletic Training Programs

The Commission on Accreditation of Athletic Training Education (CAATE) website provides a list of all the accredited programs in the United States. It provides you with the name of the college, who to contact, and a link to the institution's website. An Undergraduate Athletic Training degree can only be received at an accredited school for athletic training.

Entry-level Masters Programs

Although the majority of athletic trainers receive a bachelor's degree in athletic training before taking the Board of Certification Exam (BOC), it is not the only way to receive an education in athletic training. An entry-level masters program is a two-year program that covers the same material as an undergraduate athletic training degree. Common prerequisite classes are human anatomy, human physiology, kinesiology, biomechanics, exercise physiology, nutrition, and personal health along with a certain number of observation hours completed under the supervision of a certified athletic trainer (ATC). Prerequisites can vary by institution so be sure to research the prerequisites for your institutions of interest. There are 26 accredited entry level masters programs in the U.S.A.

Graduate School in Athletic Training and Related Fields

There are approximately 15 accredited athletic training masters programs. These programs consist of students who are already certified athletic trainers that want to advance their academic and clinical experience. These are two-year programs which culminate with a Master of Science degree (M.S.) in athletic training. Graduate programs in athletic training are not always specifically in athletic training, but in a related field. Some of these fields may include, but are not limited to, kinesiology, biomechanics, sports management, sport and exercise psychology, exercise physiology, health promotion, etc. These programs are also two years in length. While enrolled in one of these programs, the athletic trainer may gain clinical experience and receive a stipend through a make some money by obtaining a graduate assistantship.

Link to Schools

- Entry Level Masters Programs in the U.S.A.
- Post-professional Programs in Athletic Training

Graduate Assistant Position

A graduate assistant athletic trainer position is a position in which a graduate athletic training student is able to work as an assistant athletic trainer while taking graduate courses. Graduate assistant athletic trainers are responsible for providing the medical coverage of select teams at the institution where they are working. Responsibilities may vary, but include administering daily medical coverage for selected intercollegiate athletic teams (practice/event); traveling with the assigned team, evaluation and documentation of athletic injuries, administrative responsibilities, serve as Approved Clinical Instructor (ACI) or Clinical Instructor (CI) in a CAATE – accredited ATEP, and other duties as assigned by the head athletic trainer. Other responsibilities may include working at a high school, clinic, teaching, or doing research. Graduate assistant positions are generally about 10-month appointments that are renewable after the first year, and may include additional summer work. Visit the National Athletic Trainers' Association Career Center for job postings.

Accredited Programs

Athletic Training programs are evaluated by CAATE to ensure that they follow the standards for Entry-Level Athletic Training Programs. Evaluations may take place every three to seven years depending on the results of the last visit. Successfully completing the CAATE accredited education program is a part of the criteria that determines a candidate's eligibility for the Board of Certification (BOC) examination.

Organizations

"The National Athletic Trainers' Association (NATA) is the professional membership association for certified athletic trainers and others who support the athletic training profession. Founded in 1950, the NATA has grown to more than 35,000 members worldwide today. The majority of certified athletic trainers choose to be members of the NATA – to support their profession, and to receive a broad array of membership benefits. By joining forces as a group, NATA members can accomplish more for the athletic training profession than they can individually".

Before the formation of NATA, athletic trainers occupied a somewhat insecure place in the athletic program. Since that time, as a direct result of the standards and ethics established by NATA, there has been considerable professional advancement. Every year NATA works on behalf of all athletic trainers to enhance health care for both athletic trainers and those who receive care.

NATA is the professional organization for Athletic trainers across the nation. Each region of the USA has their own district under NATA but within their area, they have their own agendas and board members. Each district also has a director that serves on the NATA Board of Directors.

There are 10 districts.

Every state has their own state athletic training association that acts similar to the district associations as they have their own board members. The state associations answer to the district associations and the National Athletic Trainers' Association. Links to the state associations can be found through the regional websites.

Current Topics

Due to the physicality of athletics and the campaign for healthy well-being, there are issues that become hot topics in the media. Athletic trainers have to continually be aware of changes in laws, position statements of the National Athletic Trainers Association, and institutional policies.

Current hot topics and topics to keep an eye on include:

- NATA Press Room
- Concussion laws, position statements, and policies.
- Youth Sports Legislation
- Guidelines in Prevention of Chronic Overuse Injury in Pediatric Patients
- Athletic Trainers as Physician Extenders
- Education on Public Safety in the Workplace
- Certified Athletic Trainer as a partner in the Athletic Department

Audiology

Audiology is a branch of science that studies hearing, balance, and related disorders. Its practitioners, who treat those with hearing loss and proactively prevent related damage are audiologists. Employing various testing strategies (e.g. hearing tests, otoacoustic emission measurements, videonystagmography, and electrophysiologic tests), audiology aims to determine whether someone can hear within the normal range, and if not, which portions of hearing (high, middle, or low frequencies) are affected and to what degree. If an audiologist determines that a hearing loss or vestibular abnormality is present he or she will provide recommendations to a patient as to what options (e.g. hearing aid, cochlear implants, appropriate medical referrals) may be of assistance.

In addition to testing hearing, audiologists can also work with a wide range of clientele in rehabilitation (individuals with tinnitus, auditory processing disorders, cochlear implant users and/or hearing aid users), from pediatric populations to veterans and may perform assessment of tinnitus and the vestibular system.

Audiologist

An audiologist is a health-care professional specializing in identifying, diagnosing, treating and monitoring disorders of the auditory and vestibular system portions of the ear. Audiologists are trained to diagnose, manage and/or treat hearing, tinnitus, or balance problems. They dispense, manage, and rehabilitate hearing aids and assess candidacy for and map cochlear implants. They counsel families through a new diagnosis of hearing loss in infants, and help teach coping and compensation skills to late-deafened adults. They also help design and implement personal and industrial hearing safety programs, newborn hearing screening programs, school hearing screening programs, and provide special fitting ear plugs and other hearing protection devices to help prevent hearing loss. Audiologists are trained to evaluate peripheral vestibular disorders originating from inner ear pathologies. They also provide treatment for certain vestibular and balance disorders such as Benign Paroxysmal Positional Vertigo (BPPV). In addition, many audiologists work as auditory scientists in a research capacity.

Audiologists have training in anatomy and physiology, hearing aids, cochlear implants, electrophysiology, acoustics, psychophysics, neurology, vestibular function and assessment, balance disorders, counseling and sign language. Audiologists also run neonatal hearing screening programme which has been made compulsory in many hospitals in US, UK and India. An Audiologist usually graduates with one of the following qualifications: MSc(Audiology), Au.D., STI, PhD, or ScD, depending the program and country attended.

History

The use of the terms "Audiology" and "Audiologist" in publications has been traced back only as far as 1946. The original creator of the term remains unknown, but Berger identified possible originators as Mayer BA Schier, Willard B Hargrave, Stanley Nowak,

Norman Canfield, or Raymond Carhart. In a biographical profile by Robert Galambos, Hallowell Davis is credited with coining the term in the 1940s, saying the then-prevalent term "auricular training" sounded like a method of teaching people how to wiggle their ears.

The first US university course for audiologists was offered by Carhart at Northwestern University, in 1946. Audiology was born of hearing aid dispensers to address the hearing damage from World War II veterans.

Requirements

Australia

In Australia Audiologists must hold a Masters in Audiology, Masters of Clinical Audiology or Masters of Audiology Studies or alternatively bachelor's degree from overseas certified by the VETASSESS. Audiologists in Australia are not required to be a member of any professional body. But to dispense hearing aids to eligible pensioners and eligible war veterans one must have two years clinical experience and be registered with an approved body such as Audiology Australia (AudA) or the Australian College of Audiology (ACAud). In Australia, by general definition an 'Audiologist' - is a University graduate with postgraduate qualifications in Audiology or equivalent training. Audiologists have broad responsibilities and expertise in all non-medical areas of hearing services including complex hearing assessment and rehabilitation of hearing impairment (which includes hearing aid prescription, fitting and management). An 'Audiometrist' - has completed a TAFE Certificate Course in hearing aid audiometry and/or received in-house training from the hearing aid industry.

Audiology Australia via The Code of Ethics and the Practice Standards, governs the professional practice of audiology for members of Audiology Australia. To meet these high standards Members undertake professional development to enable them to maintain appropriate skills and learning in their areas of professional practice. The purpose of the Continuing Professional Development (CPD) program is to provide a structure that enables members to formally document the ways in which they manage and extend their professional skills and knowledge. The Audiology Australia CPD program provides recognition and encouragement for the continuing participation of the members in high quality professional development. The CPD program enable members to demonstrate to external stakeholders (clients, employers, government, the community and other professional groups) their commitment to the highest standards of professional competence for Audiologists. The CPD program is focused on maintaining a high quality practice of audiology and is tied to the Certificate of Clinical Practice (CCP). Audiology Australia members who are not engaged in clinical practice are not required to formally document their CPD and will not be issued with a Certificate of Clinical Practice. ACAud Members are required to demonstrate their professional competence and are assessed against ACAud's Professional Competency Standards. Recognised

Competencies are shown on a Member's Certificate of Competency that is prominently displayed in the Member's clinic and renewed annually.

There are six Universities in Australia that offer graduate programs (via course work and/or research degrees) in Audiology for local and overseas students. All programs offered are recognised as eligible for membership of the Society - Audiology Australia and the International Society of Audiology (ISA).

- University of Western Australia
- University of Melbourne
- Flinders University
- La Trobe University
- Macquarie University
- University of Queensland

Canada

In Canada, a Masters of Science (M.Sc.) is the minimum requirement to practice Audiology in the country. The profession is regulated in certain provinces: New Brunswick, Quebec, Ontario, Manitoba, Saskatchewan, Alberta and British Columbia, where it is illegal to practice without being registered as a full member in the appropriate provincial regulatory body.

There are currently five universities in Canada which offer graduate programs in Audiology. Entry requirements typically include specific prerequisite course work in undergraduate studies (usually in phonetics, phonology, acoustics, developmental psychology, perception, anatomy, statistics, physics and research methods) or an additional preparatory year prior to entry into the program and a competitive GPA in the bachelor's degree. The following universities offer the MSc in audiology:

- University of British Columbia (BC)
- Université de Montréal (QC) - French instruction
- University of Western Ontario (ON)
- University of Ottawa (ON) - French instruction
- Dalhousie University (NS)

India

The Government of India established the All India Institute of Speech and Hearing, which has become the country's leading Institute in the field of communication disorders since 1966. The second Audiology & Speech Language Therapy program was started in the same year, at T.N.Medical College and BYL Nair Ch.Hospital in Mumbai. There are currently 20 Universities in India which provide Speech Pathology and Audiology programs. These programs are accredited by Rehabilitation council of India.

To practice audiology, professionals need to have either Bachelors/Master's degree in Audiology and be registered with Rehabilitation Council of India (RCI). Indian speech and hearing association (ISHA) is a professional platform of the audiologist and speech language pathologists where annual conferences are held. The educational institutions awarding degrees need to attain recognition from RCI. Presently there are around 70 institutions which offer at least a graduate degree in the field (BASLP). Approximately 20 colleges offer higher degrees such as MASLP, M.Sc Audiology and Speech Language Pathology. Few such eminent institutions in Northern India are Guru Gobind Singh Medical College located in Faridkot of Punjab, Post Graduate Institute of Medical Education and Research, Chandigarh; Ali Yavar Jung National Institute for the Hearing Handicapped, Mumbai in western India and many more. There are nearly 1000 or more private clinics in India providing speech and hearing services.

An internationally recognized degree, unique multilingual/multicultural background, excellent communication in English has increased the global demand of Indian Audiologists considering the shortage of these graduates especially in western countries. However, in recent times, the profession has been plagued by introduction of short term diploma programs which has resulted in dilution of services particularly in hearing aid dispensing and there have been mass protests by speech and hearing fraternity to stop such courses and curb malpractices.

Malaysia

There are only 3 Malaysian educational institutions offering degrees in Audiology:

- University Kebangsaan Malaysia
- University Science Malaysia
- International Islamic University Malaysia

United Kingdom

There are currently three routes to becoming a Registered Audiologist:

- BSc in Audiology
- MSc in Audiology

- Fast track conversion Diploma for those with a BSc in other relevant science subject, available at Southampton, Manchester, UCL, London and Edinburgh
- BSc(Hons) in Clinical Physiology (Audiology) available at Glasgow Caledonian University. All applicants must be NHS employees.

There are 10 United Kingdom educational institutions offering degrees in Audiology:

- Anglia Ruskin University
- De Montfort University
- University of Manchester
- University of Leeds
- Aston University
- Queen Margaret University
- University of Southampton
- Swansea University
- Middlesex University
- University College London

United States

In the United States, audiologists are regulated by state licensure or registration in all 50 states and the District of Columbia. Starting in 2007, the Doctor of Audiology (Au.D.) became the entry-level degree for clinical practice for some states, with most states expected to follow this requirement very soon, as there are no longer any professional programs in audiology which offer the master's degree. Minimum requirements for the Au.D. degree include a minimum of 75 semester hours of post-baccalaureate study, meeting prescribed competencies, passing a national exam offered by Praxis Series of the Educational Testing Service, and practicum experience that is equivalent to a minimum of 12 months of full-time, supervised experience. Most states have continuing education renewal requirements that must be met to stay licensed. Audiologists can also earn a certificate from the American Speech-Language-Hearing Association or seek board certification through the American Board of Audiology (ABA). Currently there are over 70 Au.D. programs in the United States:

Distance Au.D. Programs:

- A.T. Still University through Arizona School of Health Sciences
- University of Florida

Residential Au.D. Programs:

- A.T. Still University through Arizona School of Health Sciences
- Arizona State University
- Auburn University (AL)
- Ball State University (IN)
- Bloomsburg University of Pennsylvania
- Central Michigan University
- East Carolina University
- East Tennessee State University
- Gallaudet University (DC)
- Idaho State University
- Illinois State University
- Indiana University
- James Madison University(VA)
- Lamar University (TX)
- Long Island Au.D. Consortium (NY)
- Louisiana State University at New Orleans
- Louisiana Tech University
- Miami University (OH)
- Missouri State University
- Montclair State University
- Northeast Ohio Au.D. Consortium
- Northeastern University
- Northern Illinois University
- Northwestern University
- Nova Southeastern University (FL)
- Ohio State University
- Ohio University
- Pacific University (OR)
- Purdue University & Indiana University School of Medicine (IN)
- Rush University (IL)
- Salus University (formerly Pennsylvania College of Optometry)
- San Diego State University/University of California, San Diego(CA)
- Syracuse University
- Texas Tech University
- CUNY Graduate Center (NY)
- Towson University (MD)
- University at Buffalo (NY)
- University of Arizona
- University of Arkansas at Little Rock & University of Arkansas for Medical Sciences Consortium
- University of Cincinnati (OH)
- University of Colorado - Boulder (CO)
- University of Connecticut
- University of Florida
- University of Illinois
- University of Iowa
- University of Kansas
- University of Louisville (KY)
- University of Maryland, College Park
- University of Massachusetts - Amherst
- University of Memphis (TN)
- University of Minnesota
- University of Nebraska-Lincoln
- University of North Carolina at Chapel Hill
- University of North Texas
- University of Northern Colorado
- University of Oklahoma
- University of Pittsburgh (PA)
- University of Puerto Rico, Medical Sciences Campus
- University of South Alabama
- University of South Dakota
- University of South Florida
- University of Southern Mississippi
- University of Tennessee
- University of Texas at Austin
- University of Texas at Dallas
- University of Utah
- University of Washington - (WA)
- University of Wisconsin–Madison
- Utah State University
- Vanderbilt University (TN)
- Washington University (MO)
- Wayne State University (MI)
- West Virginia University (WV)
- Western Michigan University
- Wichita State University (KS)

In the past, audiologists have typically held a master's degree and the appropriate healthcare license. However, in the 1990s the profession began to transition to a doctoral level as a minimal requirement. In the United States, starting in 2007, audiologists were required to receive a doctoral degree (Au.D. or Ph.D.) in audiology from an accredited university graduate or professional program before practicing. All states require licensing, and audiologists may also carry national board certification from the American Board of Audiology or a certificate of clinical competence in audiology (CCC-A) from the American Speech-Language-Hearing Association.

Audiologists are autonomous practitioners and do not need physician orders or supervision. However, many audiologists work in doctor's office and hospitals. The median salary for an audiologist in the United States is approximately $65,500 in 2008 according to the Bureau of Labor Statistics. Audiologists who earn over $98,880 (top ten percentile) per annum typically have their own private practice.

Portugal

The exercise of audiologist profession in Portugal necessarily imply the qualifications Degree in Audiology or legally equivalent as defined in Decree-Law 320/99 of August 11 Article 4.

At present, the degree in Audiology is administered in two Schools:

Health Technology School of Coimbra - Polytechnic Institute of Coimbra

School of Health Sciences - Polytechnic Institute of Porto

In Portugal, research in Audiology is still undeveloped. Most work in this area is mainly on standardization and noise. At this time students of Audiology Colleges may have relevant a role in this area as well as the professionals who attend Masters degree and Doctorates degree.

Nursing

Nursing is a profession within the health care sector focused on the care of individuals, families, and communities so they may attain, maintain, or recover optimal health and quality of life. Nurses may be differentiated from other health care providers by their approach to patient care, training, and scope of practice. Nurses practice in many specialisms with differing levels of prescriber authority. Many nurses provide care within the ordering scope of physicians, and this traditional role has shaped the public image of nurses as care providers. However, nurses are permitted by most jurisdictions to practice independently in a variety of settings depending on training level. In the postwar period, nurse education has undergone a process of diversification towards advanced and specialized credentials, and many of the traditional regulations and provider roles are changing.

Nurses develop a plan of care, working collaboratively with physicians, therapists, the patient, the patient's family and other team members, that focuses on treating illness to improve quality of life. In the U.S. (and increasingly the United Kingdom), advanced practice nurses, such as clinical nurse specialists and nurse practitioners, diagnose health problems and prescribe medications and other therapies, depending on individual state regulations. Nurses may help coordinate the patient care performed by other members of an interdisciplinary health care team such as therapists, medical practitioners and dietitians. Nurses provide care both interdependently, for example, with physicians, and independently as nursing professionals.

History

Traditional

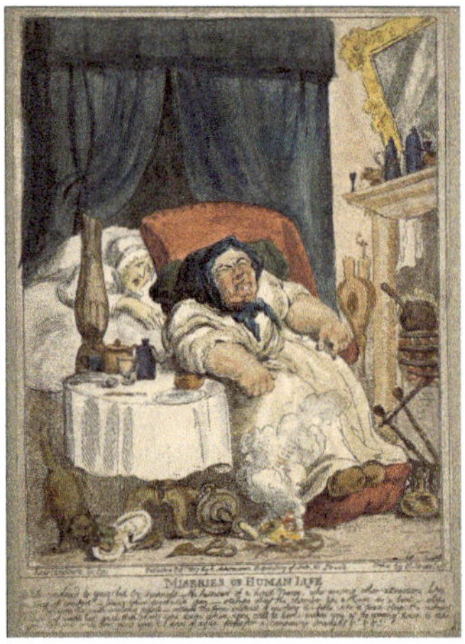

A convalescing woman trying in vain to rouse her slumbering hired nurse: the cat scavenges her food and the candle sets light to the carpet. Coloured etching by Nikolaus Heideloff (de), 1807, after Thomas Rowlandson

Nursing historians face the challenge of determining whether care provided to the sick or injured in antiquity was nursing care. In the fifth century BC, for example, the Hippocratic Collection in places describes skilled care and observation of patients by male "attendants", who may have been early nurses. Around 600 BC in India, it is recorded in Sushruta Samhita, Book 3, Chapter V about the role of nurse as "the different parts or members of the body as mentioned before including the skin, cannot be correctly described by one who is not well versed in anatomy. Hence, any one desirous of acquiring a thorough knowledge of anatomy should prepare a dead body and carefully, observe, by dissecting it, and examine its different parts."

Before the foundation of modern nursing, members of religious orders such as nuns and monks often provided nursing-like care. Examples exist in Christian, Islamic and Buddhist traditions amongst others. Phoebe, mentioned in Romans 16 has been described in many sources as "the first visiting nurse". These traditions were influential in the development of the ethos of modern nursing. The religious roots of modern nursing remain in evidence today in many countries. One example in the United Kingdom is the use of the honorific "sister" to refer to a senior nurse.

During the Reformation of the 16th century, Protestant reformers shut down the monasteries and convents, allowing a few hundred municipal hospices to remain in operation in northern Europe. Those nuns who had been serving as nurses were given pensions or told to get married and stay home. Nursing care went to the inexperienced as traditional caretakers, rooted in the Roman Catholic Church, were removed from their positions. The nursing profession suffered a major setback for approximately 200 years.

19th Century

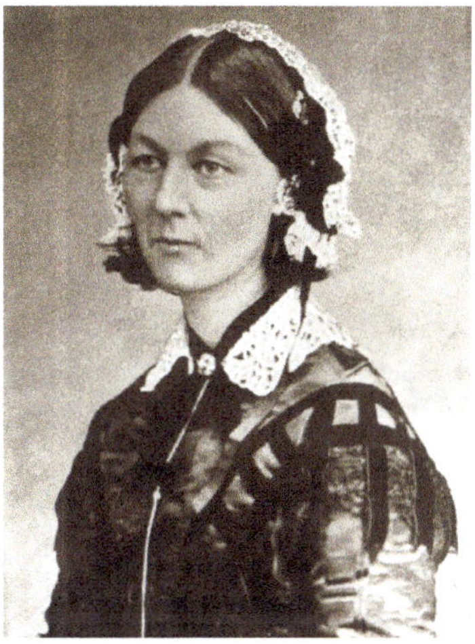

Florence Nightingale was an influential figure in the development of modern nursing. No uniform had been created when Florence Nightingale was employed during the Crimean War. Both nursing role and education were first defined by Florence Nightingale.

Florence Nightingale laid the foundations of professional nursing during the Crimean War. Her *Notes on Nursing* became popular. The Nightingale model of professional education, having set up the first school of nursing that is connected to a continuously operating hospital and medical school, spread widely in Europe and North America after 1870.

Other important nurses in the development of the profession include:

- Agnes Hunt from Shropshire was the first orthopedic nurse and was pivotal in the emergence of the orthopedic hospital The Robert Jones & Agnes Hunt Hospital in Oswestry, Shropshire.
- Agnes Elizabeth Jones and Linda Richards, who established quality nursing schools in the USA and Japan; Linda Richards was officially America's first professionally trained nurse, graduating in 1873 from the *New England Hospital for Women and Children* in Boston
- Clarissa Harlowe "Clara" Barton, a pioneer American teacher, patent clerk, nurse, and humanitarian, and the founder of the American Red Cross.

- Saint Marianne Cope, a Sister of St Francis who opened and operated some of the first general hospitals in the United States, instituting cleanliness standards which influenced the development of America's modern hospital system.

Catholic orders such as Little Sisters of the Poor, Sisters of Mercy, Sisters of St. Mary, St. Francis Health Services, Inc. and Sisters of Charity built hospitals and provided nursing services during this period. In turn, the modern deaconess movement began in Germany in 1836. Within a half century there were over 5,000 deaconesses in Europe.

Formal use of nurses in the modern military began in the latter half of the nineteenth century. Nurses saw active duty in the First Boer War, the Egyptian Campaign (1882) and the Sudan Campaign (1883).

20th Century

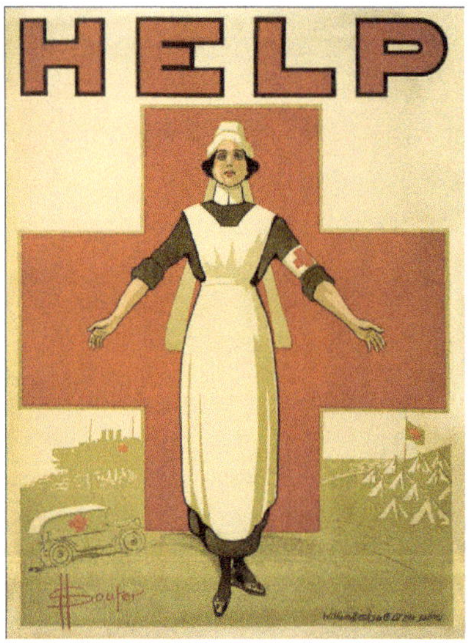

A recruiting poster for Australian nurses from World War I.

Hospital-based training came to the fore in the early 1900s, with an emphasis on practical experience. The Nightingale-style school began to disappear. Hospitals and physicians saw women in nursing as a source of free or inexpensive labor. Exploitation of nurses was not uncommon by employers, physicians and educational providers.

Many nurses saw active duty in World War I, but the profession was transformed during the second World War. British nurses of the Army Nursing Service were part of every overseas campaign. More nurses volunteered for service in the US Army and Navy than any other occupation. The Nazis had their own Brown Nurses, 40,000 strong. Two dozen German Red Cross nurses were awarded the Iron Cross for heroism under fire.

The modern era saw the development of undergraduate and post-graduate nursing degrees. Advancement of nursing research and a desire for association and organization led to the formation of a wide variety of professional organizations and academic journals. Growing recognition of nursing as a distinct academic discipline was accompanied by an awareness of the need to define the theoretical basis for practice.

In the 19th and early 20th century, nursing was considered a women's profession, just as doctoring was a men's profession. With increasing expectations of workplace equality during the late 20th century, nursing became an officially gender-neutral profession, though in practice the percentage of male nurses remains well below that of female physicians in the early 21st century.

Definition

Although nursing practice varies both through its various specialties and countries, these nursing organizations offer the following definitions:

Nursing encompasses autonomous and collaborative care of individuals of all ages, families, groups and communities, sick or well and in all settings. Nursing includes the promotion of health, prevention of illness, and the care of ill, disabled and dying people. Advocacy, promotion of a safe environment, research, participation in shaping health policy and in patient and health systems management, and education are also key nursing roles.

—*International Council of Nurses*

The use of clinical judgment in the provision of care to enable people to improve, maintain, or recover health, to cope with health problems, and to achieve the best possible quality of life, whatever their disease or disability, until death.

—*Royal College of Nursing (2003)*

Nursing is the protection, promotion, and optimization of health and abilities; prevention of illness and injury; alleviation of suffering through the diagnosis and treatment of human responses; and advocacy in health care for individuals, families, communities, and populations.

—*American Nurses Association*

The unique function of the nurse is to assist the individual, sick or well, in the performance of those activities contributing to health or its recovery (or to peaceful death) that he would perform unaided if he had the necessary strength, will or knowledge.

—*Virginia Avenel Henderson*

As a Profession

The authority for the practice of nursing is based upon a social contract that delineates professional rights and responsibilities as well as mechanisms for public accountability. In almost all countries, nursing practice is defined and governed by law, and entrance to the profession is regulated at the national or state level.

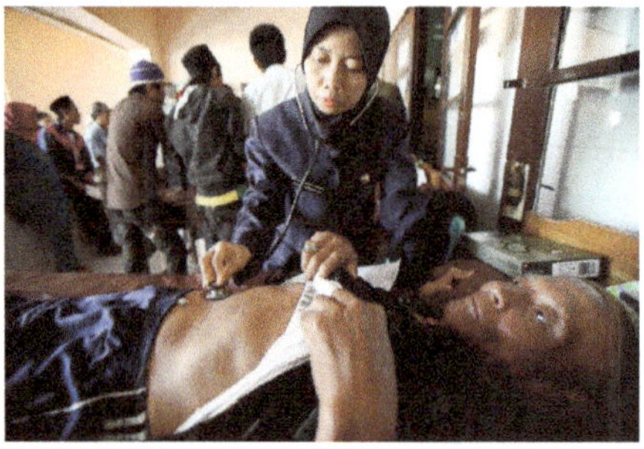

A nurse in Indonesia examining a patient

The aim of the nursing community worldwide is for its professionals to ensure quality care for all, while maintaining their credentials, code of ethics, standards, and competencies, and continuing their education. There are a number of educational paths to becoming a professional nurse, which vary greatly worldwide; all involve extensive study of nursing theory and practice as well as training in clinical skills.

Nurses care for individuals of all ages and cultural backgrounds who are healthy and ill in a holistic manner based on the individual's physical, emotional, psychological, intellectual, social, and spiritual needs. The profession combines physical science, social science, nursing theory, and technology in caring for those individuals.

To work in the nursing profession, all nurses hold one or more credentials depending on their scope of practice and education. A licensed practical nurse (LPN) (also referred to as a licensed vocational nurse, registered practical nurse, enrolled nurse, and state enrolled nurse) works independently or with a registered nurse (RN). The most significant differentiation between an LPN and RN is found in the requirements for entry to practice, which determines entitlement for their scope of practice. For example, Canada requires a bachelor's degree for the RN and a two-year diploma for the LPN. A registered nurse provides scientific, psychological, and technological knowledge in the care of patients and families in many health care settings. Registered nurses may earn additional credentials or degrees.

In the USA, multiple educational paths will qualify a candidate to sit for the licensure examination as a registered nurse. The Associate Degree in Nursing (ADN) is awarded to the nurse who has completed a two-year undergraduate academic degree awarded by community colleges, junior colleges, technical colleges, and bachelor's degree-granting colleges and universities upon completion of a course of study usually lasting two years. It is also referred to as Associate in Nursing (AN), Associate of Applied Science in Nursing (AAS), or Associate of Science in Nursing (ASN). The Bachelor of Science in Nursing (BSN) is awarded to the nurse who has earned an American four-year academic degree in the science and principles of nursing, granted by a tertiary education university or similarly accredited school. After completing either the LPN or either RN education programs in the USA, graduates are eligible to sit for a licensing examination to become a nurse, the passing of which is required for the nursing license. The National Licensure Examination (NCLEX) test is a multiple choice exam nurses take to become licensed. It costs two-hundred dollars to take the NCLEX. It examines a nurses ability to properly care for a client. Study books and practice tests are available to purchase.

Nurses may follow their personal and professional interests by working with any group of people, in any setting, at any time. Some nurses follow the traditional role of working in a hospital setting. Other options include: Pediatrics, Neonatal, Maternity, OBGYN, Geriatrics, Ambulatory, or Nurse Anesthetists. There are many other options nurses can explore depending on the type of degree and education acquired. RNs may also pursue different roles as advanced practice registered nurses.

Nurses are not truly doctor's assistants. This is possible in certain situations, but nurses more often are independently caring for their patients or assisting other nurses. Registered Nurses treat patients, record their medical history, provide emotional support, and provide follow-up care. Nurses also help doctors perform diagnostic tests. Nurses are almost always working on their own or with other nurses. Nurses will assist doctors in the emergency room or in trauma care when help is needed.

Gender Issues

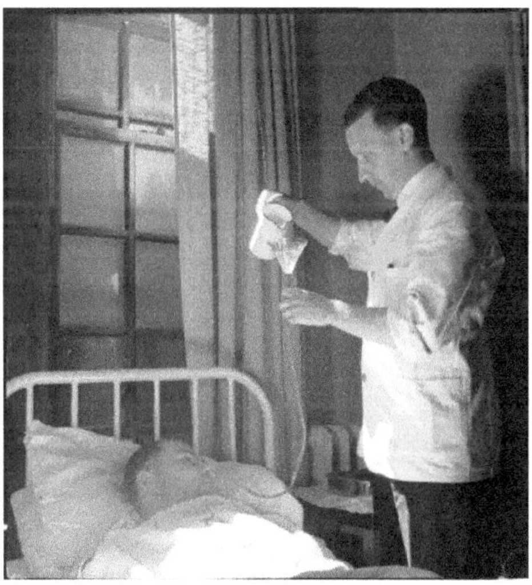

A male nurse at Runwell Hospital, Wickford, Essex, in 1943

Despite equal opportunity legislation, nursing has continued to be a female-dominated profession. For instance, the male-to-female ratio of nurses is approximately 1:19 in Canada and the United States. This ratio is represented around the world. Notable exceptions include Francophone Africa, which includes the countries of Benin, Burkina Faso, Cameroon, Chad, Congo, Côte d'Ivoire, the Democratic Republic of Congo, Djibouti, Guinea, Gabon, Mali, Mauritania, Niger, Rwanda, Senegal, and Togo, which all have more male than female nurses. In Europe, in countries such as Spain, Portugal,

Czechoslovakia and Italy, over 20% of nurses are male. The number of male-registered nurses in the United States between 1980 and 2000s doubled.

There are many myths about nursing, including the profession and the people that work as a nurse. One of the most common myths is that all nurses are females. The nursing industry is dominated by females, but there are male nurses in the profession as well. A study in 2011 shows that 91% of all nurses in the United States were female, and 9% were male. Although females are more common, male nurses receive more pay. In the same survey, male nurses average $60,700 per year and female nurses average $51,100 per year. Male nurses have the highest percentage as nurse anesthetists, rating at 41%.

Theory and Process

Nursing practice is the actual provision of nursing care. In providing care, nurses implement the nursing care plan using the nursing process. This is based around a specific nursing theory which is selected based on the care setting and population served. In providing nursing care, the nurse uses both nursing theory and best practice derived from nursing research.

In general terms, the nursing process is the method used to assess and diagnose needs, plan outcomes and interventions, implement interventions, and evaluate the outcomes of the care provided. Like other disciplines, the profession has developed different theories derived from sometimes diverse philosophical beliefs and paradigms or worldviews to help nurses direct their activities to accomplish specific goals.

Scope of Activities

Activities of Daily Living Assistance

Assisting in activities of daily living (ADL) are skills required in nursing as well as other professions such as nursing assistants. This includes assisting in patient mobility, such as moving an activity intolerant patient within bed. For hygiene, this often involves bed baths and assisting with urinary and bowel elimination.

Medication

Nurses do not have the authority to prescribe medications, with few exceptions. All medications administered by nurses must be from a medication order from a licensed practitioner. Nurses are legally responsible for the drugs they administer and there may be legal implications when there is an error in a drug order and the nurse could be expected to have noted and reported error. In the United States, nurses have the right to refuse any medication administration that they deem to be harmful to the patient. In the United Kingdom there are some nurses who have taken additional specialist training that allows them to prescribe certain medications.

Patient Education

The patient's family is often involved in the education. Effective patient education leads to fewer complications and hospital visits.

Specialities

Nursing is the most diverse of all healthcare professions. Nurses practice in a wide range of settings but generally nursing is divided depending on the needs of the person being nursed.

The major populations are:

- communities/public
- family/individual across the lifespan
- adult-gerontology
- pediatrics
- neonatal
- women's health/gender-related
- psych/mental health

There are also specialist areas such as cardiac nursing, orthopedic nursing, palliative care, perioperative nursing, obstetrical nursing, oncology nursing, nursing informatics, telenursing.

Practice Settings

Nurses practice in a wide range of settings, from hospitals to visiting people in their homes and caring for them in schools to research in pharmaceutical companies. Nurses work in occupational health settings (also called industrial health settings), free-standing clinics and physician offices, nurse-led clinics, long-term care facilities and camps. They also work on cruise ships and in military service. Nurses act as advisers and consultants to the health care and insurance industries. Many nurses also work in the health advocacy and patient advocacy fields at companies such as Health Advocate, Inc. helping in a variety of clinical and administrative issues. Some are attorneys and others work with attorneys as legal nurse consultants, reviewing patient records to assure that adequate care was provided and testifying in court. Nurses can work on a temporary basis, which involves doing shifts without a contract in a variety of settings, sometimes known as *per diem nursing*, *agency nursing* or *travel nursing*. Nurses work as researchers in laboratories, universities, and research institutions. Nurses have also been delving into the world of informatics, acting as consultants to the creation of computerized charting programs and other software.

Occupational Hazards

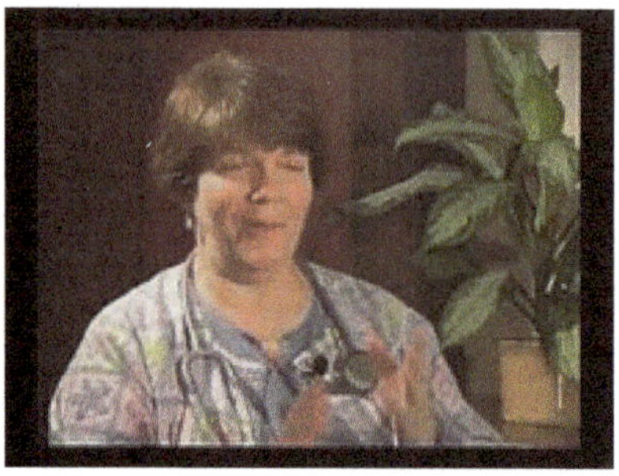

A video describing occupational hazards that exist among nurses

Internationally, there is a serious shortage of nurses. One reason for this shortage is due to the work environment in which nurses practice. In a recent review of the empirical human factors and ergonomic literature specific to nursing performance, nurses were found to work in generally poor environmental conditions. Some countries and states have passed legislation regarding acceptable nurse-to-patient ratios.

The fast-paced and unpredictable nature of health care places nurses at risk for injuries and illnesses, including high occupational stress. Nursing is a particularly stressful profession, and nurses consistently identify stress as a major work-related concern and have among the highest levels of occupational stress when compared to other professions. This stress is caused by the environment, psychosocial stressors, and the demands of nursing, including new technology that must be mastered, the emotional labor involved in nursing, physical labor, shift work, and high workload. This stress puts nurses at risk for short-term and long-term health problems, including sleep disorders, depression, mortality, psychiatric disorders, stress-related illnesses, and illness in general. Nurses are at risk of developing compassion fatigue and moral distress, which can worsen mental health. They also have very high rates of occupational burnout (40%) and emotional exhaustion (43.2%). Burnout and exhaustion increase the risk for illness, medical error, and suboptimal care provision.

In the United States, the Occupational Health Safety Network (OHSN) is an electronic surveillance system developed by the National Institute for Occupational Safety and Health (NIOSH) to address health and safety risks among health care personnel, including nurses. It focuses on three high risk and preventable events: musculoskeletal injuries from patient handling activities; slips, trips, and falls; and workplace violence. Hospitals and other healthcare facilities can upload the occupational injury data they already collect for analysis and benchmarking with other de-identified facilities, in order to identify and implement timely and targeted interventions.

Nurses are also at risk for violence and abuse in the workplace. Violence is typically perpetrated by non-staff (e.g. patients or family), whereas abuse is typically perpetrated by other hospital personnel. 57% of American nurses reported in 2011 that they had been threatened at work; 17% were physically assaulted.

Prevention

There are a number of interventions that can mitigate the occupational hazards of nursing. They can be individual-focused or organization-focused. Individual-focused interventions include stress management programs, which can be customized to individuals. Stress management programs can reduce anxiety, sleep disorders, and other symptoms of stress. Organizational interventions focus on reducing stressful aspects of the work environment by defining stressful characteristics and developing solutions to them. Using organizational and individual interventions together is most effective at reducing stress on nurses.

Worldwide

Australia

Catholic religious institutes were influential in the development of Australian nursing, founding many of Australia's hospitals - the Irish Sisters of Charity were first to arrive in 1838 and established St Vincent's Hospital, Sydney in 1857 as a free hospital for the poor. They and other orders like the Sisters of Mercy, and in aged care the Sisters of the Little Company of Mary and Little Sisters of the Poor founded hospitals, hospices, research institutes and aged care facilities around Australia.

A census in the 1800s found several hundred nurses working in Western Australia during the colonial period of history, this included Aboriginal female servants who cared for the infirm.

The state nursing licensing bodies amalgamated in Australia in 2011 under the federal body AHPRA (Australian Health Practitioner Registration Authority). Several divisions of nursing license is available and recognized around the country.

- Enrolled nurses may initiate some oral medication orders with a specific competency now included in national curricula but variable in application by agency.
- Registered nurses hold a university degree (enrolled nurses can progress to registered nurse status and do get credit for previous study)
- Nurse practitioners have started emerging from postgraduate programs and work in private practice.
- Mental health nurses must complete further training as advanced mental health practitioners in order to administer client referrals under the *Mental Health Act*.

Australia enjoys the luxury of a national curriculum for vocational nurses, trained at TAFE colleges or private RTO. Enrolled and registered nurses are identified by the department of immigration as an occupational area of need, although registered nurses are always in shorter supply, and this increases in proportion with specialization.

In 1986 there were a number of rolling industrial actions around the country, culminating when five thousand Victorian nurses went on strike for eighteen days. The hospitals were able to function by hiring casual staff from each other's striking members, but the increased cost forced a decision in the nurses' favor

European Union

In the European Union, the profession of nurse is regulated. A profession is said to be regulated when access and exercise is subject to the possession of a specific professional qualification. The regulated professions database contains a list of regulated professions for nurse in the EU member states, EEA countries and Switzerland. This list is covered by the Directive 2005/36/EC .

Iran

Nursing educational program in Iran is similar to the nursing educational program in other countries from some aspects. Holding secondary school diploma and passing the entrance exam is necessary for the admission in this course. Entrance exam to governmental universities and Azad University is held on separate basis. Duration of associate degree course of operating room and anesthesia is 2 years, bachelor's degree in nursing is 4 years and master's degree in nursing is 2- 2.5 years and PhD degree in nursing is 4–5 years.

In the beginning, nursing educational program was the part of medical educational program. On the basis of this structure, the nurse follows the instruction of physician without any question. Nowadays, nursing educational program in Iran has been progressed and after the year 1992 considering the community base care, the nursing educational program also has changed. At present nursing education is held in 43 governmental nursing colleges and 63 nursing colleges of Azad University. Governmental universities' students do not have to pay tuition fee, but in Azad University which is a private university, the students have to pay necessary expenses. PhD degree program is held only in governmental universities under the supervision of Ministry of Health and Ministry of Sciences.

In bachelor's degree program, nursing students start the clinical work from 2nd term and pass till the completion of 6th term simultaneously with theoretical subjects. 7th and 8th terms are allocated for training program. At present nursing educational program in throughout Iran is the same and is compiled under the supervision of Supreme Council of Ministry of Health, Treatment and Medical Education. Nursing students take the theoretical subjects, training and internship courses in various sections of educational hospitals and hospitals that affiliated to universities. Students' learning, in clinical sections is performed under the direct supervision and guidance of nursing instructors, but in the final year, activities of students mainly performs under the supervision of nursing personnel and alternate supervision of nursing instructors.

Students, during the years of study have opportunity to create relation with patients in the various sections especially intensive care units and to achieve experiences. Students' progress in clinical environments is from simple issues toward harder issues. At present practical nursing degree and associate degree Nursing Program has been canceled and Iranian nurses must hold bachelor's degree in order to work in Iran from accredited universities confirmed by the Ministry of Health.

Nursing Groups in Iran

- Nurse

Nurse is a person who is holding four years university degree and executes works relating to nursing profession including taking care of patients, perform health and medical services, educational, research and managerial affairs. At present annually 6000 persons are graduated in the bachelor's degree program in nursing.

- Practical Nurse

A person who is holding secondary school diploma in nursing and have completed 2 years program in nursing and cooperate in activities of nurses in medical sections under the supervision of nurses.

- Nursing Assistant

A person who is holding secondary school diploma and passing short term program for the execution of initial cares of patients under the supervision of nurses.

- Operating Room Technician

These persons after obtaining secondary school diploma and passing university's entrance exam and completing 2 years program are in charge of performing professional duties in operation room for preparing patients for surgery and necessary cooperation with surgeons at the time of surgery. These persons by passing the exam are eligible to continue uncontinuous bachelor's degree course in nursing.

- Anesthesia Technician

These persons after obtaining secondary school diploma and passing university's entrance exam and completing 2 years program in Anesthesia, are in charge of performing profession duties in the operating room in the field of anesthesia including preparing the patients for anesthesia and necessary cooperation with anesthesiologists at the time of operation. These persons by passing exam are eligible to continue uncontinuous bachelor's degree course in nursing.

- Emergency medical technician

These persons after obtaining secondary school diploma and passing entrance exam of university and obtaining technician diploma are in change of performing affairs including rendering first aid services to the patients and emergency victims resulting from accidents with motor vehicles, explosion, debris, falling from height, fractures, burns, poisonings, cuts, drowning, industrial accidents (cutting of limbs), patients with heart diseases and baby delivering.

- Master in Nursing

Nurses after obtaining bachelor's degree and passing the entrance exam are eligible to continue their study in geriatric nursing, pediatric nursing, medical surgical nursing, community health nursing, psychiatric nursing and nursing education. These persons after graduation mainly become in charge of nurses' education or management of medical sections. Duration of this program is 2.5 years. At present annually 150 persons are graduated in master's degree program in nursing.

- PhD in Nursing

Nurses by holding master's degree after passing entrance exam, are eligible to continue their study in PhD in the field of Nursing. Duration of this program is 4 years and the graduates mainly will work in educational and research sections. At present annually 20 persons are graduated in this program.

Nursing Jobs in Iran

According to the censes at present approximately 120,000 nurses are working in Iran in various sections. Most of them are working in hospitals and health centers belong to Ministry of Health, Treatment & Medical Education. Also, nurses are working in the hospitals affiliated to social security organization, armed forces, private sector and charity sector.

Within the last years of independence, nurses' activities are established in offices of consultancy and rendering nursing services at home. Nurses by establishment these centers can render consultant and care services to the client.

At present to work as a nurse only holding accredited academic degree is sufficient, but there are programs for nurses to take RN examination after graduation.

Also, upon the approval and execution of continuous educational act, the Iranian nurses should obtain score of 15 every year in various educational courses held by the Ministry of Health of Universities, Scientific Associations and Nursing organization.

Iranian Nursing Organization (INO)

Having an independent organization which can defend the rights of nurses and to follow up nurses' problems was the long time wishes of Iranian nurses. Before Islamic revolution in 1979, some efforts were taken in this respect which finally results to establishment of Iranian Nurses Association and activities were taken in this respect. After the victory of Islamic revolution, this association also canceled its activities and after that, number of associations mainly with political and professional formation was established, but the main problem of nurses was still present. Gradually in the year 1994 with the efforts of numbers of persons mostly nursing students and faculty member, the preliminary step was taken for the establishment of nursing organization. This preliminary nucleus started its work in the name of Nursing Coordination council with the instruction of students.

This council had correspondences with the president, speaker of parliament, ministry of health, treatment and medical education in connection with problems of nursing society. Also this organization had correspondence with nursing colleges for unity throughout the country.

After this date till March 2001, number of state seminars were held in various cities and finally on March 5.2001, generalities of formation of Nursing Organization which was in the agenda of Islamic Consultative Assembly and approved, was finally approved in an open session on Aug.12.2001. Finally with the procurement of comments of Guardian's Organization in Jan.2002, Establishment Act of Nursing Organization was approved by the parliament.

The first election of board of directors throughout the country was performed on Sept.20.2002 and members of 85 boards of directors of districts were elected throughout the country with the direct vote of nurses. The board of directors of the first Supreme of Organization, was elected on Dec.8.2002.

United Kingdom

To practice lawfully as a registered nurse in the United Kingdom, the practitioner must hold a current and valid registration with the Nursing and Midwifery Council. The title "Registered Nurse" can only be granted to those holding such registration. This protected title is laid down in the Nurses, Midwives and Health Visitors Act, 1997. From April 2016, nurses in the United Kingdom are expected to revalidate every three years.

First and Second Level

First-level nurses make up the bulk of the registered nurses in the UK. They were previously known by titles such as RGN (registered general nurse), RSCN (registered sick children's nurse), RMN (registered mental nurse) and RNMS (registered nurse (for the) mentally subnormal). The titles used now are similar, including RNA (registered nurse adult), RNC (registered nurse child), RNMH (registered nurse mental health) and RNLD (registered nurse learning disabilities).

Second-level nurse training is no longer provided, however they are still legally able to practice in the United Kingdom as a registered nurse. Many have now either retired or undertaken conversion courses to become first-level nurses. They are entitled to refer to themselves as registered nurses as their registration is on the Nursing & Midwifery Council register of nurses, although most refer to themselves as ENs or SENs.

Advanced Practice

- Nurse practitioners – Most of these nurses obtain a minimum of a master's degree, and a desired post grad certificate. They often perform roles similar to those of physicians and physician assistants. They can prescribe medications as independent or supplementary prescribers, although are still legally regulated, unlike physician's assistants. Most NPs have referral and admission rights to hospital specialties. They commonly work in primary care (e.g. GP surgeries), A&E departments, or pediatrics although they are increasingly being seen in other areas of practice. In the UK, the title "nurse practitioner" is legally protected.
- Specialist community public health nurses – traditionally district nurses and health visitors, this group of research and publication activities.
- Lecturer-practitioners (also called practice education facilitators) – these nurses work both in the NHS, and in universities. They typically work for 2–3 days per week in each setting. In university, they train pre-registration student nurses, and often teach on specialist courses for post-registration nurses
- Lecturers – these nurses are not employed by the NHS. Instead they work full-time in universities, both teaching and performing research.

Managers

Many nurses who have worked in clinical settings for a long time choose to leave clinical nursing and join the ranks of the NHS management. This used to be seen as a natural career progression for those who had reached ward management positions, however with the advent of specialist nursing roles, this has become a less attractive option.

Nonetheless, many nurses fill positions in the senior management structure of NHS organizations, some even as board members. Others choose to stay a little closer to their clinical roots by becoming clinical nurse managers or *modern matrons*.

Nurse Education

Nursing in the United Kingdom

Pre-registration

In order to become a registered nurse, one must complete a program recognised by the Nursing and Midwifery Council (NMC) . Currently, this involves completing a degree, available from a range of universities offering these courses, in the chosen branch specialty, leading to both an academic award and professional registration as a 1st level registered nurse. Such a course is a 50/50 split of learning in university (i.e. through lectures, assignments and examinations) and in practice (i.e. supervised patient care within a hospital or community setting).

These courses are three (occasionally four) years' long. The first year is known as the common foundation program (CFP), and teaches the basic knowledge and skills required of all nurses. Skills included in the CFP may include communication, taking observations, administering medication and providing personal care to patients. The remainder of the program consists of training specific to the student's chosen branch of nursing. These are:

- Adult nursing.
- Child nursing.
- Mental health nursing.
- Learning disabilities nursing.

As of 2013, the Nursing and Midwifery Council will require all new nurses qualifying in the UK to hold a degree qualification. However, those nurses who hold a diploma, or even a certificate in nursing are still able to legally practice in the UK, although they are able to undertake university modules to obtain enough credits to top up to a degree.

Midwifery training is similar in length and structure, but is sufficiently different that it is not considered a branch of nursing. There are shortened (18 month) programs to allow nurses already qualified in the adult branch to hold dual registration as a nurse and a midwife. Shortened courses lasting 2 years also exist for graduates of other disciplines to train as nurses. This is achieved by more intense study and a shortening of the common foundation program.

As of 2016 student nurses in the UK can apply a bursary from the government to support them during their nurse training, and may also be eligible for a student loan, although there has been speculation that this will not be available in the future.

Before Project 2000, nurse education was the responsibility of hospitals and was not based in universities; hence many nurses who qualified prior to these reforms do not hold an academic award.

Post-registration

After the point of initial registration, there is an expectation that all qualified nurses will continue to update their skills and knowledge. The Nursing and Midwifery Council insists on a minimum of 35 hours of education every three years, as part of its post registration education and practice (PREP) requirements.

There are also opportunities for many nurses to gain additional clinical skills after qualification. Cannulation, venipuncture, intravenous drug therapy and male catheterization are the most common, although there are many others (such as advanced life support) which some nurses will undertake.

Many nurses who qualified with a diploma choose to upgrade their qualification to a degree by studying part-time. Many nurses prefer this option to gaining a degree initially, as there is often an opportunity to study in a specialist field as a part of this upgrading. Financially, in England, it was also much more lucrative, as diploma students get the full bursary during their initial training, and employers often pay for the degree course as well as the nurse's salary.

In order to become specialist nurses (such as nurse consultants, nurse practitioners etc.) or nurse educators, some nurses undertake further training above bachelor's degree level. Master's degrees exist in various healthcare related topics, and some nurses choose to study for PhDs or other higher academic awards. District nurses and health visitors are also considered specialist nurses, and in order to become such they must undertake specialist training. This is a one-year full-time degree.

All newly qualifying district nurses and health visitors are trained to prescribe from the Nurse Prescribers' Formulary, a list of medications and dressings typically useful to those carrying out these roles. Many of these (and other) nurses will also undertake training in independent and supplementary prescribing, which allows them (as of 1 May 2006) to prescribe almost any drug in the British National Formulary. This has been the cause of a great deal of debate in both medical and nursing circles.

Canada

History

Canadian nursing dates all the way back to 1639 in Quebec with the Augustine nuns. These nuns were trying to open up a mission that cared for the spiritual and physical needs of patients. The establishment of this mission created the first nursing apprenticeship training in North America. In the nineteenth century there were some Catholic orders of nursing that were trying to spread their message across Canada. Most nurses were female and only had an occasional consultation with a physician. Towards the end of the nineteenth century hospital care and medical services had been improved and expanded. Much of this was due to Nightingale's influence. In 1874 the first formal nursing training program was started at the General and Marine Hospital in St. Catharines in Ontario.

Education

All Canadian nurses and prospective nurses are heavily encouraged by the Canadian Nurses Association to continue their education to receive a baccalaureate degree. They believe that this is the best degree to work towards because it results in better patient outcomes. In addition to helping patients, nurses that have a baccalaureate degree will be less likely to make small errors because they have a higher level of education. A baccalaureate degree also gives a nurse a more critical opinion, which gives him or her more of an edge in the field. This ultimately saves the hospital money because they deal with less problematic incidents. All Canadian provinces and territories except for the Yukon and Quebec require that all nurses must have a baccalaureate degree. The basic length of time that it takes to obtain a baccalaureate degree is four years. However, Canada does have a condensed program that is two years long.

Nursing specialty certification is available through the Canadian Nurses Association in nineteen practice areas. Some of those specialties are cardiovascular nursing, community health nursing, critical care nursing, emergency nursing, gerontological nursing, medical-surgical nursing, neuroscience nursing, oncology nursing, orthopedic nursing, psychiatric/mental health nursing, and rehabilitation nursing. Certification requires practice experience and passing a test that is based on competencies for that specialty.

Public Opinion

Canadian nurses hold a lot of responsibility in the medical field and are considered vital. According to the Canadian Nurses Association, "They expect RNs to develop and implement multi-faceted plans for managing chronic disease, treating complex health conditions and assisting them in the transition from the hospital to the community. Canadians also look to RNs for health education and for strategies to improve their health. RNs assess the appropriateness of new research and technology for patients and adjust care plans accordingly".

Japan

History

Nursing was not an established part of Japan's healthcare system until 1899 with the Midwives Ordinance. From there the Registered Nurse Ordinance came into play in 1915. This established a legal substantiation to registered nurses all over Japan. A new law geared towards nurses was created during World War II. This law was titled the *Public Health Nurse, Midwife and Nurse Law* and it was established in 1948. It established educational requirements, standards and licensure. There has been a continued effort to improve nursing in Japan. In 1992 the Nursing Human Resource Law was passed. This law created the development of new university programs for nurses. Those programs were designed to raise the education level of the nurses so that they could be better suited for taking care of the public.

Types of Nurses

Japan only recognizes four types of nursing and they are Public Health Nursing, Midwifery, Registered Nursing and Assistant Nursing.

Public Health

This type of nursing is designed to help the public and is also driven by the public's needs. The goals of public health nurses are to monitor the spread of disease, keep vigilant watch for environmental hazards, educate the community on how to care for and treat themselves, and train for community disasters.

Midwifery

Nurses that are involved with midwifery are independent of any organization. A midwife takes care of a pregnant woman during labour and postpartum. They assist with things like breastfeeding and caring for the child.

Nursing Assistant

Individuals who are assistant nurses follow orders from a registered nurse. They report back to the licensed nurse about a patient's condition. Assistant nurses are always supervised by a licensed registered nurse.

Education

In 1952 Japan established the first nursing university in the country. An Associate Degree was the only level of certification for years. Soon people began to want nursing degrees at a higher level of education. Soon the Bachelor's degree in Nursing (BSN) was established. Currently Japan offers doctorate level degrees of nursing in a good number of its universities.

There are three ways that an individual could become a registered nurse in Japan. After obtaining a high school degree the person could go to a nursing university for four years and earn a bachelor's degree, go to a junior nursing college for three years or go to a nursing school for three years. Regardless of where the individual attends school they must take the national exam. Those who attended a nursing university have a bit of an advantage over those who went to a nursing school. They can take the national exam to be a registered nurse, public health nurse or midwife. In the cases of become a midwife or a public health nurse, the student must take a one-year course in their desired field after attending a nursing university and passing the national exam to become a registered nurse. The nursing universities are the best route for someone who wants to become a nurse in Japan. They offer a wider range of general education classes and they also allow for a more rigid teaching style of nursing. These nursing universities train their students to be able to make critical and educated decisions when they are out in the field. Physicians are the ones who are teaching the potential nurses because there are not enough available nurses to teach students. This increases the dominance that physicians have over nurses.

Students that attend a nursing college or just a nursing school receive the same degree that one would who graduated from a nursing university, but they do not have the same educational background. The classes offered at nursing colleges and nursing schools are focused on more practical aspects of nursing. These institutions do not offer many general education classes, so students who attend these schools will solely be focusing on their nursing educations while they are in school. Students who attend a nursing college or school do have the opportunity to become a midwife or a public health nurse. They have to go through a training institute for their desired field after graduating from the nursing school or college. Japanese nurses never have to renew their licenses. Once they have passed their exam, they have their license for life.

Today

Like the United States, Japan is in need of more nurses. The driving force behind this need this is the fact that country is aging and needs more medical care for its people. The country needs a rapid increase of nurses however things do not seem to be turning around. Some of the reasons that there is a shortage are poor working conditions, an increase in the number of hospital beds, the low social status of nurses, and the cultural idea that married women quit their jobs for family responsibilities. On average, Japanese nurses will make around 280,000 yen a month, which is one of the higher paying jobs. however, physicians make twice the amount that nurses do in a year. Similar to other cultures, the Japanese people view nurses as subservient to physicians. They are considered lesser and oftentimes negative connotations are associated with nurses. According to the American Nurses Association article on Japan, "nursing work has been described using negative terminology such as 'hard, dirty, dangerous, low salary, few holidays, minimal chance of marriage and family, and poor image'".

Some nurses in Japan are trying to be advocates. They are promoting better nursing education as well as promoting the care of the elderly. There are some organizations that unite Japanese nurses like the Japanese Nursing Association (JNA). The JNA is not to be confused with a union, it is simply a professional organization for the nurses. Members of the JNA lobby politicians and produces publications about nursing. According to the American Nurses Association's article on Japan the JNA, "works toward the improvement in nursing practice through many activities including the development of a policy research group to influence policy development, a code of ethics for nurses, and standards of nursing practice". The JNA also provides certification for specialists in mental health, oncology and community health. The JNA is not the only nursing organization in Japan. There are other subgroups that are typically categorized by the nurses' specialty, like emergency nursing or disaster nursing. One of the older unions that relates to nursing is the Japanese Federation of Medical Workers Union which was created in 1957. It is a union that includes physicians as well as nurses. This organization was involved with the Nursing Human Resource Law.

Taiwan

- In Taiwan, the Ministry of Health and Welfare is in charge of the regulation of nursing. The Taiwan Union of Nurses Association (TUNA) is the union unit in Taiwan, fighting for nurses on payment and working time issues.

United States

Two nurses in Arizona, 1943

In the US, scope of practice is determined by the state or territory in which an RN is licensed. Each state has its own laws, rules, and regulations governing nursing care. Usually the making of such rules and regulations is delegated to a state board of nursing, which performs day-to-day administration of these rules, licenses nurses and nursing assistants, and makes decisions on nursing issues. It should be noted that in some states the terms "nurse" or "nursing" may only be used in conjunction with the practice of a registered nurse (RN) or licensed practical or vocational nurse (LPN/LVN).

In the hospital setting, registered nurses often delegate tasks to LPNs and unlicensed assistive personnel.

RNs are not limited to employment as bedside nurses. They are employed by physicians, attorneys, insurance companies, governmental agencies, community/public health agencies, private industry, school districts, ambulatory surgery centers, among others. Some registered nurses are independent consultants who work for themselves, while others work for large manufacturers or chemical companies. Research nurses conduct or assist in the conduct of research or evaluation (outcome and process) in many areas such as biology, psychology, human development, and health care systems.

Many employers offer flexible work schedules, child care, educational benefits, and bonuses. About 21 percent of registered nurses are union members or covered by union contract.

Nursing is the nation's largest health care profession, with more than 3.1 million registered nurses nationwide. Of all licensed RNs, 2.6 million or 84.8% are employed in nursing. Nurses comprise the largest single component of hospital staff, are the primary providers of hospital patient care, and deliver most of the nation's long-term care. The primary pathway to professional nursing, as compared to technical-level practice, is the four-year Bachelor of Science in Nursing (BSN) degree . Registered nurses are prepared either through a BSN program; a three-year associate degree in nursing; or a three-year hospital training program, receiving a hospital diploma. All take the same state licensing exam. (The number of diploma programs has declined steadily -- to less than 10 percent of all basic RN education programs -- as nursing education has shifted from hospital-operated instruction into the college and university system.)

Educational and Licensure Requirements

Diploma in Nursing

The oldest method of nursing education is the hospital-based diploma program, which lasts approximately three years. Students take between 30 and 60 credit hours in anatomy, physiology, microbiology, nutrition, chemistry, and other subjects at a college or university, then move on to intensive nursing classes. Until 1996, most RNs in the US were initially educated in nursing by diploma programs. According to the Health Services Resources Administration's 2000 Survey of Nurses only six percent of nurses who graduated from nursing programs in the United States received their education at a Diploma School of Nursing.

Associate Degree in Nursing

The most common initial nursing education is a two-year Associate Degree in Nursing (Associate of Applied Science in Nursing, Associate of Science in Nursing, Associate Degree in Nursing), a two-year college degree referred to as an ADN. Some four-year colleges and universities also offer the ADN. Associate degree nursing programs have prerequisite and corequisite courses (which may include English, Math and Human Anatomy and Physiology) and ultimately stretch out the degree-acquiring process to about three years or greater.

Bachelor of Science in Nursing

The third method is to obtain a Bachelor of Science in Nursing (BSN), a four-year degree that also prepares nurses for graduate-level education. For the first two years in a BSN program, students usually obtain general education requirements and spend the remaining time in nursing courses. In some new programs the first two years can be substituted for an active LPN license along with the required general studies. Advocates for the ADN and diploma programs state that such programs have an on the job training approach to educating students, while the BSN is an academic degree that emphasizes research and nursing theory. Some states require a specific amount of clinical experience that is the same for both BSN and ADN students. A BSN degree qualifies its holder for administrative, research, consulting and teaching positions that would not usually be available to those with an ADN, but is not necessary for most patient care functions. Nursing schools may be accredited by either the Accreditation Commission for Education in Nursing (ACEN) or the Commission on Collegiate Nursing Education (CCNE).

Graduate Education

Advanced education in nursing is done at the master's and doctoral levels. It prepares the graduate for specialization as an advanced practice registered nurse (APRN) or for advanced roles in leadership, management, or education. The clinical nurse leader (CNL) is an advanced generalist who focuses on the improvement of quality and safety outcomes for patients or patient populations from an administrative and staff management focus. Doctoral programs in nursing prepare the student for work in nursing education, health care administration, clinical research, or advanced clinical practice. Most programs confer the PhD in nursing and Doctor of Nursing Practice (DNP).

Advanced practice registered nurse (APRN)

Areas of advanced nursing practice include that of a nurse practitioner (NP), a certified nurse midwife (CNM), a certified registered nurse anesthetist (CRNA), or a clinical nurse specialist (CNS). Nurse practitioners and CNSs work assessing, diagnosing and treating patients in fields as diverse as family practice, women's health care, emergency nursing, acute/critical care, psychiatry, geriatrics, or pediatrics, additionally, a CNS usually works for a facility to improve patient care, do research, or as a staff educator.

Licensure Examination

Completion of any one of these three educational routes allows a graduate nurse to take the NCLEX-RN, the test for licensure as a registered nurse, and is accepted by every state as an adequate indicator of minimum competency for a new graduate. However, controversy exists over the appropriate entry-level preparation of RNs. Some professional organizations believe the BSN should be the sole method of RN preparation and ADN graduates should be licensed as "technical nurses" to work under the supervision of BSN graduates. Others feel the on-the-job experiences of diploma and ADN graduates makes up for any deficiency in theoretical preparation.

Shortage in the United States

RNs are the largest group of health care workers in the United States, with about 2.7 million employed in 2011. It has been reported that the number of new graduates and foreign-trained nurses is insufficient to meet the demand for registered nurses; this is often referred to as the nursing shortage and is expected to increase for the foreseeable future. There are data to support the idea that the nursing shortage is a voluntary shortage. In other words, nurses are leaving nursing of their own volition. In 2006 it was estimated that approximately 1.8 million nurses chose not to work as a nurse. The Bureau of Labor Statistics reported that 296,900 healthcare jobs were created in 2011. RNs make up the majority of the healthcare work force, therefore these positions will be filled primarily by nurses. The BLS also states that by 2020, there will be 1.2 million nursing job openings due to an increase in the workforce, and replacements. (Rosseter, 2012).

Causes

The International Council Of Nursing (ICN), the largest international health professional organization in the world, recognizes the shortage of nurses as a growing crisis in the world. This shortage impacts the healthcare of everyone worldwide. One of the many reasons is that nurses who pursue to become nurses do so very late in their lives. This leads to a non-lengthy employment time. A national survey prepared by the Federation of Nurses and Health Professionals in 2001 found that one in five nurses plans to leave the profession within five years because of unsatisfactory working conditions, including low pay, severe under staffing, high stress, physical demands, mandatory overtime, and irregular hours. Approximately 29.8 percent of all nursing jobs are found in hospitals. However, because of administrative cost cutting, increased nurse's workload, and rapid growth of outpatient services, hospital nursing jobs will experience slower than average growth. Employment in home care and nursing homes is expected to grow rapidly. Though more people are living well into their 80s and 90s, many need the kind of long-term care available at a nursing home. Many nurses will also be needed to help staff the growing number of out-patient facilities, such as HMOs, group medical practices, and ambulatory surgery centers. Nursing specialties will be in great demand. There are, in addition, many part-time employment possibilities.

Levsey, Campbell, and Green voiced their concern about the shortage of nurses, citing Fang, Wilsey-Wisniewski, & Bednash, 2006 who state that over 40,000 qualified nursing applicants were turned away in the 2005-2006 academic year from baccalaureate nursing programs due to a lack of masters and doctoral qualified faculty, and that this number was increased over 9,000 from 32,000 qualified but rejected students from just two years earlier. Several strategies have been offered to mitigate this shortage including; Federal and private support for experienced nurses to enhance their education, incorporating more hybrid/blended nursing courses, and using simulation in lieu of clinical (hospital) training experiences.

Furthermore, there is a shortage of academically qualified instructors to teach at schools of nursing worldwide. The serious need for educational capacity is not being met, which is the underlying most important preparation resource for the nurses of tomorrow. The decrease in faculty everywhere is due to many factors including decrease in satisfaction with the workforce, poor salaries, and reduction in full-time equivalent. Throughout the span of 6 years the nursing faculty shortage has been written about an increasing amount. Unfortunately, there is no clear consensus or an organized plan on how to fix the ongoing issue.

Continuing Education

With health care knowledge growing steadily, nurses can stay ahead of the curve through continuing education. Continuing education classes and programs enable nurses to provide the best possible care to patients, advance nursing careers, and keep up with Board of Nursing requirements. The American Nurses Association and the American Nursing Credentialing Center are devoted to ensuring nurses have access to quality continuing education offerings. Continuing education classes are calibrated to provide enhanced learning for all levels of nurses. Many States also regulate Continuing Nursing Education. Nursing licensing boards requiring Continuing Nursing Education (CNE) as a condition for licensure, either initial or renewal, accept courses provided by organizations that are accredited by other state licensing boards, by the American Nursing Credentialing Center (ANCC), or by organizations that have been designated as an approver of continuing nursing education by ANCC. There are some exceptions to this rule including the state of California, Florida and Kentucky. National Healthcare Institute has created a list to assist nurses in determining their CNE credit hours requirements. While this list is not all inclusive, it offers details on how to contact nursing licensing boards directly.

Board Certification

Professional nursing organizations, through their certification boards, have voluntary certification exams to demonstrate clinical competency in their particular specialty. Completion of the prerequisite work experience allows an RN to register for an examination, and passage gives an RN permission to use a professional designation after their name. For example, passage of the American Association of Critical-care Nurses specialty exam allows a nurse to use the initials 'CCRN' after his or her name. Other organizations and societies have similar procedures.

The American Nurses Credentialing Center, the credentialing arm of the American Nurses Association, is the largest nursing credentialing organization and administers more than 30 specialty examinations.

Occupational Therapist

An occupational therapist works with a client to help them achieve a fulfilled and satisfied state in life through the use of "purposeful activity or interventions designed to achieve functional outcomes which promote health, prevent injury or disability and which develop, improve, sustain or restore the highest possible level of independence." A practical definition for OT can also be illustrated with the use of models such as the Occupational Performance Model (Australia), known as the OPM(A). At the core of this approach is the ideology that occupational therapists are concerned with the occupations of people and how these contribute to health. Specifically it is a person's occupational performance that influences their health and personal satisfaction of their individual needs. The OPM(A) is constructed on the following definition of Occupational Performance:

The ability to perceive, desire, recall, plan and carry out roles, routines, tasks and subtasks for the purpose of self-maintenance, productivity, leisure and rest in response to demands of the internal and/or external environment.

It can be seen that occupational performance, the roles it creates for a client, and the areas it can encompass are so far-reaching that an occupational therapist can work with a wide range of clients of various limitations who are being cared for in an array of settings. Occupational therapy is about helping people do the day-to-day tasks that "occupy" their time, sustain themselves, and enable them to contribute to the wider community. It is these opportunities to "do", which occupational therapy provides, that prove important and meaningful to the health of people.

Role

Occupational therapists (OTs) help people of all ages to improve their ability to perform tasks in their daily living and working environments. They work with individuals who have conditions that are mentally, physically, developmentally, socially or emotionally disabling. They also help them to develop, recover, or maintain daily living and work skills. Occupational therapists help clients not only to improve their basic motor functions and reasoning abilities, but also to compensate for permanent loss of function. Occupational therapists assist clients in performing activities of all types, ranging from using a computer to caring for daily needs such as dressing, cooking, and eating. Physical exercises may be used to increase strength and dexterity, while other activities may be chosen to improve visual acuity and the ability to discern patterns. For example, a client with short-term memory loss might be encouraged to make lists to aid recall, and a person with coordination problems might be assigned exercises to improve hand-eye coordination. Occupational therapists also use computer programs to help clients improve decision-making, abstract-reasoning, problem solving, and perceptual skills, as well as memory, sequencing, and coordination —- all of which are important for independent living. Occupational therapists are often skilled in psychological strategies such as cognitive behavioral therapy and Acceptance and Commitment Therapy, and may use cognitive therapy especially when introducing people to new strategies for carrying out daily activities such as activity pacing or using effective communication strategies.

Clients With Permanent Disabilities

Therapists instruct those with permanent disabilities, such as spinal cord injuries, cerebral palsy, or muscular dystrophy, in the use of adaptive equipment, including wheelchairs, orthotics, and aids for eating and dressing. They also design or make special equipment needed at home or at work. Therapists develop computer-aided adaptive equipment and teach clients with severe limitations how to use that equipment in order to communicate better and control various aspects of their environment.

Work-related Therapy

Some occupational therapists treat individuals whose ability to function in a work environment has been impaired. These practitioners arrange employment, evaluate the work environment, plan work activities, and assess the client's progress. Therapists also may collaborate with the client and the employer to modify the work environment so that the work can be successfully completed.

With Children

Occupational therapists may work exclusively with individuals in a particular age group or with particular disabilities. In schools, for example, they evaluate children's abilities, recommend and provide therapy, modify classroom equipment, and help children participate as fully as possible in school programs and activities. A therapist may work with children individually, lead small groups in the classroom, consult with a teacher, or serve on a curriculum or other administrative committee. Early intervention therapy services are provided to infants and toddlers who have, or are at the risk of having, developmental delays. Occupational therapist may specialize in the care of infants in the Neonatal Intensive Care Unit, providing developmental care, addressing specific physical problems, assessing neurological function, and providing care givers with education on the care of their infant and the specific problems of a premature infant. Specific therapies may include facilitating the use of the hands, promoting skills for listening and following directions, fostering social skills, or teaching dressing and grooming skills.

With the Elderly

Occupational therapy is very beneficial to the elderly population. Therapists help the elderly lead more productive, active, and independent lives through a variety of methods, including the use of adaptive equipment. Occupational therapists work with the elderly in many varied environments, such as in their homes in the community, in hospital, and in residential care facilities to name a few. In the home environment, occupational therapists may work with the client to assess for hazards and to identify environmental factors that contribute to falls. Occupational therapists are often instrumental in assessing for appropriate wheelchairs for the elderly. In addition, therapists with specialized training in driver rehabilitation assess an individual's ability to drive using both clinical and on-the-road tests. The evaluations allow the therapist to make recommendations for adaptive equipment, training to prolong driving independence, and alternative transport options.

Mental Health

Occupational therapists also work with people who have mental health problems and learning disabilities. In this work, therapists choose activities that help people learn to engage in and cope with daily life. Activities include time management skills, budgeting, shopping, homemaking, and the use of public transportation. Occupational therapists also may work with individuals who are dealing with alcoholism, drug abuse, depression, eating disorders, or stress-related disorders. The ultimate aim would be to help people to engage in a personally satisfying and socially adaptive range of occupations.

With Terminally ill Patients

Occupational therapists work with patients with terminal illness like cancer, Muscular dystrophy,etc. All performance areas including work, play and leisure are widely affected in these sets of patients. An occupational therapist provides various means to these patients to restore or maintain their deteriorating performance components by using their residual capacities and capabilities to give them a sense of self-importance and a measure of confidence.

With People Experiencing Chronic Pain

Occupational therapists often work within interdisciplinary or multidisciplinary teams (professionals such as nurses and doctors) to help individuals with chronic pain develop active self-management strategies. An area of specific concern to occupational therapists is the use of time but it is also common for occupational therapists to help people return to work, and to return to leisure and family activities. Occupational therapists may use a variety of interventions including biofeedback, relaxation, goal setting, problem solving, planning, and carry this out within both group and individual settings. Therapists may work within a clinic setting, or in the community including the workplace, school, home and health care centres. Occupational therapists may assess occupational performance before and after intervention, as a measure of effectiveness and reduction in disability.

Assessment

Assessing and recording a client's activities and progress is an important part of an occupational therapist's job. Accurate records are essential for evaluating clients, for billing, and for reporting to physicians and other health care providers.

Thorough and accurate assessment ensures that Occupational Therapists select appropriate and effective interventions for their clients. Assessment in Occupational Therapy is complex and multifaceted, and is an essential component of the Occupational Therapy Process. Assessment occurs at the beginning of the Process (providing the foundation for effective treatment), at the end (evaluation). Reassessment also occurs throughout intervention.

Hand Therapy

Occupational Therapy also plays a major role in the rehabilitation and recovery of patients who have hand or upper extremity injuries. They play a significant role in liaising with Hand Surgeon/Orthopeadic Surgeon and patients employers or case managers in providing the best client centered rehabilitation program. Occupational Therapist treats conditions ranging from soft tissue injuries such as Tennis Elbows to nerve neuropathies such as Cubital Tunnel Syndrome/ Carpal Tunnel Syndrome. An Array of Upper Limb assessment are utilised to provide a treatment care that is effective and appropriate. Treatment modalities such as orthosis/splints, soft braces and education are some of the common treatment tool that an occupational therapist will use during treatment. Hand Therapy is a specialised field of occupational therapy and it requires therapist to be highly skilled and knowledgeable in upper limb anatomy to be able to work in this area. It is definitely an area where Occupational Therapy is famous for due to the therapeutic models that the profession practices which focus on occupation as means and ends and their aim of returning patients to them performing their daily functions.

Orthotics

Orthotics is a specialty within the medical field concerned with the design, manufacture and application of orthoses. An *orthosis* (plural: *orthoses*) is "an externally applied device used to modify the structural and functional characteristics of the neuromuscular and skeletal system". An orthotist is the primary medical clinician responsible for the prescription, manufacture and management of orthoses. An orthosis may be used to:

- Control, guide, limit and/or immobilize an extremity, joint or body segment for a particular reason
- To restrict movement in a given direction
- To assist movement generally
- To reduce weight bearing forces for a particular purpose
- To aid rehabilitation from fractures after the removal of a cast
- To otherwise correct the shape and/or function of the body, to provide easier movement capability or reduce pain

Orthotics combines knowledge of anatomy and physiology, pathophysiology, biomechanics and engineering. Patients who benefit from an orthosis may have a condition such as spina bifida or cerebral palsy, or have experienced a spinal cord injury or stroke. Equally, orthoses are sometimes used prophylactically or to optimise performance in sport.

Manufacture and Materials

Orthoses were traditionally made by following a tracing of the extremity with measurements to assist in creating a well-fitted device. Subsequently, the advent of plastics as a material of choice for construction necessitated the idea of creating a plaster of Paris mold of the body part in question. This method is still extensively used throughout the industry. Currently, CAD/CAM, CNC machines and 3D printing are involved in orthotic manufacture.

Orthoses are made from various types of materials including thermoplastics, carbon fibre, metals, elastic, EVA, fabric or a combination of similar materials. Some designs may be purchased at a local retailer; others are more specific and require a prescription from a physician, who will fit the orthosis according to the patient's requirements. Over-the-counter braces are basic and available in multiple sizes. They are generally slid on or strapped on with Velcro, and are held tightly in place. One of the purposes of these braces is injury protection.

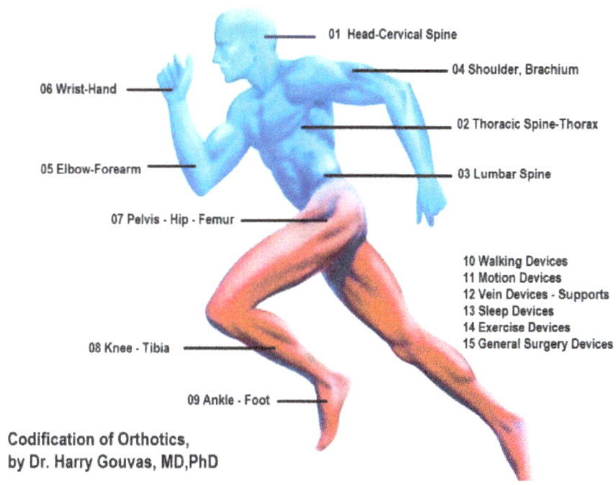

Codification of Orthotics, drawn by Harry Gouvas

Classification

Under the International Standard terminology, orthoses are classified by an acronym describing the anatomical joints which they contain. For example, an ankle foot orthosis ('AFO') is applied to the foot and ankle, a thoracolumbosacral orthosis ('TLSO') affects the thoracic, lumbar and sacral regions of the spine. It is also useful to describe the function of the orthosis. Use of the International Standard is promoted to reduce the widespread variation in description of orthoses, which is often a barrier to interpretation of research studies.

Upper-limb Orthoses

Upper-limb (or upper extremity) orthoses are mechanical or electromechanical devices applied externally to the arm or segments thereof in order to restore or improve function, or structural characteristics of the arm segments encumbered by the device. In general, musculoskeletal problems that may be alleviated by the use of upper limb orthoses include those resulting from trauma or disease (arthritis for example). They may also be beneficial in aiding individuals who have suffered a neurological impairment such as stroke, spinal cord injury, or peripheral neuropathy.

Types of Upper-limb Orthoses

- Upper-limb orthoses

    - Clavicular and shoulder orthoses
    - Arm orthoses
    - Functional arm orthoses
    - Elbow orthoses
- Forearm-wrist orthoses
- Forearm-wrist-thumb orthoses
- Forearm-wrist-hand orthoses
- Hand orthoses
- Upper-extremity orthoses (with special functions)

Lower-limb Orthoses

A lower-limb orthosis is an external device applied to a lower-body segment to improve function by controlling motion, providing support through stabilizing gait, reducing pain through transferring load to another area, correcting flexible deformities, and preventing progression of fixed deformities. The term caliper or calipers remains in widespread use for lower-limb orthoses in the United Kingdom.

Foot Orthoses

Foot orthoses comprise a custom made insert or footbed fitted into a shoe. Commonly referred to as "orthotics" these orthoses provide support for the foot by redistributing ground reaction forces as well as realigning foot joints while standing, walking or running. A great body of information exists within the orthotic literature describing the sciences that might be used to aid people with foot problems as well as the impact "orthotics" can have on foot, knee, hip, and spine deformities. They are used by everyone from athletes to the elderly to accommodate biomechanical deformities and a variety of soft tissue inflammatory conditions such as plantar fasciitis. They may also be used in conjunction with properly fitted orthopaedic footwear in the prevention of foot ulcers in the at-risk diabetic foot.

Ankle-foot Orthosis

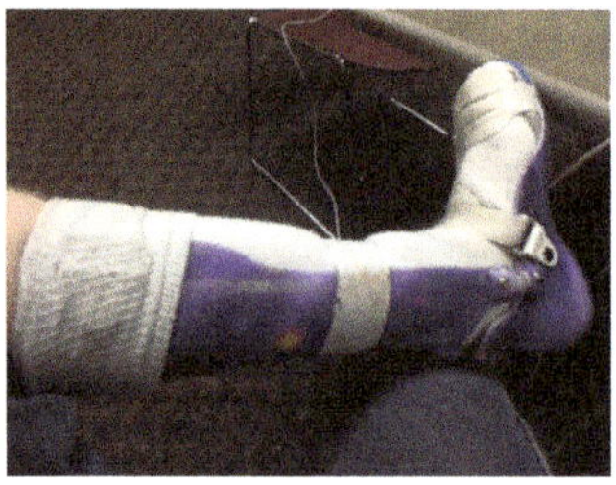

An AFO worn on the left foot with ankle hinge

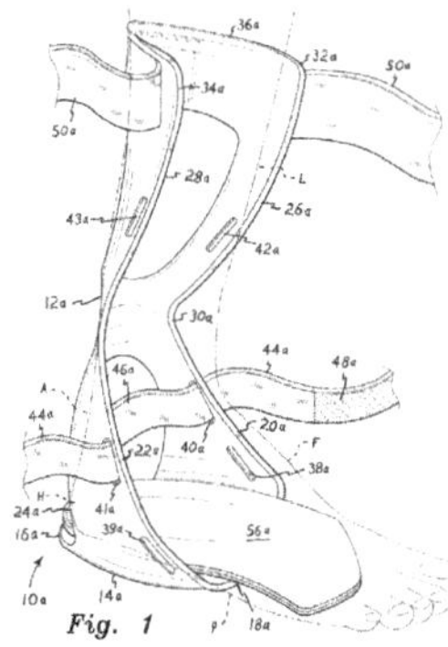

Fig. 1

Schematic ankle-foot orthosis

An ankle-foot orthosis (AFO) is an orthosis or brace that encumbers the ankle and foot. AFOs are externally applied and intended to control position and motion of the ankle, compensate for weakness, or correct deformities. AFOs can be used to support weak limbs, or to position a limb with contracted muscles into a more normal position. They are also used to immobilize the ankle and lower leg in the presence of arthritis or fracture, and to correct foot drop; an AFO is also known as a foot-drop brace. Ankle-foot orthoses are the most commonly used orthoses, making up about 26% of all orthoses provided in the United States. According to a review of Medicare payment data from 2001 to 2006, the base cost of an AFO was about $500 to $700. An AFO is generally constructed of lightweight polypropylene-based plastic in the shape of an "L", with the upright portion behind the calf and the lower portion running under the foot. They are attached to the calf with a strap, and are made to fit inside accommodative shoes. The unbroken "L" shape of some designs provides rigidity, while other designs (with a jointed ankle) provide different types of control.

Obtaining a good fit with an AFO involves one of two approaches:

1. provision of an off-the-shelf or prefabricated AFO matched in size to the end user
2. custom manufacture of an individualized AFO from a positive model, obtained from a negative cast or the use of computer-aided imaging, design, and milling. The plastic used to create a durable AFO must be heated to 400 °F., making direct molding of the material on the end user impossible.

The International Red Cross recognizes four major types of AFOs:

Flexible AFOs	Anti-Talus AFOs	Rigid AFOs	Tamarack Flexure Joint
may provide dorsiflexion assistance, but give poor stabilization of the subtalar joint.	block ankle motion, especially dorsiflexion; do not provide good stabilization for the subtalar joint.	block ankle movements and stabilize the subtalar joint; may also help control adduction and abduction of the forefoot.	provide subtalar stabilization while allowing free ankle dorsiflexion and free or restricted plantar flexion. Depending upon the design; may provide dorsiflexion assistance to correct foot drop.

The International Committee of the Red Cross published its manufacturing guidelines for ankle-foot orthoses in 2006. Its intent is to provide standardized procedures for the manufacture of high-quality modern, durable and economical devices to people with disabilities throughout the world.

Knee-ankle-foot Orthosis (KAFOs)

A knee-ankle-foot orthosis (KAFO) is an orthosis that encumbers the knee, ankle and foot. Motion at all three of these lower limb areas is affected by a KAFO and can include stopping motion, limiting motion, or assisting motion in any or all of the three planes of motion in a human joint: saggital, coronal, and axial. Mechanical hinges, as well as electrically controlled hinges have been used. Various materials for fabrication of a KAFO include but are not limited to metals, plastics, fabrics, and leather. Conditions that might benefit from the use of a KAFO include paralysis, joint laxity or arthritis, fracture, and others. Although not as widely used as knee orthoses, KAFOs can make a real difference in the life of a paralyzed person, helping them to walk therapeutically or, in the case of polio patients, on a community level. These devices are expensive and require maintenance. Some research is being done to enhance the design; even NASA helped spearhead the development of a special knee joint for KAFOs

Knee Orthosis (KO)

A knee orthosis (KO) or knee brace is a brace that extends above and below the knee joint and is generally worn to support or align the knee. In the case of diseases causing neurological or muscular impairment of muscles surrounding the knee, a KO can prevent flexion or extension instability of the knee. In the case of conditions affecting the ligaments or cartilage of the knee, a KO can provide stabilization to the knee by replacing the function of these injured or damaged parts. For instance, knee braces can be used to relieve pressure from the part of the knee joint affected by diseases such as arthritis or osteoarthritis by realigning the knee joint into valgus or varus. In this way a KO may help reduce osteoarthritis pain. However, a knee brace is not meant to treat an injury or disease on its own, but is used as a component of treatment along with drugs, physical therapy and possibly surgery. When used properly, a knee brace may help an individual to stay active by enhancing the position and movement of the knee or reducing pain.

Prophylactic, Functional and Rehabilitation Braces

Prophylactic braces are used primarily by athletes participating in contact sports. Evidence about prophylactic knee braces, the ones football lineman wear are often rigid with a knee hinge, indicates they are ineffective in reducing anterior cruciate ligament tears, but may be helpful in resisting medial and lateral collateral ligament tears.

Functional braces are designed for use by people who have already experienced a knee injury and need support to recover from it. They are also indicated to help people who are suffering from pain associated with arthritis. They are intended to reduce the rotation of the knee and support stability. They reduce the chance of hyperextension, and increase the agility and strength of the knee. The majority of these are made of elastic. They are the least expensive of all braces and are easily found in a variety of sizes.

Rehabilitation braces are used to limit the movement of the knee in both medial and lateral directions- these braces often have an adjustable range of motion stop potential for limiting flexion and extension following ACL reconstruction. They are primarily used after injury or surgery to immobilize the leg. They are larger in size than other braces, due to their function.

Spinal Orthoses

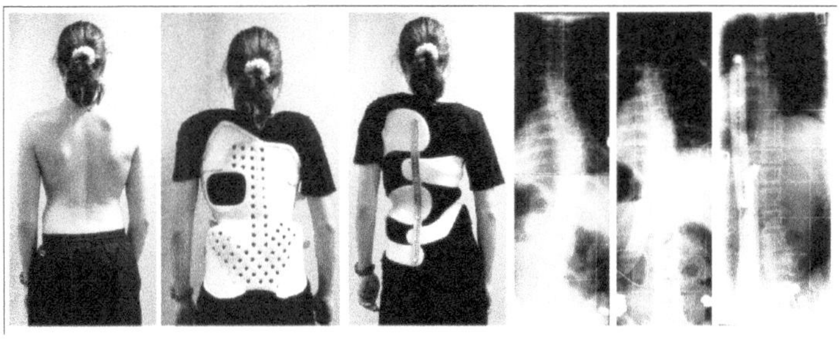

Two different spinal orthoses used to treat scoliosis

Scoliosis, a condition describing an abnormal curvature of the spine, may in certain cases be treated with spinal orthoses, such as the Milwaukee brace, the Boston brace, and Charleston bending brace. As this condition develops most commonly in adolescent females who are undergoing their pubertal growth spurt, compliance with wearing is these orthoses is hampered by the concern these individuals have about changes in appearance and restriction caused by wearing these orthoses. Spinal orthoses may also be used in the treatment of spinal fractures. A Jewett brace, for instance, may be used to facilitate healing of an anterior wedge fracture involving the T10 to L3 vertebrae. A body jacket may be used to stabilize more involved fractures of the spine. The halo brace is a cervical thoracic orthosis used to immobilize the cervical spine, usually following fracture. The halo brace allows the least cervical motion of all cervical orthoses currently in use; it was first developed by Vernon L. Nickel at Rancho Los Amigos National Rehabilitation Center in 1955.

Orthotists

Orthotists are healthcare professionals who specialize in the provision of orthoses. In the United States, orthotists work by prescription from a licensed healthcare provider. Physical therapists are not legally authorized to prescribe orthoses in the U.S. In the U.K., orthotists will often accept open referrals for orthotic assessment without a specific prescription from doctors or other healthcare professionals.

Training Around the World

Canada

In Canada, a Certified Orthotists C.O. (c) provides clinical assessment, patient management, technical design, and fabrication of custom orthoses to maximize patient outcomes. To be awarded certification by the Canadian Board for Certification of Prosthetists and Orthotists (CBCPO) an applicant must meet the following requirements and procedures: must be fluent in French or English, be a Canadian citizen or legal landed immigrant, graduated from a CBCPO approved and officially recognized post-secondary clinical Prosthetic and Orthotic school, completed a minimum 3450 hours of Residency in Orthotics under the direct supervision of a Practitioner that is Canadian certified orthotist, upon completion of the residency the person may apply to sit the national certification exams, pass all the sections of the 3-day national exam that includes written, practical and oral exams, and finally be awarded certification by CBCPO board of directors

United Kingdom

In the UK orthotists assess patients, and where appropriate design and fit orthoses for any part of the body. Registration is with the Health and Care Professions Council . The training is a B.Sc.(Hons) in Prosthetics and Orthotics at either the University of Salford or University of Strathclyde. New graduates are therefore eligible to work as an orthotist and/or prosthetist.

United States

A licensed orthotist is an orthotist who is recognized by the particular state in which they are licensed to have met basic standards of proficiency, as determined by examination and experience to adequately and safely contribute to the health of the residents of that state. An American Board of Certification certified orthotist has met certain standards; these include a degree in orthotics, completion of a one-year residency at an approved clinical site, and passing a rigorous three-part exam. A certified orthotist (CO) is an orthotist who has passed the certification standards of the American Board of Certification in Orthotics, Prosthetics and Pedorthics. Other credentialing bodies who are involved in orthotics include the Board for Orthotic Certification, the pharmaceutical industry, the Professional Footwear Association, and various of the professional associations who work with athletic trainers, physical and occupational therapists, and orthopedic technologists/cast technicians.

Iran

Four universities including the Iran University of Medical Science, Isfahan University of Medical Science, University of Social Welfare and Rehabilitation Sciences and Iran

Red Crescent University confer bachelor of science in the Prosthetics and Orthotics. Three universities including Isfahan University of Medical Science, the Iran University of Medical Science and University of Social Welfare and Rehabilitation Science also confer M.Sc. and Ph.D. New bachelor graduates are eligible to work as an orthotist and prosthetist after registration in the Medical Council of Iran.

Optometry

Optometry is a healthcare profession which involves examining the eyes and applicable visual systems for defects or abnormalities as well as the medical diagnosis and management of eye disease. Traditionally, the field of optometry began with the primary focus of correcting refractive error through the use of spectacles. Modern day optometry, however, has evolved through time so that the educational curriculum additionally includes medical training in the diagnosis and management of ocular disease in countries where the profession is established and regulated. Optometrists (also known as Doctors of Optometry for those holding the O.D. degree or ophthalmic opticians in the U.K) are healthcare professionals who provide primary eyecare through comprehensive eye examinations to detect and treat various visual abnormalities and eye diseases. Being a regulated profession, an optometrist's scope of practice may differ depending on location. Thus, disorders or diseases detected outside the treatment scope of optometry are referred out to relevant medical professionals for proper care, more commonly to ophthalmologists who are medical doctors that specialize in advanced medical and surgical care of the eye. Optometrists typically work closely together with other eye care professionals such as ophthalmologists and opticians to deliver quality and efficient eyecare to the general public.

The word entered the language when the instrument for measuring vision was called an optometer, (before the terms phoropter or refractor were used). The root word *opto* is a shortened form derived from the Greek word *ophthalmos* meaning, "eye." Like most healthcare professions, the education and certification of optometrists is regulated in most countries. Optometric professionals and optometry-related organizations interact with governmental agencies, other healthcare professionals, and the community to deliver eye- and vision-care.

History

The history of optometry can be traced back to the early studies on optics and image formation by the eye. The origins of optometric science (optics, as taught in a basic physics class) date back a few thousand years BC as evidence of the existence of lenses for decoration has been found.

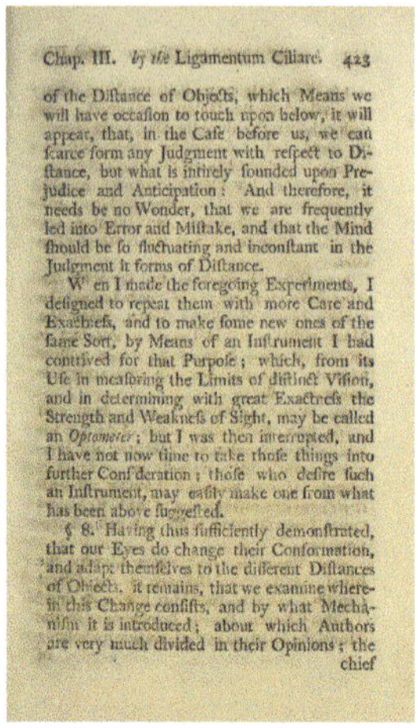

Chap. III. *by the* Ligamentum Ciliare. 423

of the Diſtance of Objects, which Means we will have occaſion to touch upon below, it will appear, that, in the Caſe before us, we can ſcarce form any Judgment with reſpect to Diſtance, but what is intirely founded upon Prejudice and Anticipation: And therefore, it needs be no Wonder, that we are frequently led into Error and Miſtake, and that the Mind ſhould be ſo fluctuating and inconſtant in the Judgment it forms of Diſtance.

When I made the foregoing Experiments, I deſigned to repeat them with more Care and Exactneſs, and to make ſome new ones of the ſame Sort, by Means of an Inſtrument I had contrived for that Purpoſe; which, from its Uſe in meaſuring the Limits of diſtinct Viſion, and in determining with great Exactneſs the Strength and Weakneſs of Sight, may be called an *Optometer*; but I was then interrupted, and I have not now time to take thoſe things into further Conſideration; thoſe who deſire ſuch an Inſtrument, may eaſily make one from what has been above ſuggeſted.

§ 8. Having thus ſufficiently demonſtrated, that our Eyes do change their Conformation, and adapt themſelves to the different Diſtances of Objects, it remains, that we examine wherein this Change conſiſts, and by what Mechaniſm it is introduced; about which Authors are very much divided in their Opinions; the chief

Page 423 from "A treatise on the eye, the manner and phaenomena of vision" by William Porterfield, Published 1759 in Edinburgh. In this book the word "optometer" appears for the first time.

Optometric history is tied to the development of

- vision science (related areas of medicine, microbiology, neurology, physiology, psychology, etc.)
- optics, optical aids
- optical instruments, imaging techniques
- other eye care professions

It is unknown when the first spectacles were made. The British scientist and historian Sir Joseph Needham, in his *Science and Civilization in China*, discusses the occasional claim that spectacles were invented in China. He states that the belief may have been based on a source that was modified during the Ming dynasty (14th - 17th century), that the original document made no references to eyeglasses, and that the references that were there stated the eyeglasses were imported.

Alternatively, research by David A. Goss in the United States shows they may have originated independently in the late 13th century in Italy as stated in a manuscript from 1305 where a monk from Pisa named Rivalto stated "It is not yet 20 years since there was discovered the art of making eyeglasses". Spectacles were manufactured in Italy, Germany, and the Netherlands by 1300.

In 1907 Professor Berthold Laufer, who was a German American anthropologist, stated in his history of spectacles 'the opinion that spectacles originated in India is of the greatest probability and that spectacles must have been known in India earlier than in Europe'.

But Joseph Needham stated in his "Science and Civilization" that the paper by Laufer had many inconsistencies, and that the references in the document used by Laufer were not in the original copies but added during the Ming dynasty.,

However, the German word *brille* (eyeglasses) is derived from Sanskrit *vaidurya*. Etymologically, *brille* is derived from beryl, Latin *beryllus*, from Greek *beryllos*, from Prakrit *verulia, veluriya*, from Sanskrit *vaidurya*, of Dravidian origin from the city of *Velur* (modern *Belur*). Medieval Latin *berillus* was also applied to eyeglasses, hence German *brille*, from Middle High German *berille*, and French *besicles* (plural) *spectacles*, altered from old French *bericle*

Benito Daza de Valdes published the third book on optometry in 1623, where he mentioned the use and fitting of eyeglasses. In 1692, William Molyneux wrote a book on optics and lenses where he stated his ideas on myopia and problems related to close-up vision. The scientists Claudius Ptolemy and Johannes Kepler also contributed to the creation of optometry. Kepler discovered how the retina in the eye creates vision. From 1773 until around 1829, Thomas Young discovered the disability of astigmatism and it was George Biddell Airy who designed glasses to correct that problem that included spherocylindrical lens.

Although the term optometry appeared in the 1759 book *A Treatise on the Eye: The Manner and Phenomena of Vision* by Scottish physician William Porterfield, it was not until the early twentieth century in the United States and Australia that it began to be used to describe the profession. By the early twenty-first century however, marking the distinction with dispensing opticians, it had become the internationally accepted term.

Training, Licensing, Representation and Scope of Practice

Optometry is officially recognized in many jurisdictions. Most have regulations concerning education and practice. Optometrists, like many other healthcare professionals, are required to participate in ongoing continuing education courses to stay current on the latest standards of care. The World Council of Optometry has a web resource that provides basic information on eye care providers for more than 46 countries.

Africa

Ghana

The Ghana Optometric Association (GOA) regulates the practise of Optometry in Ghana. After the six-year training at any of the two Universities offering the course, the O.D degree is awarded. The new Optometrist must write a qualifying exam, after which the optometrist is admitted as a member of the GOA, leading to the award of the title MGOA.

Mozambique

The first optometry course in Mozambique was started in 2009 at Universidade Lurio, Nampula. The course is part of the Mozambique Eyecare Project. University of Ulster, Dublin Institute of Technology and Brien Holden Vision Institute are supporting partners.

Nigeria

In Nigeria, optometry is regulated by the Optometry and Dispensing Opticians Registration Board of Nigeria established under the Optometry and Dispensing Opticians (Registration ETC) Act of 1989 (Cap O9 Laws of Federation of Nigeria 2004). The Boards publishes from time to time lists of approved qualifications and training institutions in the federal government gazette. The Doctor of Optometry degree is awarded after a six-year training at one of the accredited universities in Imo, Edo and Abia states.

Asia

India

In 2010 it was estimated that India needs 115,000 optometrists; whereas India has approximately 9000 optometrists (4-year trained) and 40,000 optometrists (2-year trained). In order to prevent blindness or visual impairment more well trained optometrists are required in India. It should be noted that definition of optometry differs considerably in different countries of the world. India needs more optometry schools offering four-year degree courses with a syllabus similar to that in force in those countries where practice of optometry is statutorily regulated and well established with an internationally accepted definition.

In 2013 it was reported in the Indian Journal of Ophthalmology that poor spectacle compliance amongst school children in rural Pune resulted in significant vision loss.

In 2015 it was reported in the Optometry and Vision Science that, optometrists need to be more involved in providing core optometry services like binocular vision and low vision.

Training in India

At present there are more than fifty schools of optometry in India. In 1958, two schools of optometry were established, one at Gandhi Eye Hospital, Aligarh in Uttar Pradesh and other one at Sarojini Devi Eye Hospital, Hyderabad in Andhra Pradesh, under second five-year plan by Director General of Health Services of Government of India. These schools offered diplomas in optometry courses of two years duration validated by State Medical Faculties.

Subsequently, four more schools were opened across India situated at Sitapur Eye Hospital, Sitapur in Uttar Pradesh, Chennai (formerly Madras) in Tamil Nadu, Bengalooru (formerly Bangalore) in Karnataka and Thiruvananthapuram (formerly Trivandrum) in Kerala.

The Elite School of Optometry (ESO) was established in 1985 at Chennai and was the first to offer a four-year degree course.

Academic degrees such as Bachelor of Optometry, Master of Optometry and Doctor of Philosophy in Optometry are awarded in India by the universities recognised by University Grants Commission (India), a statutory body responsible for the maintenance of standards of higher education in India.

Optometrists across India are encouraged to register with the Optometry Council of India, a self-regulatory body registered under the Indian Company Act.

Malaysia

It takes four years to complete a Degree in Optometry. Today, optometry courses are well received by citizens. More universities and higher education studies are about to implement the courses. e.g. National Institute of Ophthalmic Sciences in Petaling Jaya whereby it is the academic arm of The Tun Hussein Onn National Eye Hospital.

Pakistan

Optometry is taught as a five/four-year Doctor/ Bachelors/ Bachelors with Honors course at many institutions notable among which are Department of Optometry & Vision Sciences (DOVS) FAHS, ICBS, Lahore, Pakistan Institute of Community Ophthalmology (PICO) Peshawar, College of Ophthalmology & Allied Vision Sciences (COAVS) Lahore and Al-Shifa Institute of Ophthalmology Islamabad. After graduation the optometrists can join a four-tiered service delivery level (Centre of Excellence, Tertiary/ Teaching, District headquarter and sub-district /Tehsil headquarters). M.Phil in Optometry is also available at select institutions such as King Edward Medical University, Lahore Department of Optometry & Vision Sciences (DOVS) FAHS, ICBS, Lahore started bridging programmes for Bachelors/ Bachelors with Honors to become Doctor of Optometry OD, Post Professional Doctor of Optometry(PP-OD), Transitional Doctor of Optometry(t-OD). Optometry is not yet a regulated field in Pakistan as there is no professional licensing board or authority responsible for issuing practice licenses to qualified optometrists. This creates difficulty for Pakistani optometrists who wish to register abroad. University of Lahore has recently launched Doctor of optometry (OD)

Philippines

Optometry is regulated by the Professional Regulation Commission of the Philippines. To be eligible for licensing, each candidate must have satisfactorily completed a doctor of optometry course at an accredited institution and demonstrate good moral character with no previous record of professional misconduct. Professional organizations of optometry in the Philippines include Optometric Association of the Philippines and Integrated Philippine Association of Optometrists, Inc. (IPAO).

Saudi Arabia

In Saudi Arabia optometrists must complete a five-year doctor of optometry degree from Qassim University and King Saud University .

Singapore

Tertiary education for optometrists takes 3 years at the following institutions.

Singapore Polytechnic - Diploma in Optometry Singapore Polytechnic

Ngee Ann Polytechnic - Diploma in Optometry Ngee Ann Polytechnic

Thailand

Since later 1990, Thailand has set goal to provide more than 600 optometrists to meet the minimal public demands and international standards in vision cares. There are more than three university degree programs in Thailand. Each program accept students that have completed grade 12th or the third year in high school (following US education model.) These programs offer "Doctor of Optometry" degree to graduates from the program that will take six years to complete the courses. Practicing optometrists will also required to pass licensing examination (three parts examinations) that is administrated through a committee under the Ministry of Public Health.

Nowadays, the number of practicing optometrists in Thailand is still less than one hundred. However, it has projected that the number of practicing optometrists in Thailand will greatly increase within the next ten years. In theoretical scenario, the number of optometrists should be able to meet minimal public demands around 2030 or earlier.

Australasia

Australia

Australia currently has five recognized courses in optometry:

- Bachelor of Vision Science and Master of Optometry (BVisSci MOptom), Deakin University
- Bachelor of Medical Science (Vision Science) and Master of Optometry, Flinders University
- Bachelor of Optometry Bachelor of Science (BOptom BSc), University of New South Wales
- Bachelor of Vision Science and Master of Optometry, Queensland University of Technology
- Doctor of Optometry, Melbourne University (post-graduate)

To support these courses the Australian College of Optometry provides clinical placements to undergraduate students from Australian Universities and abroad.

in 2016, almost 5000 optometrists in general practice were licensed with their regulatory body,the Optometry Board of Australia. Of these, approximately 2300 were registered with the scheduled medicines endorsement, which enables them to prescribe some medicines for the treatment of conditions of the eye.

New Zealand

New Zealand currently has one recognised course in optometry:

- Bachelor of Optometry (BOptom), The University of Auckland

In July 2014, the Medicines Amendment Act 2013 and Misuse of Drugs Amendment Regulations 2014 came into effect. Among other things, the changes to the Act name optometrists as authorised prescribers. This change enables optometrists with a therapeutic pharmaceutical agent (TPA) endorsement to prescribe all medicines appropriate to their scope of practice, rather than limiting them to a list of medicines specified in regulation; this recognises the safe and appropriate prescribing practice of optometrists over the previous nine years.

Europe

Since the formation of the European Union, "there exists a strong movement, headed by the Association of European Schools and Colleges of Optometry (AESCO), to unify the profession by creating a European-wide examination for optometry" and presumably also standardized practice and education guidelines within EU countries. The first examinations of the new European Diploma in Optometry were held in 1998 and this was a landmark event for optometry in continental Europe.

Francc

There is no regulatory framework and optometrists are sometimes trained by completing an apprenticeship at an ophthalmologists' private office.

Germany

Optometric tasks are performed by ophthalmologists and professionally trained and certified opticians.

Greece

Hellenic Ministry of Education founded the first department of Optometry at Technological Educational Institute of Patras in 2007. After protests from the department of Optics at Technological Educational Institute of Athens (the only department of Optics in Greece, until 2006), the Government changed the names of the departments to "Optics and Optometry" and included lessons in both optics and optometry. Optometrists-Opticians have to complete a 4-year undergraduate honours degree. Then the graduates can be admitted to postgraduate courses in Optometry at universities around the world.

Since 2015, a Master of Science (MSc) course in Optometry is offered by the Technological Educational Institute of Athens.

The Institute of Vision and Optics (IVO) of the University of Crete focuses on the sciences of vision and is active in the fields of research, training, technology development and provision of medical services. Professor Ioannis Pallikaris has received numerous awards and recognitions for the Institute's contribution to ophthalmology. In 1989 he performed the first LASIK procedure on a human eye.

Hungary

Optometrists education takes 4 years in the medical universities in Hungary, and they will get a Bachelor of Science degree. They work in networks and retail stores and private optics, very few are located in the Health Care care system as ophthalmologists as an assistant.

Ireland

The profession of Optometry has been represented for over a century by the Association of Optometrists, Ireland [AOI]. In Ireland an optometrist must first complete a four-year degree in optometry at Dublin Institute of Technology. Following successful completion of the a degree, an optometrist must then complete professional qualifying examinations to enter the register of the Opticians Board [Bord na Radharcmhaistoiri]. Optometrists must be registered with the Board to practice in the Republic of Ireland.

The A.O.I. runs a comprehensive continuing education and professional development program on behalf of Irish optometrists. The legislation governing optometry was drafted in 1956. Some feel that the legislation restricts optometrists from using their full range of skills, training and equipment for the benefit of the Irish public. The amendment to the Act in 2003 addressed one of the most significant restrictions: the use of cycloplegic drugs to examine children.

Italy

The Italian Government does not legally recognise optometry as a health profession;Optometric tasks are performed by ophthalmologists and optometry has been declared illegal and not existing since July 2016. anyway before this sentence the highest court used to recognize that "optometry can be practiced, given that there are no law that prohibit it". It is taught at seven universities: Padua, Turin, Milan, Salento, Florence, Naples and Rome, as three years course (like a BSc) of "Scienze e tecnologie fisiche" as sector of the Physics Department, but you cannot practice this discipline being illegal.

Additionally, courses are available at some private institutions (as at Vinci Institute near Firenze) that offer advanced professional education for already qualified opticians (most of the Italian optometrists are also qualified opticians, i.e. "ottico abilitato"). The fitness-to-practice is granted by the study title itself (i.e.: "titolo abilitante") after an exam; there are no professional councils nor registry nor regulatory bodies, other than the government Ministry of Health itself, which does not recognize this title.

Norway

In Norway the optometric profession has been regulated as a healthcare profession since 1988. After a three-year bachelor program one can practice basic optometry. At least one year in clinical practice qualify for a post-degree half-year sandwich course in contact lens fitting, which is regulated as a healthcare specialty. A separate regulation for the use of diagnostic drugs in optometric practice was introduced in 2004.

Russia

In Russia optometry education has been accredited by the Federal Agency of Health and Social Development. There are only two educational institutions that teach optometry in Russia: Saint Petersburg Medical Technical College, formerly known as St. Petersburg College of Medical Electronics and Optics, and The Helmholtz Research Institute for Eye Diseases. They both belong and are regulated by the Ministry of Health. The optometry program is a four-year program. It includes one to two science foundation years, one year focused on clinical and proficiency skills, and one year of clinical rotations in hospitals. Graduates take college/state examinations and then receive a specialist diploma. This diploma is valid for only five years and must be renewed every five years after receiving additional training at state accredited programs.

The scope of practice for optometrists in Russia includes: refraction, contact lens fitting, spectacles construction and lens fitting (dispensing), low vision aids, foreign body removal, referrals to other specialists after clinical condition diagnoses (management of diseases in the eye).

United Kingdom

Licensing

Optometrists in the United Kingdom (also known as *ophthalmic opticians*) are regulated by the General Optical Council under the Opticians Act 1989 and distinguished from medical practitioners. Registration with the GOC is mandatory to practice optometry in the UK. Members of the College of Optometrists (incorporated by a Royal Charter granted by Her Majesty Queen Elizabeth II) may use the suffix MCOptom.

The National Health Service provides for the medical, ophthalmic (covering optometry), dental and other ancillary needs of every person in the UK.

Training

In the United Kingdom, optometrists have to complete a 3 or 4 (Scotland) year undergraduate honours degree followed by a minimum of a one-year "pre-registration period", (internship), where they complete clinical practice under the supervision of a qualified and experienced practitioner. During this year the pre-registration candidate is given a number of quarterly assessments, often including temporary posting at a hospital, and on successfully passing all of these assessments, a final one-day set of examinations (details correct for candidates from 2006 onwards). Following successful completion of these assessments and having completed one year's supervised practice, the candidate is eligible to register as an optometrist with the General Optical Council (GOC) and, should they so wish, are entitled to membership of the College of Optometrists. Ten universities offer Optometry in the UK: Anglia Ruskin, Aston, Bradford, Cardiff, City, Glasgow Caledonian, Hertfordshire, Manchester, University of Plymouth and Ulster University at Coleraine, University of Portsmouth

Additionally, the Institute of Optometry in London offers a post-graduate professional doctorate in optometry in partnership with London South Bank University.

Scope of Practice

In 1990 a survey of the opinions of British medical practitioners regarding the services provided by British optometrists was carried out by Agarwal at City University in London. A majority of respondents were in favour of optometrists extending their professional role by treating external eye conditions and prescribing broad spectrum topical antibiotics through additional training and certification.

Since 2009, optometrists in the UK have been able to undertake additional postgraduate training and qualifications that allow them to prescribe medications to treat and manage eye conditions. There are currently three registerable specialties:

- Additional supply specialty - to write orders for, and supply in an emergency, a range of drugs in addition to those ordered or supplied by a normal optometrist.
- Supplementary prescribing specialty - to manage a patient's clinical condition and prescribe medicines according to a clinical management plan set up in conjunction with an independent prescriber, such as a GP or ophthalmologist or qualified optometrist.
- Independent prescribing specialty - to take responsibility for the clinical assessment of a patient, establish a diagnosis and determine the clinical management required, including prescribing where necessary.

North America

Canada

Training

In Canada, in order to obtain their professional designation, doctor of optometry degree, optometrists typically must complete minimum three years undergraduate education, and a four or five year university program in optometry accredited by the Accreditation Council on Optometric Education. There are two schools of optometry located in Canada and 20 in the United States that are accredited and recognized in Canada. The two Canadian schools of optometry accredited are at the University of Waterloo and at Université de Montreal. Upon completion of their optometry education, they are also required to satisfy the provincial requirements of the province or territory they are intended to practice. These requirements include a national examination administered by the Canadian Examiners in Optometry, and licensure by the provincial or territorial governing body.

Licensing

In Canada, regulatory of professions is within provincial jurisdiction. Therefore, regulation of optometry is unique to individual provinces and territories. In Ontario, optometrists are licensed by the College of Optometrists of Ontario.

Representation

In Canada the profession is represented by the Canadian Association of Optometrists. In the province of Ontario, the Ontario Association of Optometrists is the designated representative of optometrists to the provincial government.

Scope of Practice

Optometrists in Canada are licensed to prescribe topical and oral medications; however, the exact medications that they are licensed to prescribe varies province by province. In Ontario, optometrists are able to prescribe drugs to treat normal tension glaucoma (a type of primary glaucoma), transient intraocular pressure elevations, an acute glaucoma crisis, and dacryocystitis. In Alberta, optometrists will soon have their scope of practice increased to include prescribing certain oral and topical drugs, ordering lab tests, ordering and applying ultrasound tests, and treating certain types of glaucoma.

United States

Optometrists in the United States are doctors of optometry (O.D.) who function as primary eye care providers. While optometrists traditionally specialize in refractive vision correction through eyeglasses and contact lenses, the practice of optometry has now developed significant overlap with general ophthalmology, the branch of medicine involving the health of the eyes and visual system. Optometrists are licensed to diagnose and treat many common diseases of the eye through oral, topical, diagnostic, and therapeutic medications. Doctors of optometry are also currently able to perform certain types of laser surgery in three states, Oklahoma, Kentucky, and Louisiana.

Scope of Practice

Within the United States healthcare system, optometrists function as primary eye care providers who are especially experienced in fitting contact lenses and eyeglass prescriptions while also treating and managing common eye diseases such as glaucoma and dry eye syndrome. Optometrists are also known as optometric physicians (O.D.), held to the same standard as other government regulated health care practitioners participating in Medicare. Ophthalmologists are medical eye physicians and surgeons (M.D. or D.O.) who have completed medical school, ophthalmology residency, and specialty fellowship in certain divisions of ocular surgery (example: cornea, retina, glaucoma, etc.). Opticians are eye care professionals who fit and dispense vision correcting lens prescriptions written by optometrists and ophthalmologists.

Today's optometrists manage the majority of primary eye care and medical eye care in the United States. They conduct routine comprehensive eye exams, prescribe refractive eyeglass and contact lens prescriptions, and manage many common eye diseases and conditions (example: glaucoma, diabetic retinopathy, dry eye syndrome, red eye, anterior uveitis, etc.). When their patients require tertiary care and surgical management, optometrists often refer and co-manage with ophthalmology. When systemic conditions are suspect, today's optometrists will also co-manage medical cases with other medical specialties including internal medicine, emergency medicine, neurology, rheumatology, dermatology, pediatrics, oncology, and radiology.

Optometrists in the United States are licensed to treat eye diseases with:

- Oral medications such as antibiotics, antivirals, steroids, and short term narcotics.)
- Topical medications such as prescription eye drops to treat eye infections, anterior uveitis, and glaucoma.

Optometrists in the United States may also be trained in certain surgical procedures, including ocular foreign body removal, corneal epithelial debridement, removal of "lumps and bumps" around the eyes, ocular injections, and even certain laser surgeries including yag capsulotomy, laser trabeculoplasty, and peripheral iridotomy.

The scope of practice in optometry varies state to state and is individually regulated. For example:

- In Oklahoma and Louisiana, the state optometry board also allows state-certified optometrists to perform surgeries limited to the anterior segment of the eye.
- In Kentucky, recent legislation permits Optometrists to perform a multitude of laser procedures.

Regulation

Doctors of optometry in the United States are currently regulated by state boards that determine their scope of practice, which may vary from state to state. The Association of Regulatory Boards of Optometry (ARBO) assists these state board licensing agencies in regulating the practice of optometry.

Licensing

The American Optometric Association (AOA) represents optometrists nationally in the United States. Prior to admittance into optometry school, optometrists typically complete four years of undergraduate study, culminating in a bachelor's degree. Required undergraduate coursework for pre-optometry students covers a variety of health, science, and mathematics courses. These courses include: four semesters of chemistry (including general, organic, and biochemistry + laboratories), two semesters of physics and biology + laboratories, as well as one semester of calculus, statistics, physiology, anatomy, microbiology, and psychology. Additional requirements are imposed by specific institutions. Once completing these courses, admission to an optometry doctorate program requires that candidates score well on the O.A.T., Optometry Admission Tests. There are currently 21 optometry schools in the United States, and admission into these schools is highly competitive.

Education and Training

Optometrists are required to complete a four-year postgraduate degree program to earn their doctor of optometry (O.D.) titles. The four-year program includes classroom and clinical training in geometric, physical, physiological and ophthalmic optics, specialty contact lens evaluation and fitting, ocular anatomy, ocular disease, ocular pharmacology, neuroanatomy and neurophysiology of the vision system, pediatric visual development, gerontology, binocular vision, color, form, space, movement and vision perception, design and modification of the visual environment, and vision performance and vision screening. In addition, an optometric education also includes human anatomy, systemic diseases, general pharmacology, general pathology, microbiology, sensory and perceptual psychology, biochemistry, statistics and epidemiology.

Upon completion of an accredited program in optometry, graduates hold the doctor of optometry degree (O.D.) and are able to apply for licensure to practice optometry in the state of their choosing after passing three national board examinations. Optometrists must pass all national board examinations administered by the National Board of Examiners in Optometry (NBEO) during their four years of postgraduate education. This three-part examination includes applied basic science, patient assessment and management, and clinical skills performance testing. Some optometrists go on to complete one to two-year residency and fellowship training in a specific sub-specialty such as ocular disease, cornea and specialty contact lens, pediatric eye care, vision therapy and rehabilitation, refractive and ocular surgical co-management, low vision, neuro-optometry, and traumatic brain injury vision rehabilitation. All optometrists are required to fulfill continuing education requirements to stay current regarding the latest standards of care.

South America

Argentina

In Argentina optometrists are required to register with the local Ministry of Public Information, but licensing is not required. Anyone holding a bachelor's degree may register as an optometrist after completing a written exam. Fees for the exam are set by the provincial government and vary from province to province.

Brazil

The Brazilian Government does not state rules about optometry, and the Brazilian Council of Ophthalmology recommends against its official legal recognition.

The CBOO (Brazilian Council of Optics and Optometry), which is affiliated to the WCO (World Council of Optometry), represents Brazilian optometrists. In conjunction with organizations representative weight of Brazilian companies, including the National Commerce Confederation for goods, services and tourism (CNC), through the CBÓptica/CNC, its defense arm of optometric and optical industry, are defending the right of free and independent practice of optometrists, even if it is against the interests of ophthalmologists.

The Federal Supreme Court (STF), the Brazilian Court of Justice and the Superior Court of Justice (STJ), another important National Court, ruled several processes granting inquestionable victories to optometrists.

Opticals, Optometry Centres and Optometry Clinics have nowadays operating permission granted by the health authorities since 2008, when the first Judgement in Supreme Courts grateful for the work of the professionals of optometry.

In Brazilian law, however, there is an explicit recommendation that the one prescribing corrective lenses are prohibited to sell them. This restricting rule to the ophthalmologists has keeping the optic shops away from Hospitals and Eye Care Clinics since 1930, and it has to be reviewed before any further regulation for the optometrists.

Colombia

In Colombia optometry education has been accredited by the Ministry of Health. The last official revision to the laws regarding healthcare standards in the country was issued in 1992 through the Law 30. Currently there are eight official universities that are entitled by ICFES to grant the optometrist certification. The first optometrists arrived in the country from North America and Europe circa 1914. These professionals specialized in optics and refraction. In 1933, under Decrees 449 and 1291, the Colombian Government officially set the rules for the formation of professionals in the field of optometry. In 1966 La Salle University opened its first Faculty of Optometry after recommendation from a group of professionals. At the present time optometrists are encouraged to keep up with new technologies through congresses and scholarships granted by the government or the private sector (such as Bausch & Lomb).

Prosthetist

A prosthetist, as defined by The American Board for Certification in Orthotics, Prosthetics and Pedorthics, Inc., is a person who measures, designs, fabricates, fits, or services a prosthesis as prescribed by a licensed physician, and who assists in the formulation of the prosthesis prescription for the replacement of external parts of the human body lost due to amputation or congenital deformities or absences.

A prosthetist is a person who has been certified to fit prostheses to residual limbs of the upper and lower extremities. The fitting of lower extremity prostheses, for example, involves making a socket that fits the residuum as a first step. The socket is usually manufactured by glass or carbon fiber infused with acrylic resin or from thermoplastics over a positive model of the residuum. The socket is connected to a foot or ankle assembly and in the case of above knee amputation, an artificial knee. The connecting components are usually an aluminum tube with two part pyramid alignment devises one at each end. One of the devices connects to the ankle and the other one to the socket. They allow the foot to be placed in proper position to support the person's weight with the least possible lateral forces acting through the system. Prostheses are aligned with the client walking, while the prosthetist observes the gait and corrects for any deviations from optimized movement when the leg is in the air and for its position at heel strike and toe off.

In the United States, a Certified Prosthetist (CP) is a prosthetist who has passed the psychometrically validated certification standards and met the established educational criteria of The American Board for Certification in Orthotics, Prosthetics and Pedorthics, Inc. and maintains certification through mandatory continuing education program and adherence to the Code of Professional Responsibility. The Board for Orthotic Certification also has a designation (boco) for people who have passed their test.

Iran

Four universities including the Iran University of Medical Science, Isfahan University of Medical Science, University of Social Welfare and Rehabilitation Sciences and Iran Red Crescent University confer bachelor of science in the Prosthetics and Orthotics. Three universities including Isfahan University of Medical Science , the Iran University of Medical Science and University of Social Welfare and Rehabilitation Science also confer M.Sc. and Ph.D. New bachelor graduates are eligible to work as an orthotist and prosthetist after registration in the Medical Council of Iran.

Psychiatric Rehabilitation

Psychiatric rehabilitation, also known as psychosocial rehabilitation, and sometimes simplified to psych rehab by providers, is the process of restoration of community functioning and well-being of an individual diagnosed in mental health or mental or emotional disorder and who may be considered to have a psychiatric disability.

Society affects the psychology of an individual by setting a number of rules, expectations and laws. Psychiatric rehabilitation work is undertaken by rehabilitation counselors (especially the individuals educated in psychiatric rehabilitation), licensed professional counselors (who work in the mental health field), psych rehab consultants or specialists (in private businesses), university level Masters and PhD levels, classes of related disciplines in mental health (psychiatrists, social workers, psychologists, occupational therapists) and community support or allied health workers represented in the new direct support professional workforce in the United States (e.g., psychiatric aides).

These workers seek to affect changes in a person's environment and in a person's ability to deal with his/her environment, so as to facilitate improvement in symptoms or personal distress and life outcomes. These services often "combine pharmacologic treatment (often required for program admission), independent living and social skills training, psychological support to clients and their families, housing, vocational rehabilitation and employment, social support and network enhancement and access to leisure activities." There is often a focus on challenging stigma and prejudice to enable social inclusion, on working collaboratively in order to empower clients, and sometimes on a goal of full recovery. The latter is now widely known as a recovery approach or model. Recovery is a process rather than an outcome. It is a personal journey that is about the rediscovery of self in the process of learning to live with the debilitations of the illness rather than being defined by illness with hope, planning and community engagement.

Yet, new in these fields is a person-centered approach to recovery and client-centered therapy based upon Carl Rogers. and user-service direction (as approved in the US by the Centers for Medicare and Medicaid Services).

Definition

Psychiatric rehabilitation is not a practice but a field of academic study or discipline, similar to social work or political science; other definitions may place it as a specialty of community rehabilitation or physical medicine and rehabilitation. It is aligned with the community support development of the National Institute on Mental Health begun in the 1970s, and is marked by a rigorous tradition of research, training and technical assistance, and information dissemination regarding a critical population group (e.g., psychiatric disability) in the US and worldwide. The field is responsible for developing and testing new models of community service for this population group.

The Psychiatric Rehabilitation Association provides this definition of psychiatric rehabilitation:

Psychiatric rehabilitation promotes recovery, full community integration, and improved quality of life for persons who have been diagnosed with any mental health condition that seriously impairs their ability to lead meaningful lives. Psychiatric rehabilitation services are collaborative, person-directed and individualized. These services are an essential element of the health care and human services spectrum, and should be evidence-based. They focus on helping individuals develop skills and access resources needed to increase their capacity to be successful and satisfied in the living, working, learning, and social environments of their choice.

The term was added to the U.S. National Library of Medicine's Medical Subject Headings (MeSH) in 2016. There, psychiatric rehabilitation is defined as a:

Specialty field that promotes recovery, community functioning, and increased well-being of individuals diagnosed with mental disorders that impair their ability to live meaningful lives.

History

From the 1960s and 1970s, the process of de-institutionalization meant that many more individuals with mental health problems were able to live in their communities rather than being confined to mental institutions. Medication and psychotherapy were the two major treatment approaches, with little attention given to supporting and facilitating daily functioning and social interaction. Therapeutic interventions often had little impact on daily living, socialization and work opportunities. There were often barriers to social inclusion in the form of stigma and prejudice.

Psychiatric rehabilitation work emerged with the aim of helping the community integration and independence of individuals with mental health problems. "Psychiatric rehabilitation" and "psychosocial rehabilitation" became used interchangeably, as terms for the same practice. These approaches may merge with or conflict with approaches based in the psychiatric survivors movement, including the concept of user-controlled personal assistance services.

In the 1980s, the US Department of Education, National Institute on Disability Research and Rehabilitation, revised a Rehabilitation Research and Training Center program to meet the new needs in the community of special population groups. A priority center, published in the Federal Register, was the Rehabilitation Research and Training Center in Psychiatric Disabilities (awarded to William Anthony's Boston University Center). As of 2015, it remains a priority center, providing nationwide assistance and serving as flagship center internationally.

With the founding of Psychosocial Rehabilitation Canada in 2004, the professional organization International Association of Psychosocial Rehabilitation Services (IAPSRS) changed its name to United States Psychiatric Rehabilitation Association (USPRA) and the trend is toward the use of "psychiatric rehabilitation." In 2013, USPRA removed the national designation from its name, becoming the Psychiatric Rehabilitation Association (PRA).

Academic Discipline

In 2012, Temple University was funded in the field of psychiatric disabilities for a national center with the National Institute on Disability and Rehabilitation Research (NIDRR), United States Department of Education, having this population group as a priority. Boston University's Center on Psychiatric Rehabilitation's director is President-Elect of the NAARTC program and Boston University College of Health and Rehabilitation Sciences (Sargent College) awards a Rehabilitation Science Doctor of Science (ScD) degree in the field in which it awards no separate mental health specialty degree (such as occupational therapy). Master' program in psychiatric rehabilitation was part of a MA degree in rehabilitation counseling in the School of Education, Syracuse University and courses were funded in part through the federal Rehabilitation Research and Training Program (now part of National Institute on Disability, Independent Living and Rehabilitation Research).

Theory

The theoretical base for psychosocial then psychiatric rehabilitation is community support theory as the foundational theory; it is aligned with integration and community integration theories, psychosocial theories, and the rehabilitation and educational paradigms. Its fluid nature is due to variability in development and integration into other essential fields such as family support theories (for this population group) which has already developed its own evidence-based parent education models.

The concept of psychiatric rehabilitation is associated with the field of community rehabilitation and later on social psychiatry and is not based on a medical model of disability or the concept of mental illness which is often associated with the words "mental health". However, it can also incorporate elements of a social model of disability as part of progressive professional community field. The academic field developed concurrently with the formation of new mental health agencies in the US, now often offerring supported housing services.

The *Journal of Psychosocial Rehabilitation*, then renamed the *Journal of Psychiatric Rehabilitation*, traces the development of the field over a period of several decades. The academic discipline psychiatric rehabilitation has contributed new models of services such as supported education, has cross-validated models from other fields (e.g., supported employment), has developed the *first university-based community living models for populations with "severe mental illness"*, developed institutional to community training and technical assistance, developed the degree programs at the university levels, offers leadership institutes, and worked collaboratively to expand and upgrade older models such as clubhouses and transitional employment services, among others.

Psychiatric rehabilitation was developed and formulated as a new profession of community workers (not medical psychiatry which is a MD awarded by a Medical School) which could assist both in deinstitutionalization (e.g., systems conversion) and in community development in the US. It represents the first Master's and Ph.D. classes in the US to specialize in a rehabilitation discipline focused on community versus institutions or campuses. In the US, it also represents a movement toward evidence-based practices, critical for the development of viable community support services.

Psychosocial services, in contrast, have been associated with the term "mental health" as part of community support movement nationwide since the 1970s which has an academic and political base. These services, which have roots in education, psychology and mental health (and community services) administration, were basic funded services of new community mental health agencies offering community living and professionalized community support since the 1970s. Mental health service agencies or multi-service agencies in the non-profit and voluntary sectors form a critical delivery system for psychosocial services. In the 2000s, a sometime similar but sometimes alternative approach (variability and fidelity of provider implementation in the field) employs the concept of psychosocial recovery.

Psychiatric rehabilitation was promulgated in the US through Boston University's Rehabilitation Research and Training Center on Psychiatric Rehabilitation led by Dr. William Anthony and Dr. Marianne Farkas, as well as other professors and teachers such as Julie Ann Racino, Steve Murphy and Bonnie Shoultz of Syracuse University (1989-1991) who also support a generic community approach to education. The concept has been integrated with a community support approach, including supported housing/housing and support, recreation, employment and support, culture/gender and class, families and survivors, family support, and community and systems change.

Problems experienced by people with psychiatric disabilities are thought to include difficulties understanding or dealing with interpersonal situations (e.g., misinterpreting social cues, not knowing how to respond), prejudice or bullying from others because they may seem different, problems coping with stress (including daily hassles such as travel or shopping), difficulty concentrating and finding energy and motivation. People leaving psychiatric centers after long-term hospitalizations, an outdated practice, may also have need to assist with injuries that may have occurred and community integration.

Psychiatric rehabilitation is distinct from the concept of independent living and consumer-controlled services which have been written about and promoted by psychiatric survivors. The psychiatric rehabilitation concept is separated from the psychiatric survivor concept, in education and training of individuals with psychiatric disorders, in that psychiatric survivors tend to operate services and control funding.

Services

Psychiatric rehabilitation services may include: community residential services, workplace accommodations, supported employment or education, social firms, assertive community (or outreach) teams assisting with social service agencies, medication management (e.g., self-medication training and support), housing, programs, employment, family issues, coping skills and activities of daily living and socialising. Traditionally, "24-hour" service programs (supervised and regulated options) were based upon the concept of instrumental and daily living skills as formulated in the World Health Organization (WHO) definition.

Psychiatric rehabilitation is illustrated by agency models which are offerred by traditional and non-traditional service providers, and may be considered to be integrated (e.g., dispersed sites in the community) or segregated (e.g., campus-based facilities or villages). (e.g., Fountain House Model of New York City, MHA Village in Long Beach, CA)or Transitional Living Services of Buffalo or Transitional Living Services of Onondaga County, New York. Agencies supporting integration may align with normalization or integration philosophy, as opposed to the older sheltered workshop or day care models which have been criticized for underpayment of wages at the US Congressional level in the late 2000s.

Agencies may deliver cross-field best practices (e.g., supported work), consumer voices (e.g., Rae Unzicker), multiple disabilities (e.g., chemical dependency), training of its own community residential, employment, education and support service professionals, rehabilitation outcomes, and management and evaluation of its own services.

Core principles of effective psychiatric rehabilitation (how services are delivered) must include:

- providing hope when the client lacks it,
- respect for the client wherever they are in the recovery process,
- empowering the client,
- teaching the client wellness planning, and
- emphasizing the importance for the client to develop social support networks.

Psychiatric rehabilitation (what services are delivered) varies by provider and may consist of eight main areas:

- Psychiatric (symptom management; relaxation, meditation and massage; support groups and in-home assistance)
- Health and Medical (maintaining consistency of care; family physician and mental health counseling)
- Housing (safe environments; supported housing; community residential services; group homes; apartment living)
- Basic Living Skills (personal hygiene or personal care, preparing and sharing meals, home and travel safety and skills, goal and life planning,

chores and group decision-making, shopping and appointments)

- Social (relationships, recreational and hobby, family and friends, housemates and boundaries, communications & community integration)
- Vocational and/or Educational (vocational planning, transportation assistance to employment, preparation programs (e.g., calculators), GED classes, televised education, coping skills, motivation)
- Financial (personal budget), planning for own apartment (startup funds, security deposit), household grocery; social security disability; banking accounts (savings or travel)
- Community and Legal (resources; health insurance, community recreation, memberships, legal aid society, homeownership agencies, community colleges, houses of worship, ethnic activities and clubs; employment presentations; hobby clubs; special interest stores; summer city schedules)

As of 2013, it is expected that areas such as supported housing, household management, quality medical plans, advocacy for rights, counseling, and community participation be part of the available package of options for services. Modernization in these fields includes better health care, such as women and men's health (e.g., heart disease), public and private counseling services in mental health, integrated services (for dual and multiple diagnoses), new specialized treatments (e.g., eating disorders), and understanding of trauma services and mental health. Psychiatric rehabilitation is typically associated with long term services and supports (LTSS) in the community including post secondary education as supported education.

Educational and Professional Organizations

Canada

In Canada, Psychosocial Rehabilitation/Réadaptation Psychosociale (PSR/RPS) Canada promotes education, research and knowledge exchange in relation to evidence-based psychosocial rehabilitation and recovery-oriented practices for service-providers and those receiving services for mental health challenges. A framework of competencies for service providers (individuals and organizations) was developed and announced at the 2013 Annual National Conference in Winnipeg, Manitoba.

United States

- Boston University, Center for Psychiatric Rehabilitation
- Psychiatric Rehabilitation Association, formerly the United States Psychiatric Rehabilitation Association and International Association for Psychosocial Rehabilitation; a professional organization founded in 1975.
- Rutgers School of Health Related Professions, Department of Psychiatric Rehabilitation and Counseling Professions

Respiratory Therapist

A respiratory therapist is a specialized healthcare practitioner trained in pulmonary medicine in order to work therapeutically with people suffering from pulmonary disease, who has graduated from a university and passed a national board certifying examination. Respiratory therapists work most often in intensive care and operating rooms, but are also found in outpatient clinics and home-health environments.

Respiratory therapists are specialists and educators in cardiology and pulmonology. Respiratory therapists are clinicians trained in advanced airway management; establishing and maintaining the airway during management of trauma, intensive care, and may administer anaesthesia for surgery or conscious sedation.

Respiratory therapists initiate and manage life support for people in intensive care units and emergency departments, stabilizing, treating and managing pre-hospital and hospital-to-hospital patient transport by air or ground ambulance.

In the outpatient setting Respiratory Therapists work as educators in asthma clinics, ancillary clinical staff in pediatric clinics, and sleep-disorder diagnosticians in sleep-clinics. They also serve as clinical providers in cardiology clinics and cath-labs.

Clinical Practice

Intensive care and operating room

Respiratory therapists educate, diagnose, and treat people who are suffering from heart and lung problems. Specialized in both cardiac and pulmonary care, Respiratory Therapists often collaborate with specialists in pulmonology and anaesthesia in various aspects of clinical care of patients. Respiratory therapists provide a vital role in both medicine and nursing. A vital role in ICU is the initiation and maintenance of mechanical ventilation and the care of artificial airways.

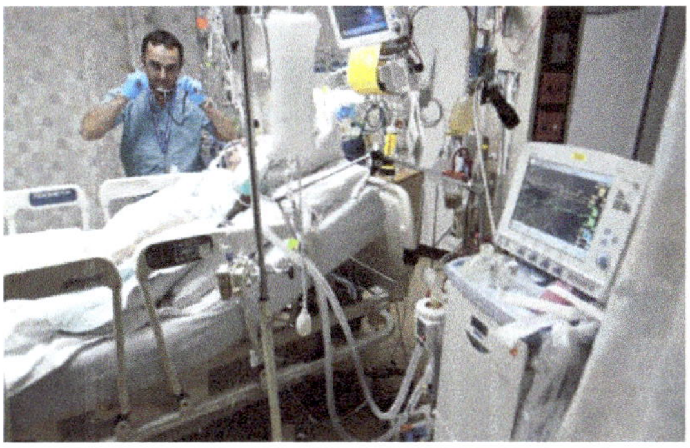

Respiratory Therapist in an intensive care unit

Outpatient clinical practice

Respiratory therapists are also primary clinicians in conducting tests to measure lung function and teaching people to manage asthma, chronic obstructive pulmonary disorder among other cardiac and lung functions.

Internationally, Respiratory Therapists that provide lung function testing are termed respiratory scientists, but in North America, they may be a Respiratory Therapist or may also be a certified pulmonary function technician in the United States.

Home-health care

Outside of clinics and hospitals, Respiratory Therapists often manage home oxygen needs of patients and their families, providing around the clock support for home ventilators and other equipment for conditions like sleep apnea.

In the clinic or outpatient setting Respiratory Therapists assist with diagnosis and serve as an educator for patients suffering from cardiac and respiratory illness. In the United States, Respiratory Therapists with certification as Registered Respiratory Therapists evaluate and treat patients with a great deal of autonomy under the direction of a pulmonologist. In facilities that maintain critical care transport teams Respiratory Therapists are a preferred addition to all types of surface or air transport.

Public education

In other settings Respiratory Therapists are found in schools as asthma educators, working with teachers and coaches about childhood symptoms of asthma and how to spot an emergency. In the United States, legislation has been introduced several times to allow Respiratory Therapists certified as asthma specialists with registered Respiratory Therapist certification to prescribe and manage previously diagnosed respiratory patients in physician clinics. In sleep clinics, Respiratory Therapists work with physicians in the diagnosis of sleep-related illnesses. Respiratory Therapists in the United States are migrating toward a role with autonomy similar to the nurse practitioner, or as an extension of the physician like the physician assistant. Respiratory Therapists are frequently utilized as complete cardiovascular specialists being utilized to place and manage arterial accesses along with peripherally-inserted central catheters.

A Respiratory Therapist gives an immunization shot to a patient

Pulmonary rehabilitation

Pulmonary rehabilitation may be initiated as a treatment as a source for continuity of improvement after a hospital stay or as a therapeutic way to increase quality of life. Pulmonary rehabilitation is intended to educate the patient, the family, and improve the overall quality of life and prognosis for the patient. Pulmonary Rehabilitation involves therapies and evaluations by Respiratory Therapists, Occupational Therapists and Physical Therapists.

Credentialing and Licensure

United States and Canada

In the United States and Canada, Respiratory Therapists are healthcare practitioners who after receiving at least an Associate of Science in Respiratory Care, complete a credentialing process.

After satisfactorily completing the required examinations and added to a registry, the practitioner is then eligible to apply for a license to practice in the region governed by their respective licensing body.

In the United States, specialist Respiratory Therapists are clinicians who hold National Board for Respiratory Care specialty credentials, which may include neonatal/pediatric specialist (CRT-NPS or RRT-NPS), adult critical care specialist (RRT-ACCS), sleep disorder specialist (CRT-SDS or RRT-SDS), and pulmonary function technologist (CPFT or RPFT). The NBRC's RRT-ACCS examination is the newest NBRC examination that was launched in 2012.

Professional credentials denoted as a certified Asthma Educator (AE-C) may also be earned by passing the National Asthma Educator Certification Board (NAECB).

In some parts of Canada, one may practice as a Provisional Respiratory Therapist after graduating, until writing and passing the CBRC exam. In Canada, similar credentialing and advanced training exists.

International Respiratory Care

Except for the United States and Canada, very few countries have a dedicated professional role for respiratory health. In these countries, respiratory care is provided by physiotherapists, nurses and physicians that have chosen to specialize in this field. In many countries this recognition is in a transition stage; as an example, in 2011, hospitals in Beijing, China began a recruitment drive to acquire Respiratory Therapists for their intensive care units where previously nurses were the only clinician.

Canada

Upon graduation from an accredited school of respiratory therapy, the graduate is then eligible to write the national exam administered by the Canadian Board for Respiratory Care.

Success on this examination will then allow the Respiratory Therapist to register with any licensing body in Canada. Alberta, Manitoba, New Brunswick, Newfoundland and Labrador, Nova Scotia, Ontario, Quebec and Saskatchewan are the Canadian provinces with provincial licensing bodies; in these provinces, it is illegal to practice the profession of Respiratory Care without first being licensed as a full or provisional member with the provincial licensing body.

These provinces are so-called regulated provinces. In some provinces, one may work provisionally upon graduating, until writing and passing the exam. In all other jurisdictions, the licensing body for the profession of Respiratory Care is the Canadian Society for Respiratory Therapy.

Registration as a full member is optional for Respiratory Therapists living in regulated provinces, however, for Respiratory Therapists living in non-regulated provinces, registration as a full member with the CSRT is compulsory. Registration with the provincial regulatory body or the CSRT (in non-regulated provinces) confers upon the Respiratory Therapist the title of Registered Respiratory Therapist (RRT). Canada and the United States recognize each their cardio-pulmonary education structure as equal, however a qualifying exam must be written in order to practice in either nation.

There is pressure for the program to become a degree, as other therapies (Physical Therapy, Occupational Therapy) now require a master's degree or greater. However, in some places such as Alberta, Canada the cardio-pulmonary course work are only offered at technical schools which are unable to grant a formal degree.

France

Respiratory therapy is a sub-specialty of physical therapy in France. Respiratory care as a specialty is regulated by the Fédération Française des Masseurs Kinésithérapeutes Rééducateurs.

Germany

The German Respiratory Society first issued a resolution to develop the dedicated Respiratory Therapist (RT) role in 2004 as a means to increase the quality of patient care, delegate physician duties and respond to the observed increase in respiratory conditions and diseases. In 2006-2006, a year-long pilot training program was offered to established nurses and physiotherapists. Researchers report that significant additional work is necessary to define and position the role of the Respiratory Therapist within the current healthcare system.

Philippines

In Philippines Respiratory Therapists are clinicians who have been awarded at minimum a Bachelor of Science in Respiratory Care degree. Licenses to practice respiratory care are regulated by the Professional Regulatory Board of Respiratory Therapy and Professional Regulation Commission which is established and legally maintained by the Philippine Respiratory Therapy Act (Republic Act No. 10024).

United Arab Emirates

In United Arab Emirates Respiratory Therapists must have been awarded a Bachelor of Science in Respiratory Care. An additional two-years of experience is required for foreign applicants. Licenses are maintained and awarded by the Dubai Health Authority. The Dubai Health Authority restricts Respiratory Therapists to working only in physical medicine and rehabilitation Centers, in hospitals, in surgical clinics with cardio-thoracic surgeons and with physicians in family/general practice or pulmonology.

Saudi Arabia

Saudi Arabia utilizes Respiratory Therapists in a similar fashion to Canada and the U.S. Some Respiratory Therapists from North America travel to Saudi Arabia for temporary need.

United States

A Respiratory Therapist teaches students about the dangers of smoking.

In the United States a Respiratory Therapist is a clinician who has at a minimum completed an Associate of Science in Respiratory Care degree along with a certification process. After satisfactorily completing required examinations either administered by the National Board for Respiratory Care or directly by the individual state licensing board (either the medical examiners board or a special state respiratory care board).

There are two recognized governing bodies in the United States; the State Board of Respiratory Care in the state in which a Respiratory Therapist is licensed to practice and the other is the National Board for Respiratory Care (NBRC) a non-profit organization which regulates two levels of certification along with some additional specialist certifications.

The Certified Respiratory Therapist (CRT) and the Registered Respiratory Therapist

(RRT). The CRT is the certification given after successfully passing the entry-level examination NBRC-ELE; The RRT certification is given after first becoming a CRT and then passing the NBRC-WRE and NBRC-CSE.

Most state boards of respiratory care require proof of the appropriate NBRC credential and award various license titles; including (but not limited to) Respiratory Care Practitioner, Licensed Registered Respiratory Therapist, and Licensed Certified Respiratory Therapist.

There has been a substantial push to standardize the state licensure by the American Association for Respiratory Care. The NBRC credential is renewed every 5 years for a fee in addition to fees assessed by the state boards of respiratory care.

United Kingdom

Respiratory therapy in the UK is not a recognized specific profession, but a specialisation route available to physicians, nurses, physiotherapists and occupational therapists.

Common titles include Cardio-Respiratory Physiotherapist, Clinical Respiratory Physiologist, Respiratory Nurse and Cardio-Respiratory Occupational Therapist.

All UK trained Physiotherapists receive advanced training in Respiratory Therapy theory and practice as a core component of their pre-registration Physiotherapy degree programme. Following qualification and a period of rotations throughout the core areas of Physiotherapy practice, they may then follow a career pathway specialising in Respiratory Physiotherapy. Areas of practice include Critical Care, respiratory medicine, Cystic Fibrosis, Asthma, Hyperventilation Syndrome, general and specialised surgery, non-invasive ventilation, ventilation weaning, cardiac and pulmonary rehab, respiratory therapy outpatient clinics and community respiratory therapy. The Association of Chartered Physiotherapists interested in Respiratory Care is the specialist interest group for UK Physiotherapists working within the field of Respiratory Therapy. All Physiotherapists working within the United kingdom must be registered with the Health and Care Professions Council, regardless of their area of clinical practice, in order to be allowed to work in both the public and private sectors. Respiratory Physiotherapy postgraduate master's degree and PhD programs exist within the United Kingdom for suitably qualified and experienced therapists.

For Respiratory Physiologists, a Bachelor of Science in Clinical Physiology is issued with a specialist option in respiratory physiology. Beyond degree level, Master of Science programs in Respiratory Care, Respiratory Disease Management, Advanced Cardiology and Clinical Respiratory Physiology are available.

Specialist Respiratory Therapists

Anesthesia Assistants

The traditional role of the operating room Respiratory Therapist has included providing technical support to the anesthesiologist for the proper use and maintenance of the anesthetic gas machine, in addition to also providing airway management. This role in the operating room has evolved to include a more advanced and specialized role with increasing responsibilities to the Respiratory Therapist. Respiratory Therapists are academically prepared to perform activities such as sedation by administration of anesthetic gases and medications, insertion and management of vascular (arterial and venous) access and assessment of the depth of anesthesia under the guidance of an anesthesiologist or nurse anesthetist. This role is similar to the nurse anesthetist, except that an Anaethestia Assistant must have an anesthesiologist supervising them and a nurse anesthetist, does not.

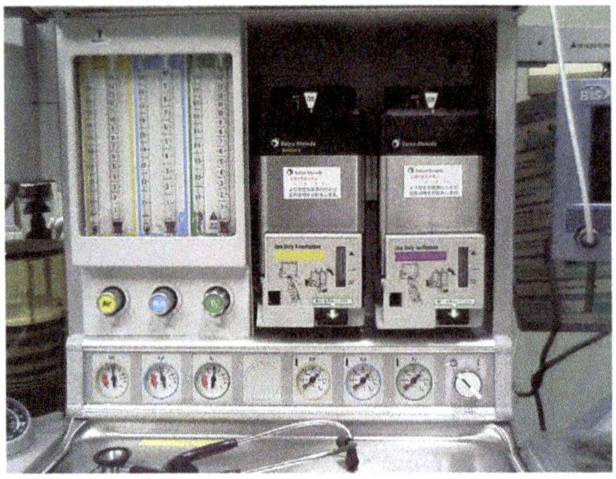

Anesthesia vaporizer

Asthma Specialists

Asthma specialists work with clinics, hospitals and schools as an educator for teachers, parents, patients and practitioners on asthma and allergies. Respiratory Therapists in the role as an Asthma Educator additionally help diagnose and treat asthma and other respiratory illness. Additionally, an Asthma Educator is the resource clinician in inpatient and outpatient environments for evaluating and advising physicians on treatment plans and helping facilitate patient understanding and compliance with the plan. In the United States, Certified Asthma Educators (AE-C) are credentialed by the National Asthma Education Certification Board (NAECB).

In Canada, the Canadian Network for Respiratory Care administers two certifications for the specialization as Respiratory Therapist Asthma Educator, the Certified Asthma Educator (CAE) (preferred by practitioners with a pediatric focus) and the Certified Respiratory Educator (CRE), which comprises the CAE program with additional training in COPD.

Cystic Fibrosis

Respiratory Therapists work with people suffering from cystic fibrosis in clinics and hospitals by educating them about their disease and working with them on a treatment plan. While admitted to a hospital, patients with cystic fibrosis have their treatment schedule modified and maintained by Respiratory Therapists. Maintaining a healthy schedule for pharmokonetic and physical therapeutic airway clearance typically more frequent than home treatment plans because admissions are usually due to an increased need for therapy during the stay.

Cardiovascular Perfusionist

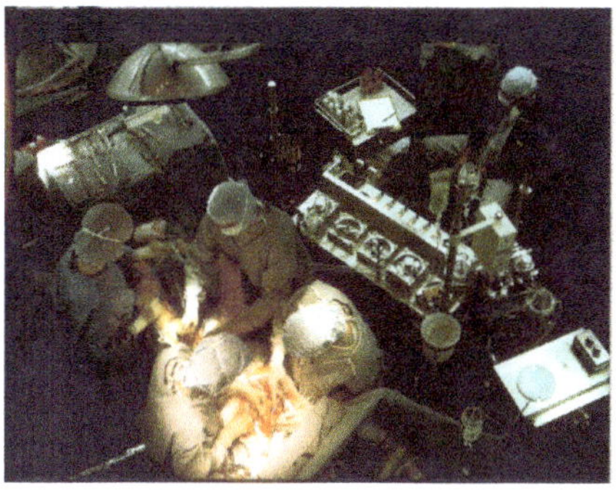

CABG surgery with CPB

Respiratory Therapists are able to fulfill the role of Perfusionist with appropriate training. The perfusionist is a highly trained member of the cardiothoracic surgical team (often time an RT with extra training) which consists of cardiac surgeons, anesthesiologists, physician assistants, surgical technicians, other Respiratory Therapists, and nurses. The perfusionist's main responsibility is to support the physiological and metabolic needs of the cardiac surgical patient so that the cardiac surgeon may operate on a still, unbeating heart. Perfusionist certifications are maintained and awarded by The American Academy of Cardiovascular Perfusion.

Extra-corporeal Membrane Oxygenation

A Respiratory Therapist takes a blood sample from a 3-day-old in preparation for transfer to an Extracorporeal Membrane Oxygenation unit

Extracorporeal membrane oxygenation (ECMO) is a modified cardiopulmonary bypass technique used for the treatment of life-threatening cardiac or respiratory failure. An ECMO Clinical Specialist is a technical specialist trained to manage the ECMO system including blood pump, tubing, artificial oxygenator, and related equipment.

The ECMO Specialist is also responsible for the clinical needs of the patient on ECMO which may include bedside management of oxygenation and carbon dioxide removal, maintenance of normal acid-base balance, administration of medications, blood and blood products, and maintenance of appropriate anticoagulation therapies for the blood. This ECMO Clinical Specialist may be the bedside critical care nurse specifically trained in ECMO patient and circuit management, or the ECMO system may be primarily managed by a registered Respiratory Therapist, or physicians with training as ECMO clinical specialists.

Neonatal & Pediatric Intensive Care

Much like adult intensivist Respiratory Therapists, neonatal and pediatric specialists deal primarily with managing life support for the pediatric or neonatal patient. Pediatric Respiratory Therapists are trained extensively in antenatal and intrapartum patients and family. In the United States a specialist certification exists and is awarded by the National Board for Respiratory Care. Available to Respiratory Therapists holding certification as a certified Respiratory Therapist or registered Respiratory Therapist however the registered Respiratory Therapist is preferred by most institutions.

Sleep Disorder Specialist

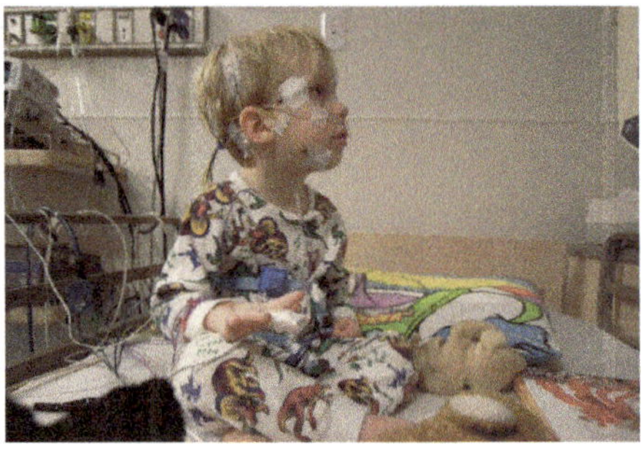

A pediatric patient prepared for a polysomnogram by a Respiratory Therapist.

Respiratory Therapists monitor, interpret and diagnose findings from a sleep study, as well as the medical history and physical exam to make the diagnosis and decide on treatment related to sleep-disorders. A sleep study can also help diagnose narcolepsy.

In the United States a sleep disorder specialist can be a Registered Respiratory Therapist with the sleep disorder specialist certification (RRT-SDS) whom performs sleep disorders testing and therapeutic intervention along with diagnosis of sleep related disease such as Obstructive Sleep Apnea or Central Apnea. In Canada it is often an RT with additional training to become a Registered Polysomnography Technician (RPSGT)

Case Management

Case management is a collaborative process that assesses, plans, implements, coordinates, monitors, and evaluates the options and services required to meet the client's health and human services needs. It is characterized by advocacy, communication, and resource management and promotes quality and cost-effective interventions and outcomes. Eligibility and certification is maintained by the Commission for Case Management Certification, a body certifying healthcare professionals in the United States.

Surface & Air Transport Specialist

Respiratory Therapists work with nurses, physicians, and paramedics in emergency flight and ground transport. They are a vital practitioner delivering care inside helicopters, air ambulance or ground ambulance working to pick up a patient and move them to a facility that has what they need. In the United States certification for transport (C-NPT) is currently awarded by The National Certification Corporation.

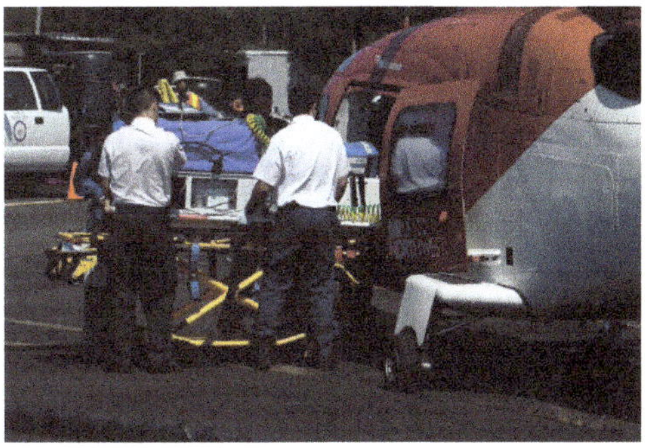

A premature infant on ECMO, a form of heart/lung machine, is being transferred between hospitals

The University of Maryland includes Respiratory Therapists as qualifying for the advanced credentialing as a critical care paramedic CCEMT-P

Pulmonary Research and Science

Respiratory Therapists are sometimes referred to as Respiratory Scientists who are specialists in pulmonary function. Respiratory Therapists work with Pulmonologists in both clinical and general research of the respiratory system, ranging from the anatomy of the respiratory epithelium to the most effective treatment of pulmonary hypertension in pediatrics. Scientific research also takes place to look for causes and possible treatment in diseases such as asthma and lung cancer.

History of Respiratory Care

The profession of respiratory care was officially established in the United States c. 1930; and respiratory research has officially existed since the early 1900s. During the early years, Respiratory Therapists were referred to as "oxygen technicians", and most of their activities involved moving cylinders of compressed gas and administering oxygen via nasal catheter or oxygen tent. Most oxygen technicians were trained on the job, although brief training programs began to appear in the late 1940s and 1950s.

Today the profession hardly resembles what it was in the 1940s. Respiratory Therapists provide direct care, patient education, and care coordination. They are academically trained in respiratory nursing and respiratory medicine. They practice in acute care facilities, long-term acute care facilities, skilled nursing facilities, assisted-living centers, subacute care units, rehabilitation centers, diagnostics units, and in the home. Respiratory Therapist training has also dramatically changed. Current accreditation standards require Respiratory Therapists to have, at minimum, an Associate of Science in Respiratory Care degree from an accredited program. Legal requirements to practice respiratory therapy have also dramatically changed. 49 states now legally recognize Respiratory Therapists. Limited permits or state licenses are now required in all states except Alaska, which has no statutory authority over the practice of respiratory care. Most states that have a licensure requirement also require continuing education.

In 2007 the American Association for Respiratory Care (AARC) began developing recommendations for the promotion of the field of respiratory care in the United States in response to increased concern regarding licensure and credentialing issues as well as international recognition of those practicing in the United States. The task force decided to recommend that by 2015 the minimum education requirement for licensure and certification as a Respiratory Therapist be a bachelor of science in respiratory therapy (BSRT). The AARC task force also recommended the American Respiratory Care Foundation change its scholarship policies and only award assistance and grants to those working toward a bachelor's degree. The Committee on Accreditation for Respiratory Care (CoARC) was asked by the AARC task force to change its accreditation standards and no longer accredit associates level respiratory care programs. The CoARC replied by a press release rejecting the recommendation. In 2011 legislation introduced by the AARC will help improve the use of Respiratory Therapists in clinical applications by allowing them to manage patients suffering from asthma and COPD seeing a clinic for routine checkups. Similar bills have been introduced before and have died in committee.

Speech-language Pathology

Speech-language pathology is a field of expertise practiced by a clinician known as a speech-language pathologist (SLP), also called speech and language therapist, or speech therapist, who specializes in the evaluation and treatment of communication disorders, cognition, voice disorders, and swallowing disorders.

A common misconception is that speech-language pathology is restricted to correcting pronunciation difficulties, such as helping English speaking individuals enunciate their "s" and "r" sounds, and helping people who stutter to speak more fluently. In fact, speech-language pathology is concerned with a broad scope of speech, language, swallowing, and voice issues involving communication, some of which are:

- Word-finding issues, either as a result of a specific language problem such as a language delay or a more general issue such as dementia.
- Social communication difficulties involving how people communicate ideas with others (pragmatics).
- Structural language impairments, including difficulties creating sentences that are grammatical (syntax) and meaningful (semantics).

- Literacy impairments (reading and writing) related to the letter-to-sound relationship (phonics), the word-to-meaning relationship (semantics), and understanding the ideas presented in a text (reading comprehension).
- Voice difficulties, such as a raspy voice, a voice that is too soft, or other voice difficulties that negatively impact a person's social or professional performance.
- Cognitive impairments (e.g., attention, memory, executive function) to the extent that they interfere with communication.

The components of speech production include:

- phonation (producing sound);
- resonance;
- fluency;
- Intonation,
- Pitch variance;
- Voice (including aeromechanical components of respiration)

The components of language include:

- phonology (manipulating sound according to the rules of a language);
- Morphology (understanding and using minimal units of meaning);
- syntax (constructing sentences according to languages' grammar rules);
- semantics (interpreting signs or symbols of communication to construct meaning);
- pragmatics (social aspects of communication).

Primary pediatric speech and language disorders include receptive and expressive language disorders, speech sound disorders, childhood apraxia of speech, stuttering, and language-based learning disabilities.

Swallowing disorders include difficulties in any system of the swallowing process (i.e. oral, pharyngeal, esophageal), as well as functional dysphagia and feeding disorders. Swallowing disorders can occur at any age and can stem from multiple causes.

The Profession

Speech-language pathologists (SLPs) provide a wide range of services, mainly on an individual basis, but also as support for individuals, families, support groups, and providing information for the general public. Speech-language pathologists work to prevent, assess, diagnose, and treat speech, language, social communication, cognitive-communication, and swallowing disorders in children and adults. Speech services begin with initial screening for communication and swallowing disorders and continue with assessment and diagnosis, consultation for the provision of advice regarding management, intervention and treatment, and provision counseling and other follow up services for these disorders. Services are provided in the following areas:

- cognitive aspects of communication (e.g., attention, memory, problem solving, executive functions).
- speech (phonation, articulation, fluency, resonance, and voice including aeromechanical components of respiration);
- language (phonology, morphology, syntax, semantics, and pragmatic/social aspects of communication) including comprehension and expression in oral, written, graphic, and manual modalities; language processing; preliteracy and language-based literacy skills, phonological awareness.
- swallowing or other upper aerodigestive functions such as infant feeding and aeromechanical events (evaluation of esophageal function is for the purpose of referral to medical professionals);
- voice (hoarseness (dysphonia), poor vocal volume (hypophonia), abnormal (e.g. rough, breathy, strained) vocal quality. Research demonstrates voice therapy to be especially helpful with certain patient populations; individuals with Parkinson's Disease often develop voice issues as a result of their disease.
- sensory awareness related to communication, swallowing, or other upper aerodigestive functions.

Speech, language, and swallowing disorders result from a variety of causes, such as a stroke, brain injury, hearing loss, developmental delay, a cleft palate, cerebral palsy, or emotional issues.

Multi-discipline Collaboration

Speech-language pathologists collaborate with other health care professionals, often working as part of a multidisciplinary team, providing referrals to audiologists and others; providing information to health care professionals (including physicians, dentists, nurse practitioners, nurses, occupational therapists, dietitians), educators, behavior consultants (applied behavior analysis) and parents as dictated by the individual client's needs.

In relation to auditory processing disorders, collaborating in the assessment and providing intervention where there is evidence of speech, language, and/or other cognitive-communication disorders.

The treatment for patients with cleft lip and palate has an obvious interdisciplinary character. The speech therapy outcome is even better when the surgical treatment is performed earlier.

Working Environments

Speech-language pathologists work in a variety of clinical and educational settings. SLPs work in public and private hospitals, skilled nursing facilities (SNFs), long-term acute care (LTAC) facilities, hospice, and home healthcare. Speech-language pathologists may also work as part of the support structure in the education system, working in both public and private schools, colleges, and universities. Some speech-language pathologists also work in community health, providing services at prisons and young offenders' institutions or providing expert testimony in applicable court cases.

Subsequent to the American Speech-Language-Hearing Association's (ASHA's) 2005 approval of the delivery of Speech-Language Pathology services via video conference, or telepractice, SLPs have begun delivering services via this service delivery method.

Research

Speech-language pathologists conduct research related to communication sciences and disorders, swallowing disorders, or other upper aerodigestive functions.

Education and Training

United States

In the United States, speech-language pathology is a Master's entry-level professional degree field. Clinicians must hold a master's degree in Communicative Disorders/ Speech-Language Pathology (e.g. M.A., M.S., or M.Ed.) that is from a university that holds regional accreditation and from a communicative sciences and disorders program that is accredited by the American Speech-Language-Hearing Association (ASHA), the profession's national governing body as well as individual state's governing board. Programs that offer the M.Ed. degree are often housed within a university's College of education, but offer the same education and training as programs with a M.A. or M.S. degree. Beyond the master's degree, some SLPs may choose to earn a clinical doctorate in Speech Language Pathology (e.g. CScD or SLP.D), or a doctoral degree that has a research and/or professional focus (e.g., Ph.D., or Ed.D.). All degrees must be from a university that holds regional accreditation, but only the master's degree is accredited by the American Speech-Language-Hearing Association (ASHA).

All clinicians are required to complete 400 clinical hours (25 observation hours often completed during the undergraduate degree and 375 hours of graduate Clinical Practicum). They must pass multiple comprehensive exams also called Knowledge and Skills Acquisition (KASA) exams.

After all the above requirements have been met during the SLP's path to earning the graduate degree:

- State licensure and national certification by:
- Passing score on the National Speech-Language Pathology board exam (Praxis).
- Successful completion of a clinical fellowship year (CFY) as a clinical fellow (CF) under the mentorship of a fully licensed mentor clinician. The CFY is no less than 36 weeks of full-time experience, totaling a minimum of 1260 hours. During the CFY, the CF cannot earn CFY hours unless they work more than 5 hours in a week and cannot earn any CFY hours beyond 35 hours in a week.
- American Speech-Language-Hearing Association (ASHA) Certificate of Clinical Competence (CCC) and full state licensure to practice, following successful completion of clinical fellowship year(CFY).
- States are responsible for licensure of clinicians and other professionals and, as far as the new SLP, these requirements are often similar of that of the CFY. Following the state licensure procedures and national certification requirements are usually done simultaneously.

Maintaining licensure through continuing education:

- To maintain licensure, SLPs participate in periodic earning of Continuing Educational Units (CEU).

Continuing education and training obligations:

- Educate, supervise, and mentor future Speech-Language Pathologists.
- Participate in continuing education.
- Educate and provide in-service training to families, caregivers, and other professionals.
- Train, supervise, and manage Speech-Language Pathology Assistants and other support personnel.
- Educating and counseling individuals, families, co-workers, educators, and other persons in the community regarding acceptance, adaptation, and decisions about communication and swallowing.

Professional suffix:

- Credentials of a clinical fellow typically read as: MA, MS, or M.Ed, CF-SLP (e.g., Jane Doe, MA, CF-SLP).
- Credentials of a fully licensed SLP commonly read as: MA, MS, or M.Ed, CCC-SLP (e.g., Jane Doe, MA, CCC-SLP), indicating a practitioner's graduate degree and

successful completion of the fellowship year/board exams to obtain the "three Cs" the Certification of Clinical Competence, in speech-language pathology.

Salary Information

Salaries of SLPs depend on a variety of factors. These include: educational background, work experience, and location. According to the ASHA 2014 Schools Survey, the median salary for a speech-language pathologist working during the academic year at a school was $61,000. However, salaries can range from $40,000–90,000. In Australia, it has been found that the basic salary that a speech pathologist/therapist would earn in Australia is an estimate of $59,500 Australian dollars.

Methods of Assessment

For many parents, the decision of whether or not to enroll students into school-based speech therapy or privately practiced therapy is challenging. Because school-based speech therapy is run under state guidelines and funds, the process of assessment and qualification is more strict. To qualify for in-school speech therapy, students must meet the state's criteria on language testing and speech standardization. Due to such requirements, some students may not be assessed in an efficient time frame or their needs may be undermined by criteria. For a private clinic, students are more likely to qualify for therapy because it is a paid service with more availability.

Clients and Patients

Speech-language pathologists work with clients and patients who may be present with a wide range of issues.

Infants and Children

- Infants with injuries due to complications at birth, feeding and swallowing difficulties, including dysphagia
- Children with mild, moderate or severe:
    - Genetic disorders that adversely affect speech, language and/or cognitive development including cleft palate, Down syndrome, DiGeorge syndrome
    - Attention deficit hyperactivity disorder
    - Autism spectrum disorders, including Asperger syndrome
    - Developmental delay
    - Feeding disorders, including oral motor deficits
    - Cranial nerve damage

- Hearing loss
- Craniofacial anomalies that adversely affect speech, language and/or cognitive development
- Language delay
- Specific language impairment
- Specific difficulties in producing sounds, called articulation disorders, (including vocalic /r/ and lisps)
- Pediatric traumatic brain injury
- Developmental verbal dyspraxia
- Cleft palate

In the US, some children are eligible to receive speech therapy services, including assessment and lessons through the public school system. If not, private therapy is readily available through personal lessons with a qualified Speech-Language Pathologist or the growing field of telepractice. Teleconferencing tools such as Skype are being used more commonly as a means to access remote locations in private therapy practice, such as in the geographically diverse south island of New Zealand. More at-home or combination treatments have become readily available to address specific types of articulation disorders. The use of mobile applications in speech therapy is also growing as an avenue to bring treatment into the home.

In the UK, children are entitled to an assessment by local NHS Speech and Language Therapy teams, usually after referral by health visitors or education settings, but parents are also entitled to request an assessment directly. If treatment is appropriate, a care plan will be drawn up. Speech therapists often play a role in multi-disciplinary teams where a child has speech delay or disorder as part of a wider health condition.

Children and Adults

• Puberphonia
• Cerebral Palsy
• Head Injury (Traumatic brain injury)
• Hearing loss and impairments
• Learning difficulties including
  ○ Dyslexia
  ○ Specific language impairment (SLI)
  ○ Auditory processing disorder
	• Physical disabilities
	• Speech disorders (such as cluttering)
	• Stammering, stuttering (disfluency)
	• Stroke
	• Voice disorders (dysphonia)
	• Language delay
	• Motor speech disorders (dysarthria or Developmental verbal dyspraxia)
		• Naming difficulties (anomia)
		• Dysgraphia, agraphia
		• Cognitive communication disorders
		• Pragmatics
		• Laryngectomies
		• Tracheostomies
		• Oncology (Ear, nose or throat cancer)

Adults

- Adults with mild, moderate, or severe eating, feeding and swallowing difficulties, including dysphagia
- Adults with mild, moderate, or severe language difficulties as a result of:
  - Motor neuron diseases,
  - Alzheimer's disease,
  - Dementia,
  - Huntington's disease,
  - Multiple sclerosis,
  - Parkinson's disease,
  - Traumatic brain injury,
  - Mental health issues
  - Stroke
  - Progressive neurological conditions such as cancer of the head, neck and throat (including laryngectomy)
  - Aphasic
- Adults desiring transgender voice therapy (usually for male-to-female individuals)

References

- Coulehan J. L., Block M. R. (2005): The Medical Interview: Mastering skills for clinical practice, 5th Ed. F. A. Davis. ISBN 0-8036-1246-X. OCLC 232304023.
- Dunphy L. M., Winland-Brown J. E. (2011): Primary care: The art and science of advanced practice nursing. F.A. Davis. ISBN 9780803626478.
- O'Lynn, CE (2007). "History of men in nursing: a review". In O'Lynn, CE; Tranbarger, RE. Men in Nursing: History, Challenges, and Opportunities. New York: Springer Pub. pp. 6–8. ISBN 9780826103499.
- Gelfand, Stanley A. (2009). Essentials of Audiology (3 ed.). New York: Thieme Medical Publishers, Inc. p. ix. ISBN 978-1-60406-044-7. Retrieved 17 March 2015.
- Prentice, William (2011). Principles of Athletic Training: A Competency-Based Approach. New York, NY: McGraw Hill. p. 29. ISBN 9780073523736.
- Ferngren, GB (2009). Medicine & health care in early Christianity. Baltimore: Johns Hopkins University Press. p. 121. ISBN 9780801895227.

- Sachedina, Abdulaziz (2009). Islamic biomedical ethics: principles and application. Oxford: Oxford University Press. pp. 93–94. ISBN 9780195378504.
- de Bary, WT, ed. (2011). The Buddhist tradition in India, China & Japan (Unabridged. ed.). New York: Vintage eBooks. pp. 35–36. ISBN 9780307778796.
- Egenes, KJ (2009). "History of nursing". In Halstead, J; Roux, G. Issues and Trends in Nursing: Essential Knowledge for Today and Tomorrow. Sudbury, MA: Jones and Bartlett. p. 2. ISBN 9780763752255.
- Leonard, AE (2008). "Female religious orders". In Hsia, RP. A Companion to the Reformation World (1st paperback ed.). Oxford: Blackwell Publishers. p. 244. ISBN 978-1405149624.
- Lundy, KS (2014). "A history of health care and nursing". In Masters, K. Role Development in Professional Nursing Practice (3rd ed.). Burlington, MA: Jones & Bartlett Learning. pp. 11–12. ISBN 9781449681982.
- Quinn, Shawna M. "Agnes Warner and the Nursing Sisters of the Great War" (PDF). Goose Lane editions and the New Brunswick Military Heritage Project (2010) ISBN 978-0-86492-633-3. Retrieved 29 November 2014.

6

Injuries Cured by Physical Medicine and Rehabilitation

The injuries cured by physical medicine and rehabilitation is head injury, sprain, tennis elbow, wound, cramp and bruise. Any damage done to the body is known as an injury, it can be caused by falls, hits or by accidents. Injuries can cause disability or death and some of the injuries can be cured by physical medicine and rehabilitation. This topic is of great importance as it helps the readers in broadening their existing knowledge on physical medicine.

Head Injury

Any injury that results in trauma to the skull or brain can be classified as a head injury. The terms *traumatic brain injury* and *head injury* are often used interchangeably in the medical literature. This broad classification includes neuronal injuries, hemorrhages, vascular injuries, cranial nerve injuries, and subdural hygromas, among many others. These classifications can be further categorized as open (penetrating) or closed head injuries. This depends on if the skull was broken or not. Because head injuries cover such a broad scope of injuries, there are many causes—including accidents, falls, physical assault, or traffic accidents—that can cause head injuries. Many of these are minor, but some can be severe enough to require hospitalization.

The incidence (number of new cases) of head injury is 1.7 million people in the United States alone each year, with about 3% of these incidents leading to death. Adults suffer head injuries more frequently than any age group resulting from falls, motor vehicle crashes, colliding or being struck by an object, or assaults. Children, however, may experience head injuries from accidental falls or intentional causes (such as being struck or shaken) leading to hospitalization.

Unlike a broken bone where trauma to the body is obvious, head trauma can sometimes be conspicuous or inconspicuous. In the case of an open head injury, the skull is cracked and broken by an object that makes contact with the brain. This leads to bleeding. Other obvious symptoms can be neurological in nature. The person may become sleepy, behave abnormally, lose consciousness, vomit, develop a severe headache, have mismatched pupil sizes, and/or be unable to move certain parts of the body. While these symptoms happen right after head injury occurs, many problems can develop later in life. Alzheimer's disease, for example, is much more likely to develop in a person who has experienced a head injury.

Classification

Head injuries include both injuries to the brain and those to other parts of the head, such as the scalp and skull. Head injuries can be closed or open. A closed (non-missile) head injury is where the dura mater remains intact. The skull can be fractured, but not necessarily. A penetrating head injury occurs when an object pierces the skull and breaches the dura mater. Brain injuries may be diffuse, occurring over a wide area, or focal, located in a small, specific area. A head injury may cause skull fracture, which may or may not be associated with injury to the brain. Some patients may have linear or depressed skull fractures.If intracranial hemorrhage occurs, a hematoma within the skull can put pressure on the brain. Types of intracranial hemorrage include subdural, subarachnoid, extradural, and intraparenchymal hematoma. Craniotomy surgeries are used in these cases to lessen the pressure by draining off blood.

Brain injury can occur at the site of impact, but can also be at the opposite side of the skull due to a *contrecoup* effect (the impact to the head can cause the brain to move within the skull, causing the brain to impact the interior of the skull opposite the head-impact). If the impact causes the head to move, the injury may be worsened, because the brain may ricochet inside the skull causing additional impacts, or the brain may stay relatively still (due to inertia) but be hit by the moving skull (both are contrecoup injuries).

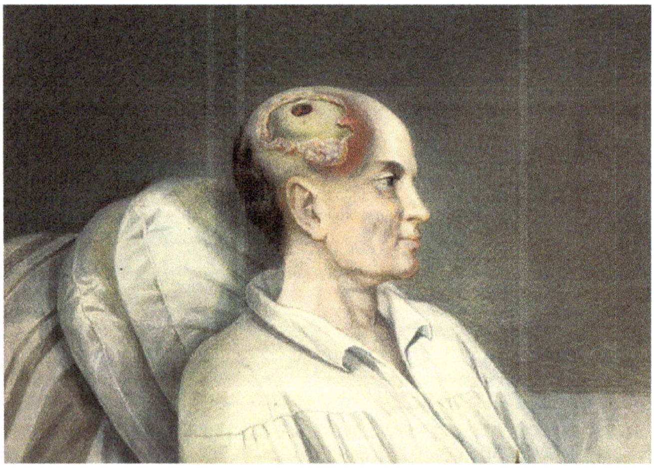

Private Patrick Hughes, Co. K, 4th New York Volunteers, wounded at the Battle of Antietam on September 17, 1862.

Specific problems after head injury can include

- Skull fracture
- Lacerations to the scalp and resulting hemorrhage of the skin

- Traumatic subdural hematoma, a bleeding below the dura mater which may develop slowly
- Traumatic extradural, or epidural hematoma, bleeding between the dura mater and the skull
- Traumatic subarachnoid hemorrhage
- Cerebral contusion, a bruise of the brain
- Concussion, a loss of function due to trauma
- Dementia pugilistica, or "punch-drunk syndrome", caused by repetitive head injuries, for example in boxing or other contact sports
- A severe injury may lead to a coma or death
- Shaken baby syndrome — a form of child abuse

Concussion

Traumatic brain injury (TBI) is an exchangeable word used for the word concussion. This term refers to a mild brain injury. This injury is a result due to a blow to the head that could make the person's physical, cognitive, and emotional behaviors irregular. Symptoms may include clumsiness, fatigue, confusion, nausea, blurry vision, headaches, and others. Mild concussions are associated with sequelae. Severity is measured using various concussion grading systems.

A slightly greater injury is associated with both anterograde and retrograde amnesia (inability to remember events before or after the injury). The amount of time that the amnesia is present correlates with the severity of the injury. In all cases the patients develop post-concussion syndrome, which includes memory problems, dizziness, tiredness, sickness and depression. Cerebral concussion is the most common head injury seen in children.

Intracranial Hemorrhage

Types of intracranial hemorrhage are roughly grouped into intra-axial and extra-axial. The hemorrhage is considered a focal brain injury; that is, it occurs in a localized spot rather than causing diffuse damage over a wider area.

Intra-axial Hemorrhage

Intra-axial hemorrhage is bleeding within the brain itself, or cerebral hemorrhage. This category includes intraparenchymal hemorrhage, or bleeding within the brain tissue, and intraventricular hemorrhage, bleeding within the brain's ventricles (particularly of premature infants). Intra-axial hemorrhages are more dangerous and harder to treat than extra-axial bleeds.

Extra-axial Hemorrhage

Hematoma type	Epidural	Subdural
Location	Between the skull and the outer endosteal layer of the dura mater	Between the *dura* and the arachnoid
Involved vessel	Temperoparietal locus (most likely) - Middle meningeal artery Frontal locus - anterior ethmoidal artery Occipital locus - transverse or sigmoid sinusesVertex locus - superior sagittal sinus	Bridging veins
Symptoms(depend on severity)	Lucid interval followed by unconsciousness	Gradually increasing headache and confusion
CT appearance	Biconvex lens	Crescent-shaped

Extra-axial hemorrhage, bleeding that occurs within the skull but outside of the brain tissue, falls into three subtypes:

- Epidural hemorrhage (extradural hemorrhage) which occur between the dura mater (the outermost meninx) and the skull, is caused by trauma. It may result from laceration of an artery, most commonly the middle meningeal artery. This is a very dangerous type of injury because the bleed is from a high-pressure system and deadly increases in intracranial pressure can result rapidly. However, it is the least common type of meningeal bleeding and is seen in 1% to 3% cases of head injury .
    - Patients have a loss of consciousness (LOC), then a lucid interval, then sudden deterioration (vomiting, restlessness, LOC)
    - Head CT shows lenticular (convex) deformity.
- Subdural hemorrhage results from tearing of the bridging veins in the subdural space between the dura and arachnoid mater.
    - Head CT shows crescent-shaped deformity
- Subarachnoid hemorrhage, which occur between the arachnoid and pia meningeal layers, like intraparenchymal hemorrhage, can result either from trauma or from ruptures of aneurysms or arteriovenous malformations. Blood is seen layering into the brain along sulci and fissures, or filling cisterns (most often the suprasellar cistern because of the presence of the vessels of the circle of Willis and their branchpoints within that space). The classic presentation of subarachnoid hemorrhage is the sudden onset of a severe headache (a thun-

derclap headache). This can be a very dangerous entity, and requires emergent neurosurgical evaluation, and sometimes urgent intervention.

Cerebral Contusion

Cerebral contusion is bruising of the brain tissue. The majority of contusions occur in the frontal and temporal lobes. Complications may include cerebral edema and transtentorial herniation. The goal of treatment should be to treat the increased intracranial pressure. The prognosis is guarded.

Diffuse Axonal Injury

Diffuse axonal injury, or DAI, usually occurs as the result of an acceleration or deceleration motion, not necessarily an impact. Axons are stretched and damaged when parts of the brain of differing density slide over one another. Prognoses vary widely depending on the extent of damage.

Signs and Symptoms

Presentation varies according to the injury. Some patients with head trauma stabilize and other patients deteriorate. A patient may present with or without neurological deficit. Patients with concussion may have a history of seconds to minutes unconsciousness, then normal arousal. Disturbance of vision and equilibrium may also occur. Common symptoms of head injury include coma, confusion, drowsiness, personality change, seizures, nausea and vomiting, headache and a lucid interval, during which a patient appears conscious only to deteriorate later.

Symptoms of skull fracture can include:

- leaking cerebrospinal fluid (a clear fluid drainage from nose, mouth or ear) may be and is strongly indicative of basilar skull fracture and the tearing of sheaths surrounding the brain, which can lead to secondary brain infection.
- visible deformity or depression in the head or face; for example a sunken eye can indicate a maxillar fracture
- an eye that cannot move or is deviated to one side can indicate that a broken facial bone is pinching a nerve that innervates eye muscles
- wounds or bruises on the scalp or face.
- Basilar skull fractures, those that occur at the base of the skull, are associated with Battle's sign, a subcutaneous bleed over the mastoid, hemotympanum, and cerebrospinal fluid rhinorrhea and otorrhea.

Because brain injuries can be life-threatening, even people with apparently slight injuries, with no noticeable signs or complaints, require close observation; They have a chance for severe symptoms later on. The caretakers of those patients with mild trauma who are released from the hospital are frequently advised to rouse the patient several times during the next 12 to 24 hours to assess for worsening symptoms.

The Glasgow Coma Scale (GCS) is a tool for measuring degree of unconsciousness and is thus a useful tool for determining severity of injury. The Pediatric Glasgow Coma Scale is used in young children. The widely used PECARN Pediatric Head Injury/Trauma Algorithm helps physicians weigh risk-benefit of imaging in a clinical setting given multiple factors about the patient - including mechanism/location of injury, age of patient, and GCS score.

Causes

Common causes of head injury are motor vehicle traffic collisions, home and occupational accidents, falls, and assaults. Wilson's disease has also been indicative of head injury. According to the United States CDC, 32% of traumatic brain injuries (another, more specific, term for head injuries) are caused by falls, 10% by assaults, 16.5% by being struck or against something, 17% by motor vehicle accidents, 21% by other/unknown ways. In addition, the highest rate of injury is among children ages 0–14 and adults age 65 and older.

Diagnosis

The need for imaging in patients who have suffered a minor head injury is debated. A non-contrast CT of the head should be performed immediately in all those who have suffered a moderate or severe head injury,an MRI is also an option. Computed tomography (CT) has become the diagnostic modality of choice for head trauma due to its accuracy, reliability, safety, and wide availability. The changes in microcirculation, impaired auto-regulation, cerebral edema, and axonal injury start as soon as head injury occurs and manifest as clinical, biochemical, and radiological changes.

Management

Most head injuries are of a benign nature and require no treatment beyond analgesics and close monitoring for potential complications such as intracranial bleeding. If the brain has been severely damaged by trauma, neurosurgical evaluation may be useful. Treatments may involve controlling elevated intracranial pressure. This can include sedation, paralytics, cerebrospinal fluid diversion. Second line alternatives include decompressive craniectomy (Jagannathan et al. found a net 65% favorable outcomes rate in pediatric patients), barbiturate coma, hypertonic saline and hypothermia. Although all of these methods have potential benefits, there has been no randomized study that has shown unequivocal benefit.

Clinicians will often consult clinical decision support rules such as the Canadian CT Head Rule or the New Orleans/Charity Head injury/Trauma Rule to decide if the patient needs further imaging studies or observation only. Rules like these are usually studied in depth by multiple research groups with large patient cohorts to ensure accuracy given the risk of adverse events in this area.

Prognosis

In children with uncomplicated minor head injuries the risk of intra cranial bleeding over the next year is rare at 2 cases per 1 million. In some cases transient neurological disturbances may occur, lasting minutes to hours. Malignant post traumatic cerebral swelling can develop unexpectedly in stable patients after an injury, as can post traumatic seizures. Recovery in children with neurologic deficits will vary. Children with neurologic deficits who improve daily are more likely to recover, while those who are vegetative for months are less likely to improve. Most patients without deficits have full recovery. However, persons who sustain head trauma resulting in unconsciousness for an hour or more have twice the risk of developing Alzheimer's disease later in life.

Head injury may be associated with a neck injury. Bruises on the back or neck, neck pain, or pain radiating to the arms are signs of cervical spine injury and merit spinal immobilization via application of a cervical collar and possibly a long board.If the neurological exam is normal this is reassuring. Reassessment is needed if there is a worsening headache, seizure, one sided weakness, or has persistent vomiting.

To combat overuse of Head CT Scans yielding negative intracranial hemorrhage, which unnecessarily expose patients to radiation and increase time in the hospital and cost of the visit, multiple clinical decision support rules have been developed to help clinicians weigh the option to scan a patient with a head injury. Among these are the Canadian Head CT rule, the PECARN Head Injury/Trauma Algorithm, and the New Orleans/ Charity Head Injury/Trauma Rule all help clinicians make these decisions using easily obtained information and noninvasive practices.

Epidemiology

Head injury is the leading cause of death in many countries.

Sprain

A sprain, also known as a torn ligament, is damage to one or more ligaments in a joint, often caused by trauma or the joint being taken beyond its functional range of motion. The severity of sprain ranges from a minor injury which resolves in a few days to a major rupture of one or more ligaments requiring surgical fixation and a period of immobilisation. Sprains can occur in any joint but are most common in the ankle and wrist.

Signs and Symptoms

- Pain
- Swelling
- Bruising
- Decreased ability to move the limb
- If a ligament ruptures, one may hear a popping sound
- Difficulty using the affected extremity

Causes

Sprains typically occur when the joint is taken beyond its functional range of motion.

There are certain factors which increase risk of sprains. Fatigue of muscles generally leads to sprains. When one suddenly starts to exercise after a sedentary lifestyle, sprains are quite common. While scientific studies are lacking, it is often thought that not warming-up is a common cause of sprains in athletes. Warming-up is thought to loosen the joint, increases blood flow and makes the joint more flexible.

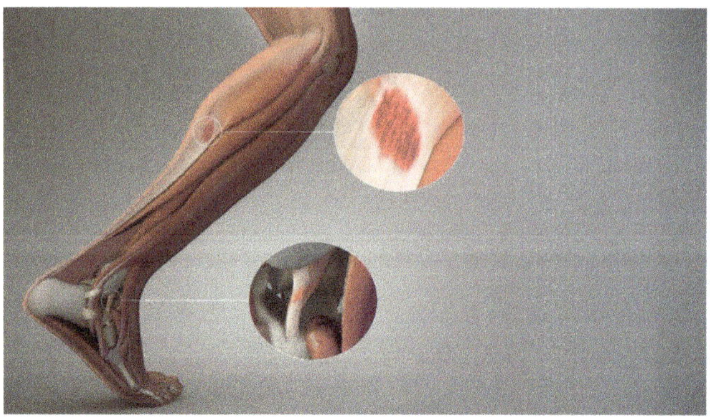

A 3D medical animation still shot illustrating a sprain

Diagnosis

A diagnosis of a sprain can often be made with a good degree of certainty by physical examination based on the clinical presentation and method of injury. In some cases, X-rays are obtained to ensure that there is no fracture. In some cases, particularly if the injury is prolonged or does not appear to be resolving as expected, magnetic resonance imaging (MRI) is performed to look at surrounding soft tissues and the ligament.

Classification

1. First degree sprain – the fibres of the ligament are stretched but intact.

2. Second degree sprain – is a tear of part of a ligament, from a third to almost all its fibres.

3. Third degree sprain – is a complete rupture of the ligament, sometimes avulsing a piece of bone.

Joints Involved

Although any joint can experience a sprain, some of the more common include:

- The ankle. It is the most common, and has been said that sprains such as serious ankle sprains are more painful and take longer to heal than actually breaking the bones in that area.
- The knee. One of the more talked about sprains is that to the anterior cruciate ligament (ACL) of the knee. This is a disabling sprain common to athletes, especially in American football, football (soccer), basketball, pole vaulting, softball, baseball and some styles of martial arts.
- Ligaments between the spinal vertebrae
- The fingers.
- The wrist.
- The toes.

Treatment

The first modality for a sprain can be remembered using the acronym RICE. The treatment of sprains depends on the extent of injury and the joint involved. Medications like non-steroidal anti-inflammatory drugs can relieve pain. Topical NSAIDs appear to be as good as those taken by mouth.

- Rest: The sprain should be rested. No additional force should be applied on site of the sprain. In case of, for example, a sprained ankle, walking should be kept to a minimum.
- Ice: Ice should be applied immediately to the sprain to reduce swelling and pain. It can be applied for 10–15 minutes at a time (longer application of ice may cause damage instead of healing), 3-4 times a day. Ice can be combined with a wrapping to minimize swelling and provide support.
- Compression: Dressings, bandages, or ace-wraps should be used to immobilize the sprain and provide support. When wrapping the injury, more pressure should be applied at the far end of the injury and decrease in the direction of the heart; the reason for this is that it more easily causes unnecessary fluid to be

flushed back up the blood stream in order to be recycled. Compression should not cut off the circulation of the limb.

- Elevation: Keeping the sprained joint elevated (in relation to the rest of the body) will also help minimize swelling.

Ice and compression (cold compression therapy) will not completely stop swelling and pain, but will help to minimize them as the sprain begins to heal itself. Careful management of swelling is critical to the healing process as additional fluid may pool in the sprained area.

The joint should be exercised again fairly soon, in milder cases from 1 to 3 days after injury. Special exercises are sometimes needed in order to regain strength and help reduce the risk of ongoing problems. The joint may need to be supported by taping or bracing, helping protect it from re-injury.

Functional Rehabilitation

Prolonged immobilization delays the healing of a sprain, as it usually leads to muscle atrophy and stiff joint. The components of an effective rehabilitation for all sprain injuries include increasing range of motion and progressive muscle strengthening exercise. These should be taken care of without delay.

Tennis Elbow

Tennis elbow or lateral epicondylitis is a condition in which the outer part of the elbow becomes sore and tender. The forearm muscles and tendons become damaged from overuse – repeating the same strenuous motions again and again. This leads to pain and tenderness on the outside of the elbow.

Any activity, including playing tennis, which involves the repetitive use of the extensor muscles of the forearm can cause acute or chronic tendonitis of the tendinous insertion of these muscles at the lateral epicondyle of the elbow. The condition is common in carpenters and laborers who swing a hammer or other tool with the forearm,continuing activity after onset of the condition and avoiding mandatory rest may lead to permanent onset of pain and only treatable via surgery. Dr. F. Runge (a German physician) is usually credited for the first description of the condition in 1873; he called it "writer's cramp" (*Schreibekrampf*). Later, it was called "washer women's elbow". As it also occurred in tennis, it soon was called "tennis elbow" after British surgeon Henry Morris published an article in *The Lancet* describing "the lawn tennis arm," 1883. The term "tennis elbow" first appeared in an 1883 paper by H.P. Major as "lawn-tennis elbow".

Signs and Symptoms

- Pain on the outer part of the elbow (lateral epicondyle)
- Point tenderness over the lateral epicondyle—a prominent part of the bone on the outside of the elbow
- Pain from gripping and movements of the wrist, especially wrist extension and lifting movements
- Pain from activities that use the muscles that extend the wrist (e.g. pouring a container of liquid, lifting with the palm down, sweeping, especially where wrist movement is required)

Symptoms associated with tennis elbow include, but are not limited to: radiating pain from the outside of the elbow to the forearm and wrist, pain during extension of wrist, weakness of the forearm, a painful grip while shaking hands or torquing a doorknob, and not being able to hold relatively heavy items in the hand. The pain is similar to the condition known as *golfer's elbow*, but the latter occurs at the medial side of the elbow.

Causes

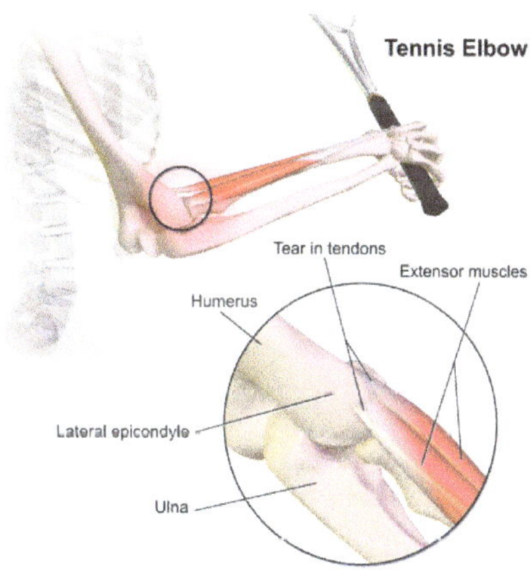

Tennis elbow

Tennis elbow is a type of repetitive strain injury, resulting from tendon overuse and failed healing of the tendon. In addition, the extensor carpi radialis brevis muscle plays a key role.

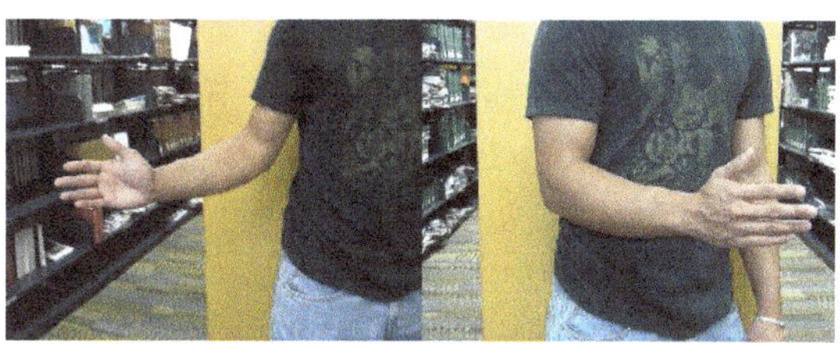

Example of repetitive movement that may cause tennis elbow

Early experiments suggested that tennis elbow was primarily caused by overexertion. However, studies show that trauma such as direct blows to the epicondyle, a sudden forceful pull, or forceful extension cause more than half of these injuries. It has also been known that incorrectly playing tennis may cause early stages of tennis elbow as shock is received when mishitting the ball.

Cyriax proposes one explanation of how tennis elbow may come about. The hypothesis states that there are microscopic and macroscopic tears between the common extensor tendon and the periosteum of the lateral humeral epicondyle. An operation conducted in this study showed that 28 out of 39 patients showed tearing at the tendon cuff. Kaplan stated that the radial nerve was significantly involved in tennis elbow. He noted the constriction of the radial nerve by adhesions to the capsule of the radiohumeral joint and the short extensor muscle of the wrist. He found evidence that many differed in how they contracted tennis elbow. Disorders such as calcification of the rotator cuff, bicipital tendinitis, or carpal tunnel syndrome may increase chances of tennis elbow.

Pathophysiology

Histological findings include granulation tissue, microrupture, degenerative changes, and there is no traditional inflammation. As a consequence, "lateral elbow tendinopathy or tendinosis" is used instead of "lateral epicondylitis".

Examination of tennis elbow tissue reveals noninflammatory tissue, and therefore, the term "angio-fibroblastic tendinosis" is used.

Longitudinal sonogram of the lateral elbow displays thickening and heterogeneity of the common extensor tendon that is consistent with tendinosis, as the ultrasound reveals calcifications, intrasubstance tears, and marked irregularity of the lateral epicondyle. Although the term "epicondylitis" is frequently used to describe this disorder, most histopathologic findings of studies have displayed no evidence of an acute, or a chronic inflammatory process. Histologic studies have demonstrated that this condition is the result of tendon degeneration, which causes normal tissue to be replaced by a disorganized arrangement of collagen. Therefore, the disorder is more appropriately referred to as "tendinosis" or "tendinopathy" rather than "tendinitis."

Colour Doppler ultrasound reveals structural tendon changes, with vascularity and hypo-echoic areas that correspond to the areas of pain in the extensor origin.

The pathophysiology of lateral epicondylitis is degenerative. Non-inflammatory, chronic degenerative changes of the origin of the extensor carpi radialis brevis (ECRB) muscle are identified in surgical pathology specimens. It is unclear if the pathology is affected by prior injection of corticosteroid.

Tennis players generally believe tennis elbow is caused by the repetitive nature of hitting thousands of tennis balls, which leads to tiny tears in the forearm tendon attachment at the elbow.

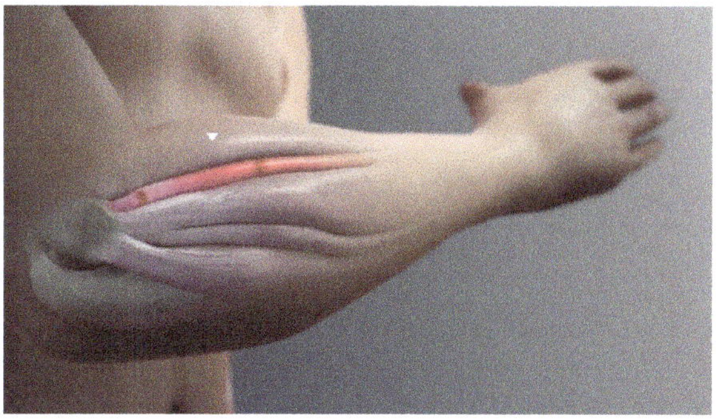

A 3D medical animation still shot illustrating the medical condition known as Tennis Elbow

The extensor digiti minimi also has a small origin site medial to the elbow that this condition can affect. The muscle involves the extension of the little finger and some extension of the wrist allowing for adaption to “snap” or flick the wrist—usually associated with a racquet swing. Most often, the extensor muscles become painful due to tendon breakdown from over-extension. Improper form or movement allows for power in a swing to rotate through and around the wrist—creating a moment on that joint instead of the elbow joint or rotator cuff. This moment causes pressure to build impact forces to act on the tendon causing irritation and inflammation.

The following speculative rationale is offered by proponents of an overuse theory of etiology: The extensor carpi radialis brevis has a small origin and does transmit large forces through its tendon during repetitive grasping. It has also been implicated as being vulnerable during shear stress during all movements of the forearm.

While it is commonly stated that lateral epicondylitis is caused by repetitive microtrauma/overuse, this is a speculative etiological theory with limited scientific support that is likely overstated. Other speculative risk factors for lateral epicondylitis include taking up tennis later in life, unaccustomed strenuous activity, decreased mental chronometry and speed and repetitive eccentric contraction of muscle (controlled lengthening of a muscle group).

Prevention

Another factor of tennis elbow injury is experience and ability. The proportion of players who reported a history of tennis elbow had an increased number of playing years. As for ability, poor technique increases the chance for injury much like any sport. Therefore, an individual must learn proper technique for all aspects of their sport. The competitive level of the athlete also affects the incidence of tennis elbow. Class A and B players had a significantly higher rate of tennis elbow occurrence compared to class C and novice players. However, an opposite, but not statistically significant, trend is observed for the recurrence of previous cases, with an increasingly higher rate as ability level decreases.

Other ways to prevent tennis elbow:

- Decrease the amount of playing time if already injured or feeling pain in outside part of the elbow.
- Stay in overall good physical shape.
- Strengthen the muscles of the forearm: (pronator quadratus, pronator teres, and supinator muscle)—the upper arm: (biceps, triceps)—and the shoulder (deltoid muscle) and upper back (trapezius). Increased muscular strength increases stability of joints such as the elbow.
- Like other sports, use equipment appropriate to your ability, body size, and muscular strength.
- Avoid any repetitive lifting or pulling of heavy objects (especially over your head)

Vibration dampeners (otherwise known as "gummies") are not believed to be a reliable preventative measure. Rather, proper weight distribution in the racket is thought to be a more viable option in negating shock.

Diagnosis

To diagnose tennis elbow, the physician performs a battery of tests in which he places pressure on the affected area while asking the patient to move the elbow, wrist, and fingers. X-rays can confirm and distinguish possibilities of existing causes of pain that are unrelated to tennis elbow, such as fracture or arthritis. Medical ultrasonography and magnetic resonance imaging (MRI) are other valuable tools for diagnosis but are frequently avoided due to the high cost. MRI screening can confirm excess fluid and swelling in the affected region in the elbow, such as the connecting point between the forearm bone and the extensor carpi radialis brevis.

Diagnosis is made by clinical signs and symptoms that are discrete and characteristic. With the elbow fully extended, the patient feels points of tenderness over the affected point on the elbow—which is the origin of the extensor carpi radialis brevis muscle from the lateral epicondyle (extensor carpi radialis brevis origin). There is also pain with passive wrist flexion and resistive wrist extension (Cozen's test). Resisted middle finger extension might indicate the involvement of Extensor Digitorum also. These tests shall be used to measure the prognosis of the condition.

Depending upon severity and quantity of multiple tendon injuries that have built up, the extensor carpi radialis brevis may not be fully healed by conservative treatment. Nirschl defines four stages of lateral epicondylitis, showing the introduction of permanent damage beginning at Stage 2.

1. Inflammatory changes that are reversible

2. Nonreversible pathologic changes to origin of the extensor carpi radialis brevis muscle
3. Rupture of ECRB muscle origin
4. Secondary changes such as fibrosis or calcification.

Treatment

Evidence for the treatment of lateral epicondylitis before 2010 was poor. There were clinical trials addressing many proposed treatments, but the trials were of poor quality.

A 2009 study looked at using eccentric exercise with a rubber bar in addition to standard treatment: the trial was stopped after 8 weeks because the improvement using the bar for therapy was so significant. Based on small sample size and a follow-up only 7 weeks from commencement of treatment, the study shows short-term improvements. This along with other studies allowed doctors to conclude that approximately 80-95% of all tennis elbow cases can be treated without surgery. However, long-term results have not yet been determined.

In some cases, severity of tennis elbow symptoms mend without any treatment, within six to 24 months. Tennis elbow left untreated can lead to chronic pain that degrades quality of daily living.

Physical

There are several recommendations regarding prevention, treatment, and avoidance of recurrence that are largely speculative including stretches and progressive strengthening exercises to prevent re-irritation of the tendon and other exercise measures.

One way to help treat minor cases of tennis elbow is to simply relax the affected arm. The rest will allow the stress and tightness within the forearm to slowly relax and eventually have the arm in working condition once again in a day or two, depending on the case.

Evidence from the Tyler study suggests that eccentric exercise using a rubber bar is highly effective at eliminating pain and increasing strength. The exercise involves grasping a rubber bar, twisting it, then slowly untwisting it.

Moderate evidence exists demonstrating that joint manipulation directed at the elbow and wrist and spinal manipulation directed at the cervical and thoracic spinal regions results in clinical changes to pain and function. There is also moderate evidence for short-term and mid-term effectiveness of cervical and thoracic spine manipulation as an add-on therapy to concentric and eccentric stretching plus mobilisation of wrist and forearm. Although not yet conclusive, the short-term analgesic effect of manipulation techniques may allow more vigorous stretching and strengthening exercises, resulting in a better and faster recovery process of the affected tendon in lateral epicondylitis.

Low level laser therapy, administered at specific doses and wavelengths directly to the lateral elbow tendon insertions, offers short-term pain relief and less disability in tennis elbow, both alone and in conjunction with an exercise regimen. Of late, dry needling has been gaining popularity in various types of tendinopathies and pain of muscular origin. Even in lateral epicondylitis, dry needling is widely employed by many physical therapists across the world. It is believed that dry needling would cause a tiny local injury in order to bring about various desirable growth factors in the vicinity. Dry needling is also aimed at eliciting local twitch response (LTR) in the extensor muscles, as in some cases of tennis elbow the extensor muscles of the forearm would harbor trigger points, which itself could be a major source of pain.

Orthotic Devices

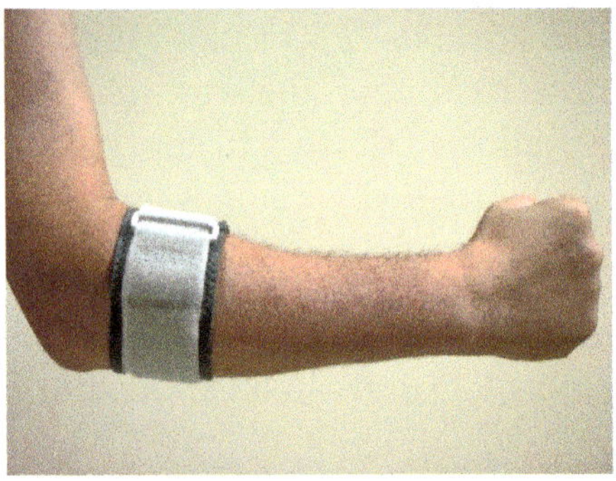

Counterforce orthosis reduces the elongation within the musculotendinious fibers

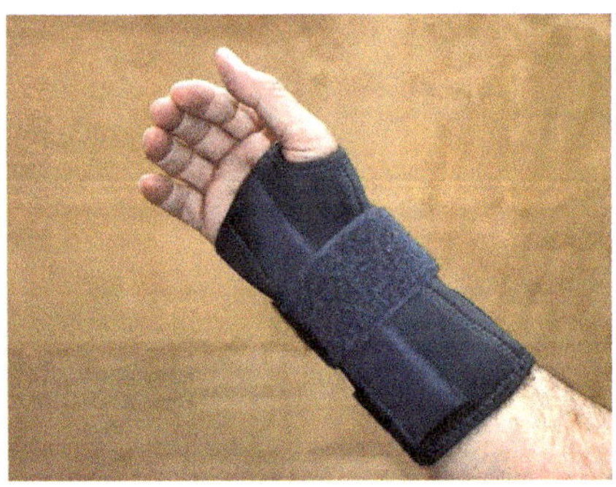

Wrist extensor orthosis reduces the overloading strain at the lesion area

Orthosis is a device externally used on the limb to improve the function or reduce the pain. Orthotics are useful therapeutic interventions for initial therapy of tennis elbow. There are two main types of orthoses prescribed for this problem: counterforce elbow orthoses and wrist extension orthoses.

Counterforce orthosis has a circumferential structure surrounding the arm. This orthosis usually has a strap which applies a binding force over the origin of the wrist extensors. The applied force by orthosis reduces the elongation within the musculotendinious fibers. Wrist extensor orthosis maintains the wrist in the slight extension. This position reduces the overloading strain at the lesion area.

Studies indicated both type of orthoses improve the hand function and reduce the pain in people with tennis elbow.

Medication

Although anti-inflammatories are a commonly prescribed treatment for tennis elbow, the evidence for their effect is usually anecdotal with only limited studies showing a benefit. A systematic review found that topical non-steroidal anti-inflammatory drugs (NSAIDs) may improve pain in the short term (up to 4 weeks) but was unable to draw firm conclusions due to methodological issues. Evidence for oral NSAIDs is mixed.

Evidence is poor for an improvement from injections of any type, be it corticosteroids, botulinum toxin, prolotherapy or other substances. Corticosteroid injection may be effective in the short term however are of little benefit after a year. A recent randomized control trial comparing the effect of cor-ticosteroid injection, physiotherapy, or a combination of corticosteroid injection and physiotherapy found that patients treated with corticosteroid injection versus placebo had lower complete recovery or improvement at 1 year (Relative risk 0.86). Patients that received corticosteroid injection also had a higher recurrence rate at 1 year versus placebo (54% versus 12%, relative risk 0.23). Complications from repeated steroid injections include skin problems such as hypopigmentation and fat atrophy leading to indentation of the skin around the injection site. Botulinum toxin type A to paralyze the forearm extensor muscles in those with chronic tennis elbow that has not improved with conservative measures may be reasonable.

Surgery

In recalcitrant cases, surgery may be an option. Surgical methods include:

- Lengthening, release, debridement, or repair of the origin of the extrinsic extensor muscles of the hand at the lateral epicondyle
- Rotation of the anconeus muscle
- Denervation of the lateral epicondyle
- Decompression of the posterior interosseous nerve

Surgical techniques for lateral epicondylitis can be done by open surgery, percutaneous surgery or arthroscopic surgery, with no evidence that any particular type is better or worse than another.

Prognosis

Response to initial therapy is common, but so is relapse (25% to 50%) and/or prolonged, moderate discomfort (40%).

Epidemiology

In tennis players, about 39.7% have reported current or previous problems with their elbow. Less than one quarter (24%) of these athletes under the age of 50 reported that the tennis elbow symptoms were "severe" and "disabling," while 42% were over the age of 50. More women (36%) than men (24%) considered their symptoms severe and disabling. Tennis elbow is more prevalent in individuals over 40, where there is about a four-fold increase among men and two-fold increase among women. Tennis elbow equally affects both sexes and, although men have a marginally higher overall prevalence rate as compared to women, this is not consistent within each age group, nor is it a statistically significant difference.

Playing time is a factor in tennis elbow occurrences. However, increased incidence with increased playing time is statistically significant only for respondents under 40. Individuals over 40 who played over two hours had a two-fold increase in chance of injury. Those under 40 had a 3.5 times increase compared to those who played less than two hours per day.

Tendinosis

Tendinosis, sometimes called chronic tendinitis, chronic tendinopathy, or chronic tendon injury, is damage to a tendon at a cellular level (the suffix "osis" implies a pathology of chronic degeneration without inflammation). It is thought to be caused by microtears in the connective tissue in and around the tendon, leading to an increase in tendon repair cells. This may lead to reduced tensile strength, thus increasing the chance of tendon rupture. Tendinosis is often misdiagnosed as tendinitis because of the limited understanding of tendinopathies by the medical community. Classic characteristics of "tendinosis" include degenerative changes in the collagenous matrix, hypercellularity, hypervascularity, and a lack of inflammatory cells which has challenged the original misnomer "tendinitis".

Causes

Tendinosis of the common extensor tendon of the elbow ("tennis elbow") is a common cause of elbow pain for adults.

The general opinion is that tennis elbow tendinosis is due to tendon overuse, and failed healing of the tendon. In addition, the extensor carpi radialis brevis muscle plays a key role.

Tendinosis of the tensor fasciae lateralis where it arises from the anterior part of the outer lip of the iliac crest; from the outer surface of the anterior superior iliac spine, and part of the outer border of the notch below it, between the gluteus medius and sartorius; and from the deep surface of the fascia lata. Pain in the hip area is a common symptom which is often misdiagnosed as hip pain.

Diagnosis

Symptoms can vary from an ache or pain and stiffness to the local area of the tendon, or a burning that surrounds the whole joint around the affected tendon. With this condition, the pain is usually worse during and after activity, and the tendon and joint area can become stiffer the following day as swelling impinges on the movement of the tendon. Many patients report stressful situations in their life in correlation with the beginnings of pain, which may contribute to the symptoms.

Swelling in a region of micro damage or partial tear may be detected visually or by touch.

Medical Imaging

Ultrasound imaging can be used to evaluate tissue strain, as well as other mechanical properties.

Ultrasound-based techniques are becoming more popular because of its affordability, safety, and speed. Ultrasound can be used for imaging tissues, and the sound waves can also provide information about the mechanical state of the tissue.

Increased water content and disorganized collagen matrix in tendon lesions may be detected by ultrasonography or magnetic resonance imaging.

Pathophysiology

Histological findings include granulation tissue, microrupture, degenerative changes, and there is no traditional inflammation. As a consequence, "lateral elbow tendinopathy or tendinosis" is used instead of "lateral epicondylitis".

Examination of tennis elbow tissue reveals noninflammatory tissue, so the term "angiofibroblastic tendinosis" is used.

Cultures from tendinopathic tendons contain an increased production of type III collagen.

Longitudinal sonogram of the lateral elbow displays thickening and heterogeneity of the common extensor tendon that is consistent with tendinosis, as the ultrasound reveals calcifications, intrasubstance tears, and marked irregularity of the lateral epicondyle. Although the term "epicondylitis" is frequently used to describe this disorder, most histopathologic findings of studies have displayed no evidence of an acute, or a chronic inflammatory process. Histologic studies have demonstrated that this condition is the result of tendon degeneration, which causes normal tissue to be replaced by a disorganized arrangement of collagen. Therefore, the disorder is more appropriately referred to as "tendinosis" or "tendinopathy" rather than "tendinitis."

Colour Doppler ultrasound reveals structural tendon changes, with vascularity and hypo-echoic areas that correspond to the areas of pain in the extensor origin.

Load-induced non-rupture tendinopathy in humans is associated with an increase in the ratio of collagen III:I proteins, a shift from large to small diameter collagen fibrils, buckling of the collagen fascicles in the tendon extracellular matrix, and buckling of the tenocyte cells and their nuclei.

Treatment

An injured tendon is very slow to heal. Partial tears heal by the rapid production of disorganized type-III collagen which is weaker than normal tendon. Recurrence of injury in the damaged region of the tendon is common.

Rehabilitation, rest, and gradual return to the activity in which tendinosis was experienced is a common therapy. There is evidence to suggest that tendinosis is not an inflammatory disorder; anti-inflammatory drugs are not an effective treatment; and inflammation is not the cause of this type of tendon dysfunction. There is a variety of treatment options but more research is necessary to determine their effectiveness. Initial recovery is usually within 2 to 3 months, and full recovery usually within 3 to 6 months. About 80% of patients will fully recover within 12 months. If the conservative therapy doesn't work, then surgery can be an option. This surgery consists of the excision of abnormal tissue. Time required to recover from surgery is about 4 to 6 months. Studies with a rat model of fatigue-damaged tendons suggested that delaying exercise until after the initial inflammatory stage of repair could promote remodelling more rapidly.

Research

Both eccentric loading and extracorporeal shockwave therapy are currently being researched as possible treatments for tendinosis. One study found both modalities to be equally effective in treating tendinosis of the Achilles tendon and more effective than a 'wait and see' approach. Other treatments for which research is on-going includes vitamin E, vitamin B6, nitric oxide, Platelet Rich Plasma (PRP), and stem cell injections.

Vitamin C

One study found increased achilles tendon healing in rats supplemented with high doses of vitamin C, which is needed for collagen synthesis.

Vitamin E

Vitamin E has been found to increase the activity of fibroblasts, leading to increased collagen fibrils and synthesis, which seems to speed up the regeneration and increase the regenerative capacity of tendons.

Nitric Oxide

Nitric oxide (NO) also appears to play a role in tendon healing and inhibition of its synthesis impairs tendon healing. The use of a nitric oxide delivery system (glyceryl trinitrate patches) applied over the area of maximal tenderness was tested in three clinical trials for the treatment of tendinopathies and was found to significantly reduce pain and increase range of motion and strength.

One study found that arginine supplementation, which may possibly increase NO signaling, was able to increase the speed of tendon healing

Soft Tissue Mobilization

Augmented Soft Tissue Mobilization (ASTM) is a form of manual therapy that has been shown in studies on rats to speed the healing of tendons by increasing fibroblast activity. One case study showed ASTM resulting in full recovery in the case of an athlete suffering from chronic ankle pain and fibrosis, after an unsuccessful course of surgery and conventional physical therapy.

Eccentric Loading

A promising line of therapy involves eccentric loading exercises involving lengthening muscular contractions.

Inflatable Brace

The use of an inflatable brace (AirHeel) was shown to be as effective as eccentric loading in the treatment of chronic Achilles tendinopathy. Both modalities produced significant reduction in pain scores, but their combination was no more effective than either treatment alone.

Shock-wave Therapy

Shock-wave therapy (SWT) may be effective in treating calcific tendinosis in both humans and rats. In rat subjects, SWT increased levels of healing hormones and proteins leading to increased cell proliferation and tissue regeneration in tendons. Another study found no evidence that SWT was useful in treating chronic pain in the Achilles tendon.

Tendon Bioengineering

The future of non-surgical care for tendinosis is likely bioengineering. Ligament reconstruction is possible using mesenchymal stem cells and a silk scaffold. These same stem cells were capable of seeding repair of damaged animal tendons. Autologous tenocyte implantation is currently being tested for tendinosis. There is a large randomized, double-blind, placebo controlled trial being conducted in the Netherlands to test the safety and efficacy of tenocyte therapy. Results from the trial are expected by April 2013.

Autologous Tenocyte Injection

A study investigated autologous tenocyte injection for the treatment of severe, chronic resistant lateral epicondylitis. A needle biopsy was used on the patellar tendon, and the extracted tendon cells were expanded by in vitro culture. The autologous tenocytes were sorted and purified by real-time polymerase chain reaction, and amplified by flow cytometry. The tenocytes were then injected into the injured tendinopathy site, which was the origin of the extensor carpi radialis brevis tendon, under the guidance of an ultrasound. After the autologous tenocyte injection treatment, patients with chronic lateral epicondylitis showed improved clinical function and structural repair at the origin of the common extensor tendon.

Nonbulbar Dermal Sheath Cells

RepliCel has planned a Phase 1/2 Achilles tendinosis clinical trial using fibroblasts that are isolated from the nonbulbar dermal sheath cells of a hair follicle, and is recruiting in Q1 2015. The tendon treatment will be tested in approximately 28 subjects. Nonbulbar dermal sheath cells are used because they produce more type I collagen than fibroblasts that are derived from adipose tissue. Type I collagen is the primary collagen in tendons. Nonbulbar dermal sheath cells will be replicated, and then reintroduced into the wounded tendons with ultrasound. After the injections, subjects will be assessed for pain, safety, and function, as well as changes in interstitial tears, tendon thickness, echotexture, and neovascularity.

Injections of MicroRNA

Scientists found that mir-29a, a single microRNA, through its interaction with a protein, interleukin 33, plays a key role in regulating the production of collagens in tendon disease. Loss of miR29a from human tendons results in an increase in collagen type-3 production, which is a key feature of tendon disease. The replacement of miR-29a in the damaged tendon cells in the laboratory restores collagen production to pre injury levels. A trial will put injections of microRNA – small molecules that help regulate gene expression – into the tendon to decrease the production of type 3 collagen and switch to type-1.

Allogenic Adipose-derived Mesenchymal Stem Cells

As of November 2013, researchers at the Seoul National University Hospital will be looking to recruit participants into a clinical trial to evaluate the efficacy of allogenic adipose-derived mesenchymal stem cells (ALLO-ASC) for the treatment of a lateral epicondylitis tendon injury where the duration of the symptoms is over six months. Adipose-derived mesenchymal stem cells will be administrated to the patients with lateral epicondylitis (tennis elbow) by an ultrasonographic-guided injection.

Elastography Ultrasound

Researchers have tried to analyze tissue strain and mechanical properties using elastography, which is an acoustical imaging technique that measures strain distributions in tissues that result from stress or compression of the tissue. Strain is inversely related to stiffness, so under a given amount of stress, tissue that displays less strain is assumed to be stiffer than tissue that exhibits more strain. Elastography is therefore an indirect method to estimate tissue stiffness.

One limitation of elastography is that it is inherently linear when ultrasound wave velocity and the material properties do not change during the strain measurement. This is a problem in soft tissues like tendons, as they are nonlinear in stiffness, and can undergo large deformations in activity. Elastography measures strain, and to more completely described the mechanical behavior, more data, like stiffness or stress would be required.

Acoustoelastography Ultrasound

Acoustoelastic theory is based on the principle that the acoustic properties of a material are altered as the material is loaded and deformed. The properties can be measured as a change in amplitude and wave velocity.

With the use of A-mode ultrasound, researchers have derived an acoustic relationship between reflected wave amplitude, and strain-dependent stiffness and stress in a deformed material.

As tendon tension increases, the intensity of reflected ultrasonic echoes increases. The increased intensity results in a brighter B-mode ultrasound image.

Acoustoelastography is an ultrasound technique that relates ultrasonic wave amplitude changes to the mechanical properties of a tendon.

It is an ultrasound-based model that can be used evaluate tendon function. Gradual deformations of a tendon can produce cine loops, where changes in echo intensity can be observed. By analyzing the echo intensity changes with Acoustoelastography, one can deduce the stiffness gradient, which is the rate of change of normalised stiffness as a function of strain.

EchoSoft ultrasound software from the Wisconsin Alumni Research Foundation and Echometrix applies the theory of acoustoelasticity to measure musculoskeletal (tendon and ligament) tissue. The software examines previously unused information found by ultrasound waves to quantify the extent of musculoskeletal injuries, or a patient's progress in a healing process.

Ultrasonic Percutaneous Tenotomy

Percutaneous ultrasonic tenotomy provided continued pain relief and functional improvement for recalcitrant tennis elbow at a 3-year follow-up.

Other Animals

Bowed tendon is a horseman's term for tendinitis (inflammation) and tendinosis (degeneration), most commonly seen in the superficial digital flexor tendon (SDFT) in the front leg.

Diagnosis

When the superficial digital flexor tendon of horses is damaged, there is a thickening of the tendon, giving it a bowed appearance when the leg is viewed from the side.

Medical Imaging

A study tested the repeatability and feasibility of using acoustoelastography for in vivo measurement of stiffness gradients in the superficial digital flexor tendons (SDFTs) of clinically normal horses. The results show that acoustoelastography is a repeatable and feasible technique for measuring stiffness gradients of superficial digital flexor tendons in clinically normal horses, and acoustoelastography has the potential to be used for comparing diseased and healthy tendon states.

A report describes the use of acoustoelastography to monitor the mechanical healing of an Achilles tendon laceration in a dog after suture repair. Serial acoustoelastography examinations of the tendon showed that mechanical properties improved throughout the recovery period. At 29 weeks, the mechanical properties of the repaired tendon were similar to that of the normal contralateral Achilles mechanism.

A study shows that acoustoelastography is a repeatable and feasible method for measuring stiffness gradients in equine superficial digital flexor tendons.

The acoustoelastic strain gauge is an ultrasound-based tissue evaluation technique that relates echo intensity changes that are observed during the stretching or relaxation tendons to the mechanical properties of the tissue. The method deduces stiffness gradient (the rate of change of normalized stiffness as a function of tissue strain) by evaluating the ultrasound dynamic images that are captured from tissue as it gradually deforms. Acoustoelastic strain gauge has been shown to accurately model stiffness and strain within tendons in vitro. To determine the repeatability and feasibility of in vivo ASG measurements of canine tendon function, stiffness gradients for the gastrocnemius tendons of dogs were recorded. Findings indicate that acoustoelastic strain gauge is a repeatable and feasible technique for measuring stiffness gradients in canine tendons.

Pathophysiology

Achilles tendons in rats were studied with acoustoelastography ultrasound. After a tendon injury, and during tendon healing, vascularity changes and cellular activity are vital to the formation of granular tissue in the tendon gap, and the subsequent development of neo-tendinous tissue that replaces damaged native tissue. Normal, intact tendon is composed mainly of type I collagen, and type III collagen increases after injury. Another study has recorded an association between collagen fibers and echogenicity tendon during Achilles tendon healing.

This report further indicates that a decrease in type I procollagen (and increase in type III collagen and periostin) correlates to reduced strength, echo intensity, and normalized stiffness. It shows that tissue normalized stiffness is linearly correlated to procollagen I, while echo intensity is seen to be nonlinearly correlated to type I procollagen. Furthermore, the increase in M1 macrophages, blood vessels, and proliferating cells that occur within two weeks of the injury are associated with a formation of granulation tissue. Ultimate stress, echo intensity, and normalized stiffness are all their lowest during these times. The results assert that the reduction in stress and normalized stiffness that is measured by ultrasonic and mechanical methods correlate well with the biological aspect of tendon healing.

Treatment

Mesenchymal stem cells, derived from a horse's bone marrow or fat, are currently being used for tendon repair in horses.

Confusion Between Tendonitis Versus Tendinosis

Tendonitis is a very common, but misleading term. Corticosteroids are drugs that reduce inflammation. They are typically injected along with a small amount of a numbing drug called lidocaine. By definition, anything that ends in "itis" means "inflammation of." Research shows that tendons are weaker following corticosteroid injections. Tendinitis is still a very common diagnosis, though research increasingly documents that what is thought to be tendinitis is usually tendinosis.

Chondromalacia Patellae

Chondromalacia patellae (also known as CMP) is inflammation of the underside of the patella and softening of the cartilage.

Chondromalacia patellae is a term sometimes treated synonymously with patellofemoral pain syndrome. However, there is general consensus that patellofemoral pain syndrome is a term that applies only to individuals without cartilage damage, thereby distinguishing it from chondromalacia patellae, a condition characterized by softening of the patellar articular cartilage.

The cartilage under the kneecap is a natural shock absorber, and overuse, injury, and many other factors can cause increased deterioration and breakdown of the cartilage. The cartilage is no longer smooth and therefore movement and use is painful. While it often affects young individuals engaged in active sports, it also afflicts older adults who overwork their knees.

Description

While the term *chondromalacia* sometimes refers to abnormal-appearing cartilage anywhere in the body, it most commonly denotes irritation of the underside of the kneecap (or "patella"). The patella's posterior surface is covered with a layer of smooth cartilage, which the base of the femur normally glides effortlessly against when the knee is bent. However, in some individuals the kneecap tends to rub against one side of the knee joint, irritating the cartilage and causing knee pain.

The condition may result from acute injury to the patella or chronic friction between the patella and a groove in the femur through which it passes during knee flexion. Possible causes include a tight iliotibial band, neuromas, bursitis, overuse, malalignment, core instability, and patellar maltracking.

Pain at the front or inner side of the knee is common in both young adults and those of more advanced years, especially when engaging in soccer, gymnastics, cycling, rowing, tennis, ballet, basketball, horseback riding, volleyball, running, combat sports, figure skating, snowboarding, skateboarding and even swimming. The pain is typically felt after prolonged sitting. Skateboarders most commonly experience this injury in their non-dominant foot due to the constant kicking and twisting required of it. Swimmers acquire it doing the breaststroke, which demands an unusual motion of the knee. People who are involved in an active life style with high impact on the knees are at greatest risk. Proper management of physical activity may help prevent worsening of the condition. Athletes are advised to talk to a physician for further medical diagnosis as symptoms may be similar to more serious problems within the knee. Tests are not necessarily needed for diagnosis, but in some situations it may confirm diagnosis or rule out other causes for pain. Commonly used tests are blood tests, MRI scans, and arthroscopy.

Treatment

In the absence of cartilage damage, pain at the front of the knee due to overuse can be managed with a combination of RICE (rest, ice, compression, elevation), anti-inflammatory medications, and physiotherapy.

Usually chondromalacia develops without swelling or bruising and most individuals benefit from rest and adherence to an appropriate physical therapy program. Allowing inflammation to subside while avoiding irritating activities for several weeks is followed by a gradual resumption. Cross-training activities such as swimming, strokes other than the breaststroke, can help to maintain general fitness and body composition. This is beneficial until a physical therapy program emphasizing strengthening and flexibility of the hip and thigh muscles can be undertaken. Use of nonsteroidal anti-inflammatory medication is also helpful to minimize the swelling amplifying patellar pain. Treatment with surgery is declining in popularity due to positive non-surgical outcomes and the relative ineffectiveness of surgical intervention.

Wound

A wound is a type of injury which happens relatively quickly in which skin is torn, cut, or punctured (an *open* wound), or where blunt force trauma causes a contusion (a *closed* wound). In pathology, it specifically refers to a sharp injury which damages the dermis of the skin.

Classification

According to level of contamination, a wound can be classified as:

- Clean wound - made under sterile conditions where there are no organisms present, and the skin is likely to heal without complications.
- Contaminated wound - usually resulting from accidental injury; there are pathogenic organisms and foreign bodies in the wound.
- Infected wound - the wound has pathogenic organisms present and multiplying, exhibiting clinical signs of infection (yellow appearance, soreness, redness, oozing pus).
- Colonized wound - a chronic situation, containing pathogenic organisms, difficult to heal (i.e. bedsore).

Open

Open wounds can be classified according to the object that caused the wound:

- Incisions or incised wounds - caused by a clean, sharp-edged object such as a knife, razor, or glass splinter.
- Lacerations - irregular tear-like wounds caused by some blunt trauma. Lacera-

tions and incisions may appear linear (regular) or stellate (irregular). The term *laceration* is commonly misused in reference to incisions.

- Abrasions (grazes) - superficial wounds in which the topmost layer of the skin (the epidermis) is scraped off. Abrasions are often caused by a sliding fall onto a rough surface.
- Avulsions - injuries in which a body structure is forcibly detached from its normal point of insertion. A type of amputation where the extremity is pulled off rather than cut off.
- Puncture wounds - caused by an object puncturing the skin, such as a splinter, nail or needle.
- Penetration wounds - caused by an object such as a knife entering and coming out from the skin.
- Gunshot wounds - caused by a bullet or similar projectile driving into or through the body. There may be two wounds, one at the site of entry and one at the site of exit, generally referred to as a "through-and-through."

Closed

Closed wounds have fewer categories, but are just as dangerous as open wounds:

- Hematomas (or blood tumor) - caused by damage to a blood vessel that in turn causes blood to collect under the skin.
    - Hematomas that originate from internal blood vessel pathology are petechiae, purpura, and ecchymosis. The different classifications are based on size.
    - Hematomas that originate from an external source of trauma are contusions, also commonly called bruises.
- Crush injury - caused by a great or extreme amount of force applied over a long period of time.

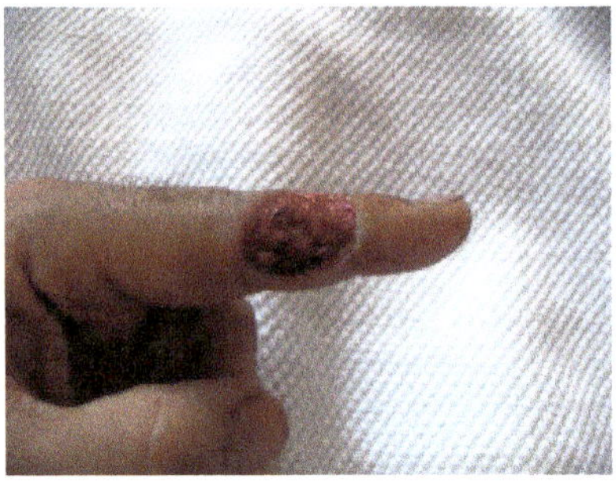

An open wound (an avulsion)

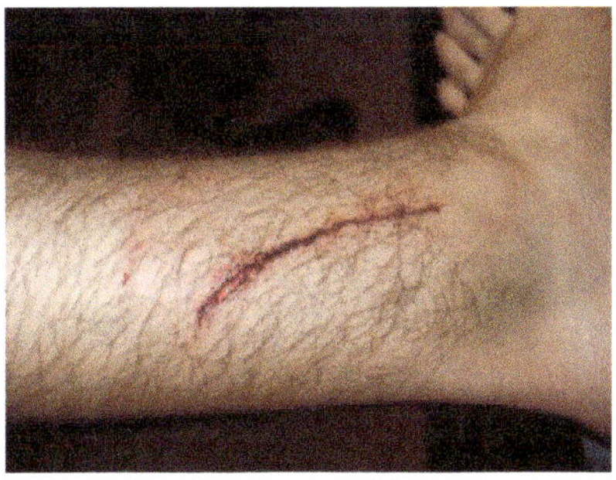
A laceration to the leg

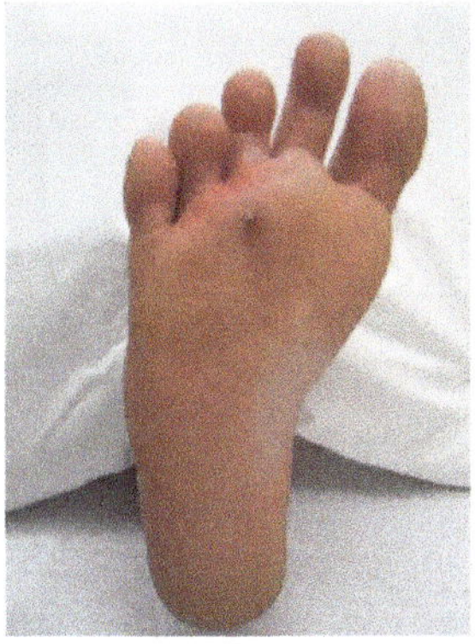
An infected puncture wound to the bottom of the forefoot.

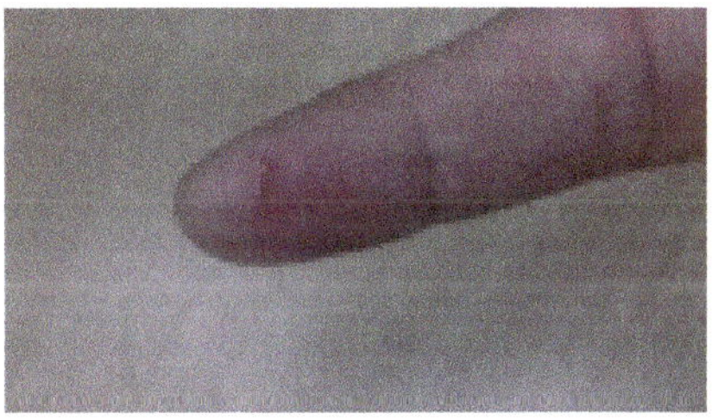
An incision: a small cut in a finger.

Pathophysiology

To heal a wound, the body undertakes a series of actions collectively known as the wound healing process.

Diagnosis

A wound may be recorded for follow-up and observing progress of healing with different techniques which include:

- Photographs, with subsequent area quantification using computer processing
- Wound tracings on acetate sheets
- Kundin wound gauge

Management

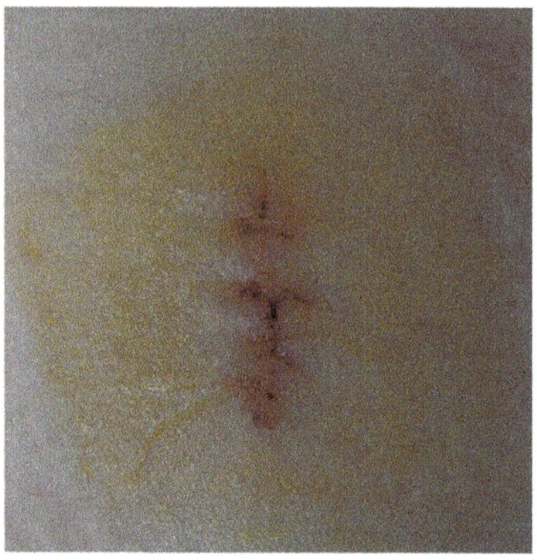

Wound, sewn with four stitches

The overall treatment depends on the type, cause, and depth of the wound, and whether other structures beyond the skin (dermis) are involved. Treatment of recent lacerations involves examining, cleaning, and closing the wound. Minor wounds, like bruises, will heal on their own, with skin discoloration usually disappearing in 1–2 weeks. Abrasions, which are wounds with intact skin (non-penetration through dermis to subcutaneous fat), usually require no active treatment except keeping the area clean, initially with soap and water. Puncture wounds may be prone to infection depending on the depth of penetration. The entry of puncture wound is left open to allow for bacteria or debris to be removed from inside.

Cleaning

Evidence to support the cleaning of wounds before closure is scant. For simple lacerations, cleaning can be accomplished using a number of different solutions, including tap water and sterile saline solution. Infection rates may be lower with the use of tap water in regions where water quality is high. Cleaning of a wound is also known as 'wound toilet'.

Closure

If a person presents to a healthcare center within 6 hours of a laceration they are typically closed immediately after evaluating and cleaning the wound. After this point in time, however, there is a theoretical concern of increased risks of infection if closed immediately. Thus some healthcare providers may delay closure while others may be willing to immediately close up to 24 hours after the injury. A single study has found that using clean non-sterile gloves is equivalent to using sterile gloves during wound closure.

If closure of a wound is decided upon a number of techniques can be used. These include bandages, a cyanoacrylate glue, staples, and sutures. Absorbable sutures have the benefit over non absorbable sutures of not requiring removal. They are often preferred in children. Buffering the pH of lidocaine makes the injection less painful.

Adhesive glue and sutures have comparable cosmetic outcomes for minor lacerations <5 cm in adults and children. The use of adhesive glue involves considerably less time for the doctor and less pain for the person. The wound opens at a slightly higher rate but there is less redness. The risk for infections (1.1%) is the same for both. Adhesive glue should not be used in areas of high tension or repetitive movements, such as joints or the posterior trunk.

Dressings

In the case of clean surgical wounds, there is no evidence that the use of topical antibiotics reduces infection rates in comparison with non-antibiotic ointment or no ointment at all. Antibiotic ointments can irritate the skin, slow healing, and greatly increase the risk of developing contact dermatitis and antibiotic resistance. Because of this, they should only be used when a person shows signs of infection and not as a preventative.

The effectiveness of dressings and creams containing silver to prevent infection or improve healing is not currently supported by evidence.

Alternative Medicine

There is moderate evidence that honey is more effective than antiseptic followed by gauze for healing wounds infected after surgical operations. There is a lack of quality evidence relating to the use of honey on other types of wounds, such as minor acute wounds, mixed acute and chronic wounds, pressure ulcers, Fournier's gangrene, venous leg ulcers, diabetic foot ulcers and Leishmaniasis.

There is no good evidence that therapeutic touch is useful in healing. More than 400 species of plants are identified as potentially useful for wound healing. Only three randomized controlled trials, however, have been done for the treatment of burns.

An electroactive material developed by NASA has been found beneficial as a wound dressing. It uses electrical activity (generated by body heat and the pressure of cell growth) to facilitate the wound healing process while protecting the wound. The bandage is fabricated from polyvinylidene fluoride, or PVDF, a thermoplastic fluoropolymer that is highly piezoelectric when poled.

Complications

Bacterial infection of wound can impede the healing process and lead to life-threatening complications. Scientists at Sheffield University have used light to rapidly detect the presence of bacteria, by developing a portable kit in which specially designed molecules emit a light signal when bound to bacteria. Current laboratory-based detection of bacteria can take hours or days.

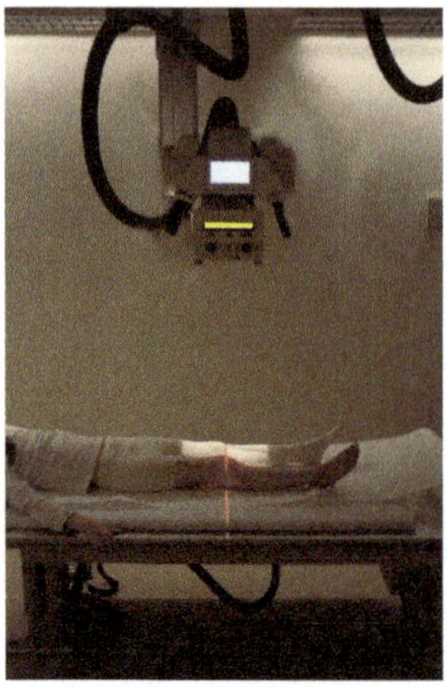

The patient has a deep wound at the knee, and radiography is used to ensure there are no hidden bone fractures.

Workup

Wounds that are not healing should be investigated to find the causes; many microbiological agents may be responsible. The basic workup includes evaluating the wound, its extent and severity. Cultures are usually obtained both from the wound site and blood. X-rays are obtained and a tetanus shot may be administered if there is any doubt about prior vaccination.

Chronic

Non-healing wounds of the diabetic foot are considered one of the most significant complications of diabetes, representing a major worldwide medical, social, and economic burden that greatly affects patient quality of life. Almost 24 million Americans—one in every 12—are diabetic and the disease is causing widespread disability and death at an epidemic pace, according to the Centers for Disease Control and Prevention. Of those with diabetes, 6.5 million are estimated to suffer with chronic or non-healing wounds. Associated with inadequate circulation, poorly functioning veins, and immobility, non-healing wounds occur most frequently in the elderly and in people with diabetes—populations that are sharply rising as the nation ages and chronic diseases increase.

Although diabetes can ravage the body in many ways, non-healing ulcers on the feet and lower legs are common outward manifestations of the disease. Also, diabetics often suffer from nerve damage in their feet and legs, allowing small wounds or irritations to develop without awareness. Given the abnormalities of the microvasculature and other side effects of diabetes, these wounds take a long time to heal and require a specialized treatment approach for proper healing.

As many as 25% of diabetic patients will eventually develop foot ulcers, and recurrence within five years is 70%. If not aggressively treated, these wounds can lead to amputations. It is estimated that every 30 seconds a lower limb is amputated somewhere in the world because of a diabetic wound. Amputation often triggers a downward spiral of declining quality of life, frequently leading to disability and death. In fact, only about one third of diabetic amputees will live more than five years, a survival rate equivalent to that of many cancers.

Many of these lower extremity amputations can be prevented through an interdisciplinary approach to treatment involving a variety of advanced therapies and techniques, such as debridement, hyperbaric oxygen treatment therapy, dressing selection, special shoes, and patient education. When wounds persist, a specialized approach is required for healing.

History

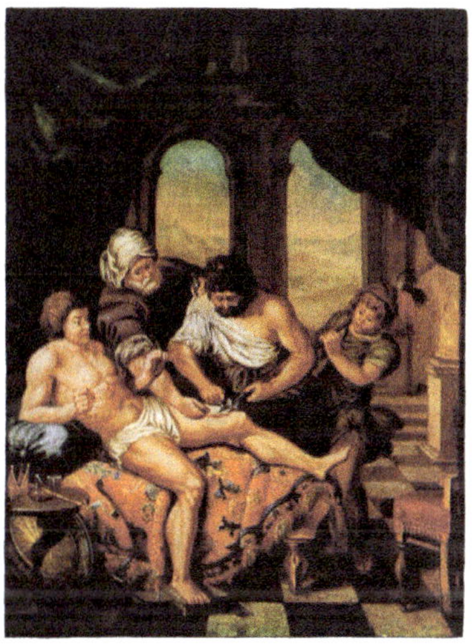

Medieval treatment of wound with lance grittings

From the Classical Period to the Medieval Period, the body and the soul were believed to be intimately connected, based on several theories put forth by the philosopher Plato. Wounds on the body were believed to correlate with wounds to the soul and vice versa; wounds were seen as an outward sign of an inward illness. Thus, a man who was wounded physically in a serious way was said to be hindered not only physically but spiritually as well. If the soul was wounded, that wound may also eventually become physically manifest, revealing the true state of the soul. Wounds were also seen as writing on the "tablet" of the body. Wounds acquired in war, for example, told the story of a soldier in a form which all could see and understand, and the wounds of a martyr told the story of their faith.

Research

In humans and mice it has been shown that estrogen might affect the speed and quality of wound healing.

Bone Fracture

A bone fracture (sometimes abbreviated FRX or Fx, F_x, or #) is a medical condition in which there is a damage in the continuity of the bone. A bone fracture can be the result of high force impact or stress, or a minimal trauma injury as a result of certain medical conditions that weaken the bones, such as osteoporosis, bone cancer, or osteogenesis imperfecta, where the fracture is then properly termed a pathologic fracture.

Although broken bone and bone break are common colloquialisms for a bone fracture, *break* is not a formal orthopedic term.

Signs and Symptoms

Although bone tissue itself contains no nociceptors, bone fracture is painful for several reasons:

- Breaking in the continuity of the periosteum, with or without similar discontinuity in endosteum, as both contain multiple pain receptors.
- Edema of nearby soft tissues caused by bleeding of torn periosteal blood vessels evokes pressure pain.
- Muscle spasms trying to hold bone fragments in place. Sometimes also followed by cramping.

Damage to adjacent structures such as nerves or vessels, spinal cord and nerve roots (for spine fractures), or cranial contents (for skull fractures) can cause other specific signs and symptoms.

Pathophysiology

The natural process of healing a fracture starts when the injured bone and surrounding tissues bleed, forming a fracture hematoma. The blood coagulates to form a blood clot situated between the broken fragments. Within a few days, blood vessels grow into the jelly-like matrix of the blood clot. The new blood vessels bring phagocytes to the area, which gradually remove the non-viable material. The blood vessels also bring fibroblasts in the walls of the vessels and these multiply and produce collagen fibres. In this way the blood clot is replaced by a matrix of collagen. Collagen's rubbery consistency allows bone fragments to move only a small amount unless severe or persistent force is applied.

At this stage, some of the fibroblasts begin to lay down bone matrix in the form of collagen monomers. These monomers spontaneously assemble to form the bone matrix, for which bone crystals (calcium hydroxyapatite) are deposited in amongst, in the form of insoluble crystals. This mineralization of the collagen matrix stiffens it and transforms it into bone. In fact, bone *is* a mineralized collagen matrix; if the mineral is dissolved out of bone, it becomes rubbery. Healing bone callus is on average sufficiently mineralized to show up on X-ray within 6 weeks in adults and less in children. This initial "woven" bone does not have the strong mechanical properties of mature bone. By a process of remodeling, the woven bone is replaced by mature "lamellar" bone. The whole process can take up to 18 months, but in adults the strength of the healing bone is usually 80% of normal by 3 months after the injury.

Several factors can help or hinder the bone healing process. For example, any form of nicotine hinders the process of bone healing, and adequate nutrition (including calcium intake) will help the bone healing process. Weight-bearing stress on bone, after the bone has healed sufficiently to bear the weight, also builds bone strength. Although there are theoretical concerns about NSAIDs slowing the rate of healing, there is not enough evidence to warrant withholding the use of this type analgesic in simple fractures.

Effects of Smoking

Smokers generally have lower bone density than non-smokers, so have a much higher risk of fractures. There is also evidence that smoking delays bone healing. Some research indicates, for example, that it delays tibial shaft fracture healing from a median healing time of 136 to 269 days. This means that the fracture healing time was approximately doubled in smokers. Although some other studies show less extreme effects, it is still shown that smoking delays fracture healing.

Diagnosis

A bone fracture may be diagnosed based on the history given and the physical examination performed. Radiographic imaging is often performed, to confirm the diagnosis. Under certain circumstances, radiographic examination of the nearby joints is indicated in order to exclude dislocations and fracture-dislocations. In situations where projectional radiography alone is insufficient, Computed Tomography (CT) or Magnetic Resonance Imaging (MRI) may be indicated.

Classification

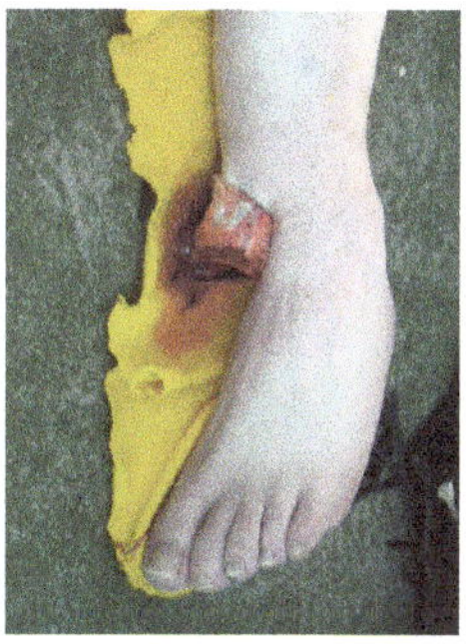

Open ankle fracture with luxation

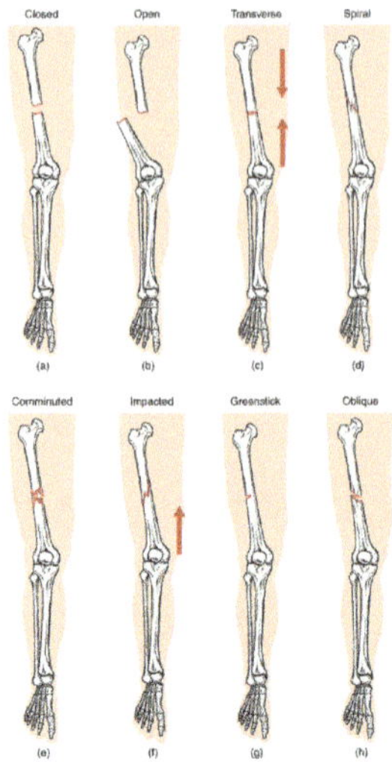

Compare healthy bone with different types of fractures:(a) closed fracture (b) open fracture (c) transverse fracture (d) spiral fracture (e) comminuted fracture (f) impacted fracture (g) greenstick fracture (h) oblique fracture

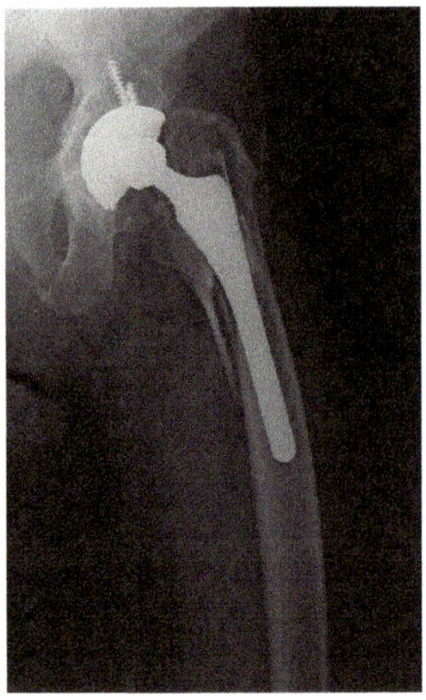

Periprosthetic fracture of left femur

In orthopedic medicine, fractures are classified in various ways. Historically they are named after the doctor who first described the fracture conditions. However, there are more systematic classifications in place currently.

Mechanism

- Traumatic fracture – This is a fracture due to sustained trauma. e.g., - Fractures caused by a fall, road traffic accident, fight etc.
- Pathologic fracture – A fracture through a bone which has been made weak by some underlying disease is called pathological fracture. e.g., - a fracture through a bone weakened by metastasis. Osteoporosis is the most common cause of pathological fracture.

- Periprosthetic fracture – A fracture at the point of mechanical weakness at the end of an implant

Soft-tissue Involvement

- Closed fracture: are those in which the overlying skin is intact
- Open fracture/Compound fracture: involve wounds that communicate with the fracture, or where fracture hematoma is exposed, and may thus expose bone to contamination. Open injuries carry a higher risk of infection.
    - Clean fracture
    - Contaminated fracture

Displacement

- Non-displaced
- Displaced
    - Translated
    - Angulated
    - Rotated
    - Shortened

Fracture Pattern

- Linear fracture: A fracture that is parallel to the bone's long axis.
- Transverse fracture: A fracture that is at a right angle to the bone's long axis .
- Oblique fracture: A fracture that is diagonal to a bone's long axis (more than 30°).
- Spiral fracture: A fracture where at least one part of the bone has been twisted.
- Compression fracture/Wedge fracture: usually occurs in the vertebrae, for example when the front portion of a vertebra in the spine collapses due to osteoporosis (a medical condition which causes bones to become brittle and susceptible to fracture, with or without trauma).
- Impacted fracture: A fracture caused when bone fragments are driven into each other.
- Avulsion fracture: A fracture where a fragment of bone is separated from the main mass.

Fragments

- Incomplete fracture: A fracture in which the bone fragments are still partially joined. In such cases, there is a crack in the osseous tissue that does not completely traverse the width of the bone
- Complete fracture: A fracture in which bone fragments separate completely.
- Comminuted fracture: A fracture in which the bone has broken into several pieces.

Anatomical Location

An anatomical classification may begin with specifying the involved body part, such as the head or arm, followed with more specific localization. Fractures that have additional definition criteria than merely localization can often be classified as subtypes of fractures that merely are, such as a Holstein-Lewis fracture being a subtype of a humerus fracture. However, most typical examples in an orthopedic classification given in previous section cannot appropriately be classified into any specific part of an anatomical classification, as they may apply to multiple anatomical fracture sites.

- Skull fracture
    - Basilar skull fracture
    - Blowout fracture – a fracture of the walls or floor of the orbit
    - Mandibular fracture
    - Nasal fracture
    - Le Fort fracture of skull – facial fractures involving the maxillary bone and surrounding structures in a usually bilateral and either horizontal, pyramidal or transverse way.
- Spinal fracture
    - Cervical fracture
        - Fracture of *C1*, including Jefferson fracture
        - Fracture of *C2*, including Hangman's fracture
        - Flexion teardrop fracture – a fracture of the anteroinferior aspect of a cervical vertebral
        - Clay-shoveler fracture – fracture through the spinous process of a vertebra occurring at any of the lower cervical or upper thoracic vertebrae

        - Burst fracture – in which a vertebra breaks from a high-energy axial load
        - Compression fracture – a collapse of a vertebra, often in the form of wedge fractures due to larger compression anteriorly.
        - Chance fracture – compression injury to the anterior portion of a vertebral body with concomitant distraction injury to posterior elements
        - Holdsworth fracture – an unstable fracture dislocation of the thoracolumbar junction of the spine
- Rib fracture
- Sternal fracture
- Shoulder fracture
    - Clavicle fracture
    - Scapular fracture
- Arm fracture
    - Humerus fracture (fracture of upper arm)
        - Supracondylar fracture
        - Holstein-Lewis fracture – a fracture of the distal third of the humerus resulting in entrapment of the radial nerve.
    - Forearm fracture
        - Ulnar fracture
            - Monteggia fracture – a fracture of the proximal third of the ulna with the dislocation of the head of the radius
            - Hume fracture – a fracture of the olecranon with an associated anterior dislocation of the radial head
        - Radius fracture
            - Essex-Lopresti fracture – a fracture of the radial head with concomitant dislocation of the distal radio-ulnar joint with disruption of the interosseous membrane.
            - Distal radius fracture

        - Galeazzi fracture – a fracture of the radius with dislocation of the distal radioulnar joint
        - Colles' fracture – a distal fracture of the radius with dorsal (posterior) displacement of the wrist and hand
        - Smith's fracture – a distal fracture of the radius with volar (ventral) displacement of the wrist and hand
        - Barton's fracture – an intra-articular fracture of the distal radius with dislocation of the radiocarpal joint.

- Hand fracture
    - Scaphoid fracture
    - Rolando fracture – a comminuted intra-articular fracture through the base of the first metacarpal bone
    - Bennett's fracture – a fracture of the base of the first metacarpal bone which extends into the carpometacarpal (CMC) joint.
    - Boxer's fracture – a fracture at the neck of a metacarpal
- Pelvic fracture
    - Fracture of the hip bone
    - Duverney fracture – an isolated pelvic fracture involving only the iliac wing.
- Femoral fracture
    - Hip fracture (anatomically a fracture of the femur bone and not the hip bone)
- Patella fracture
- Crus fracture
    - Tibia fracture
        - Pilon fracture
        - Tibial plateau fracture
        - Bumper fracture – a fracture of the lateral tibial plateau caused by a forced valgus applied to the knee

        - Segond fracture – an avulsion fracture of the lateral tibial condyle
        - Gosselin fracture – a fractures of the tibial plafond into anterior and posterior fragments
        - Toddler's fracture – an undisplaced and spiral fracture of the distal third to distal half of the tibia
    - Fibular fracture
        - Maisonneuve fracture – a spiral fracture of the proximal third of the fibula associated with a tear of the distal tibiofibular syndesmosis and the interosseous membrane.
        - Le Fort fracture of ankle – a vertical fracture of the antero-medial part of the distal fibula with avulsion of the anterior tibiofibular ligament.
        - Bosworth fracture – a fracture with an associated fixed posterior dislocation of the proximal fibular fragment which becomes trapped behind the posterior tibial tubercle. The injury is caused by severe external rotation of the ankle.
    - Combined tibia and fibula fracture
        - Trimalleolar fracture – involving the lateral malleolus, medial malleolus and the distal posterior aspect of the tibia
        - Bimalleolar fracture – involving the lateral malleolus and the medial malleolus.
        - Pott's fracture
- Foot fracture
    - Lisfranc fracture – in which one or all of the metatarsals are displaced from the tarsus
    - Jones fracture – a fracture of the proximal end of the fifth metatarsal
    - March fracture – a fracture of the distal third of one of the metatarsals occurring because of recurrent stress
    - Calcaneal fracture

OTA/AO Classification

The Orthopaedic Trauma Association Committee for Coding and Classification published its classification system in 1996, adopting a similar system to the 1987 AO Foundation system. In 2007, they extended their system, unifying the 2 systems regarding wrist, hand, foot and ankle fractures.

Classifications Named After People

- "Denis classification" for spinal fractures
- "Frykman classification" for forearm fractures (fractures of radius and ulna)
- "Gustilo open fracture classification"
- "Letournel and Judet Classification" for Acetabular fractures
- "Neer classification" for humerus fractures
- Seinsheimer classification, Evans-Jensen classification, Pipkin classification and Garden classification for hip fractures

Treatment

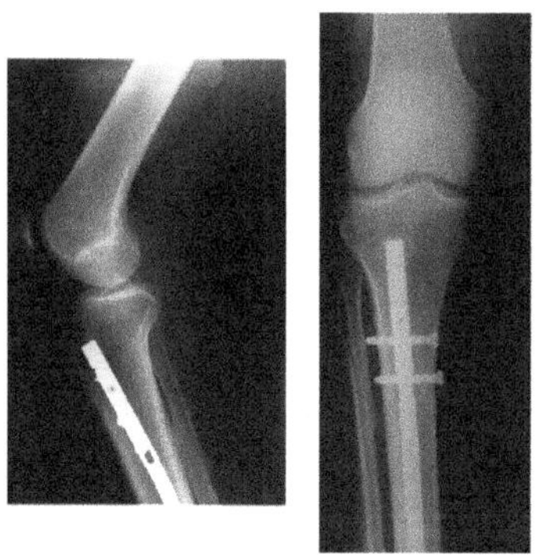

X-ray showing the proximal portion of a fractured tibia with an intramedullary nail.

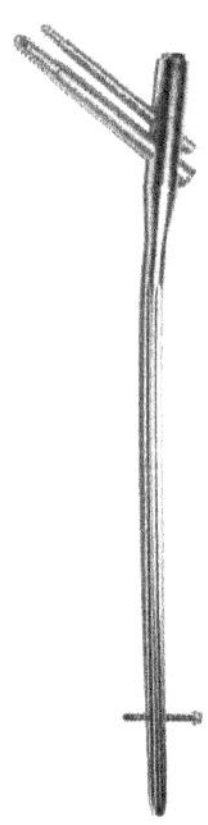

Proximal femur nail with locking and stabilisation screws for treatment of femur fractures of left thigh.

Treatment of bone fractures are broadly classified as surgical or conservative, the latter basically referring to any non-surgical procedure, such as pain management, immobilization or other non-surgical stabilization. A similar classification is *open* versus *closed treatment*, in which *open treatment* refers to any treatment in which the fracture site is surgically opened, regardless of whether the fracture itself is an open or closed fracture.

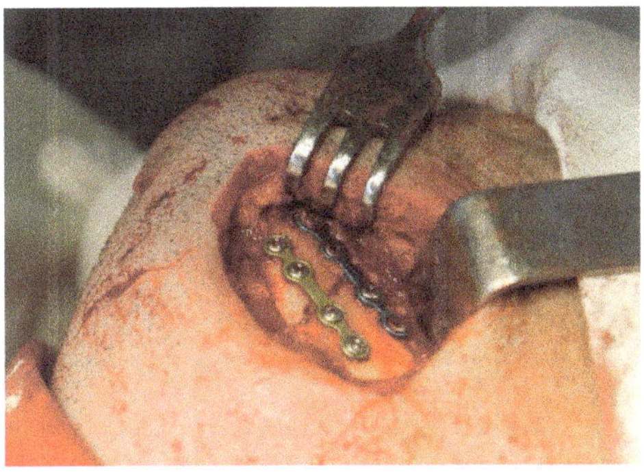

The surgical treatment of mandibular angle fracture. Fixation of the bone fragments by the plates. The principles of osteosynthesis are stability (immobility of the fragments that creates the conditions for bones coalescence) and functionality.

Pain Management

In arm fractures in children, ibuprofen has been found to be as effective as a combination of acetaminophen and codeine.

Immobilization

Since bone healing is a natural process which will most often occur, fracture treatment aims to ensure the best possible *function* of the injured part after healing. Bone fractures are typically treated by restoring the fractured pieces of bone to their natural positions (if necessary), and maintaining those positions while the bone heals. Often, aligning the bone, called reduction, in good position and verifying the improved alignment with an X-ray is all that is needed. This process is extremely painful without anesthesia, about as painful as breaking the bone itself. To this end, a fractured limb is usually immobilized with a plaster or fiberglass cast or splint which holds the bones in position and immobilizes the joints above and below the fracture. When the initial post-fracture edema or swelling goes down, the fracture may be placed in a removable brace or orthosis. If being treated with surgery, surgical nails, screws, plates and wires are used to hold the fractured bone together more directly. Alternatively, fractured bones may be treated by the Ilizarov method which is a form of external fixator.

Occasionally smaller bones, such as phalanges of the toes and fingers, may be treated without the cast, by buddy wrapping them, which serves a similar function to making a cast. By allowing only limited movement, fixation helps preserve anatomical alignment while enabling callus formation, towards the target of achieving union.

Splinting results in the same outcome as casting in children who have a distal radius fracture with little shifting.

Surgery

Surgical methods of treating fractures have their own risks and benefits, but usually surgery is done only if conservative treatment has failed, is very likely to fail, or likely to result in a poor functional outcome. With some fractures such as hip fractures (usually caused by osteoporosis), surgery is offered routinely because non-operative treatment results in prolonged immobilisation, which commonly results in complications including chest infections, pressure sores, deconditioning, deep vein thrombosis (DVT) and pulmonary embolism, which are more dangerous than surgery. When a joint surface is damaged by a fracture, surgery is also commonly recommended to make an accurate anatomical reduction and restore the smoothness of the joint.

Infection is especially dangerous in bones, due to the recrudescent nature of bone infections. Bone tissue is predominantly extracellular matrix, rather than living cells, and the few blood vessels needed to support this low metabolism are only able to bring a limited number of immune cells to an injury to fight infection. For this reason, open fractures and osteotomies call for very careful antiseptic procedures and prophylactic antibiotics.

Occasionally bone grafting is used to treat a fracture.

Sometimes bones are reinforced with metal. These implants must be designed and installed with care. *Stress shielding* occurs when plates or screws carry too large of a portion of the bone's load, causing atrophy. This problem is reduced, but not eliminated, by the use of low-modulus materials, including titanium and its alloys. The heat generated by the friction of installing hardware can easily accumulate and damage bone tissue, reducing the strength of the connections. If dissimilar metals are installed in contact with one another (i.e., a titanium plate with cobalt-chromium alloy or stainless steel screws), galvanic corrosion will result. The metal ions produced can damage the bone locally and may cause systemic effects as well.

Electrical bone growth stimulation or osteostimulation has been attempted to speed or improve bone healing. Results however do not support its effectiveness.

Complications

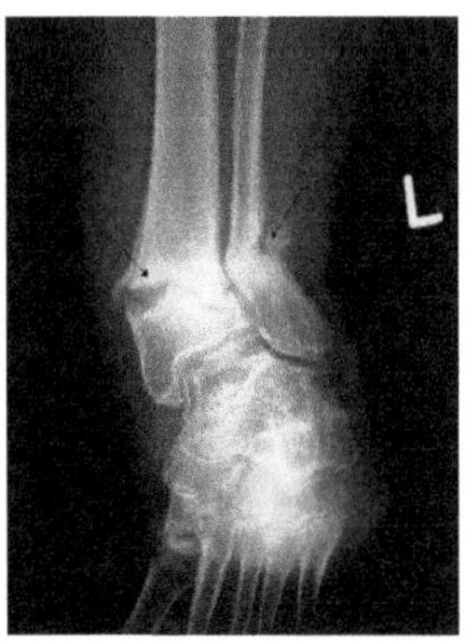

An old fracture with nonunion of the fracture fragments.

Complications of fractures can be classified into three broad groups depending upon their time of occurrence. These are as follows –

1. *Immediate* complications – occurs at the time of the fracture.
2. *Early* complications – occurring in the initial few days after the fracture.
3. *Late* complications – occurring a long time after the fracture.

Immediate complications	Early complications	Late complications
Systemic • Hypovolaemic shock	***Systemic*** • Hypovolaemic shock • ARDS – Adult respiratory distress syndrome • Fat embolism syndrome • Deep vein thrombosis • Pulmonary syndrome • Aseptic traumatic fever • Septicemia (in open fracture) • Crush syndrome	***Imperfect union of the fracture*** • Delayed union • Non union • Mal union • Cross union
Local • Injury to major vessels • Injury to muscles and tendons • Injury to joints • Injury to viscera	***Local*** • Infection • Compartment syndrome	***Others*** • Avascular necrosis • Shortening • Joint stiffness • Sudeck's dystrophy • Osteomyelitis • Ischaemic contracture • Myositis ossificans • Osteoarthritis

Children

In children, whose bones are still developing, there are risks of either a growth plate injury or a greenstick fracture.

- A greenstick fracture occurs due to mechanical failure on the tension side. That is, since the bone is not as brittle as it would be in an adult, it does not completely fracture, but rather exhibits bowing without complete disruption of the bone's cortex in the surface opposite the applied force.

- Growth plate injuries, as in Salter-Harris fractures, require careful treatment and accurate reduction to make sure that the bone continues to grow normally.
- Plastic deformation of the bone, in which the bone permanently bends but does not break, is also possible in children. These injuries may require an osteotomy (bone cut) to realign the bone if it is fixed and cannot be realigned by closed methods.
- Certain fractures are known to occur mainly in the pediatric age group, such as fracture of the clavicle & supracondylar fracture of the humerus.

Cramp

A cramp is a sudden, involuntary muscle contraction or over-shortening; while generally temporary and non-damaging, they can cause mild-to-excruciating pain, and a paralysis-like immobility of the affected muscle(s). Onset is usually sudden, and it resolves on its own over a period of several seconds, minutes, or hours. Cramps may occur in a skeletal muscle or smooth muscle. Skeletal muscle cramps may be caused by muscle fatigue or a lack of electrolytes (e.g., low sodium, low potassium, or low magnesium, although the evidence has been mixed). Cramps of smooth muscle may be due to menstruation or gastroenteritis.

Differential Diagnosis

Causes of cramping include hyperflexion, hypoxia, exposure to large changes in temperature, dehydration, or low blood salt. Muscle cramps can also be a symptom or complication of pregnancy; kidney disease; thyroid disease; hypokalemia, hypomagnesemia, or hypocalcaemia (as conditions); restless legs syndrome; varicose veins; and multiple sclerosis.

Electrolyte disturbance may cause cramping and muscle tetany, particularly hypokalemia and hypocalcaemia. This disturbance arises as the body loses large amounts of interstitial fluid through sweat. This interstitial fluid comprises mostly water and salt (sodium chloride). The loss of osmotically-active particles outside of muscle cells leads to a disturbance of the osmotic balance and therefore shrinking of muscle cells, as these contain more osmotically-active particles. This causes the calcium pump between the muscle sarcoplasm and sarcoplasmic reticulum to "short circuit"; the calcium ions remain bound to the troponin, continuing muscle contraction.

As early as 1965, researchers observed that leg cramps and restless legs syndrome can result from excess insulin, sometimes called hyperinsulinemia.

Skeletal Muscle Cramps

Skeletal muscles can be voluntarily controlled, under normal circumstances. Skeletal muscles that cramp the most often are the calves, thighs, and arches of the foot, and are sometimes called a "Charley horse" or a "corky". Such cramping is associated with strenuous physical activity and can be intensely painful; however, they can even occur while inactive and relaxed. Around 40% of people who experience skeletal cramps are likely to endure extreme muscle pain, and may be unable to use the entire limb that contains the "locked-up" muscle group. It may take up to seven days for the muscle to return to a pain-free state.

Nocturnal Leg Cramps

Nocturnal leg cramps are involuntary muscle contractions that occur in the calves, soles of the feet, or other muscles in the body during the night or (less commonly) while resting.

The duration of nocturnal leg cramps is variable, with cramps lasting anywhere from a few seconds to several minutes. Muscle soreness may remain after the cramp itself ends. These cramps are more common in older people. They happen quite frequently in teenagers and in some people while exercising at night. The precise cause of these cramps is unclear. Potential contributing factors include dehydration, low levels of certain minerals (magnesium, potassium, calcium, and sodium, although the evidence has been mixed), and reduced blood flow through muscles attendant in prolonged sitting or lying down. Nocturnal leg cramps (almost exclusively calf cramps) are considered "normal" during the late stages of pregnancy. They can, however, vary in intensity from mild to extremely painful.

A lactic acid buildup around muscles can trigger cramps; however, these happen during anaerobic respiration when a person is exercising or engaging in an activity where the heartbeat speeds up. Medical conditions associated with leg cramps are cardiovascular disease, hemodialysis, cirrhosis, pregnancy, and lumbar canal stenosis. Differential diagnoses include restless legs syndrome, claudication, myositis, peripheral neuropathy. All of these can be differentiated through careful history and physical examination.

Gentle stretching and massage, putting some pressure on the affected leg by walking or standing, or taking a warm bath or shower may help to end the cramp. If the cramp is in the calf muscle, pulling the big toe gently backwards will stretch the muscle and, in some cases, cause almost immediate relief. There is limited evidence supporting the use of magnesium, calcium channel blockers, carisoprodol, and vitamin B12.

Quinine is no longer recommended for treatment of nocturnal leg cramps due to potential fatal hypersensitivity reactions and thrombocytopenia. Arrhythmias, cinchonism, hemolytic uremic syndrome can also occur at higher dosages.

Smooth Muscle Cramps

Smooth muscle contractions may be symptomatic of endometriosis or other health problems. Menstrual cramps may also occur both before and during a menstrual cycle.

Iatrogenic Causes

Various medications may cause nocturnal leg cramps:

- Diuretics, especially potassium sparing
- Intravenous (IV) iron sucrose
- Conjugated estrogens
- Teriparatide
- Naproxen
- Raloxifene
- Long acting adrenergic beta-agonists (LABAs)
- Hydroxymethylglutaryl-coenzyme A reductase inhibitors (HMG-CoA inhibitors or statins)

Besides being painful, a nocturnal leg cramp can cause much distress and anxiety. Statins may sometimes cause myalgia and cramps among other possible side effects. Raloxifene (Evista) is a medication associated with a high incidence of leg cramps. Additional factors, which increase the probability for these side effects, are physical exercise, age, female gender, history of cramps, and hypothyroidism. Up to 80% of athletes using statins suffer significant adverse muscular effects, including cramps; the rate appears to be approximately 10–25% in a typical statin-using population. In some cases, adverse effects disappear after switching to a different statin; however, they should not be ignored if they persist, as they can, in rare cases, develop into more serious problems. Coenzyme Q10 supplementation can be helpful to avoid some statin-related adverse effects, but currently there is not enough evidence to prove the effectiveness in avoiding myopathy or myalgia.

Pathophysiology

Skeletal muscles work as antagonistic pairs. Contracting one skeletal muscle requires the relaxation of the opposing muscle in the pair. Cramps can occur when muscles are unable to relax properly due to myosin fibers not fully detaching from actin filaments. In skeletal muscle, adenosine triphosphate (ATP) must attach to the myosin heads for them to disassociate from the actin and allow relaxation; the absence of ATP in sufficient quantities means that the myosin heads remains attached to actin. An attempt to force a muscle cramped in this way to extend (by contracting the opposing muscle) can tear muscle tissue and worsen the pain. The muscle must be allowed to recover (resynthesize ATP), before the myosin fibres can detach and allow the muscle to relax.

Treatment

Stretching, massage and drinking plenty of fluid, such as water, may be helpful in treating simple muscle cramps. With exertional heat cramps due to electrolyte abnormalities (primarily sodium loss and not calcium, magnesium, and potassium), appropriate fluids and sufficient salt improves symptoms.

Medication

Quinine is likely to be effective; however, due to side effects, its use should only be considered if other treatments have failed. Vitamin B complex, naftidrofuryl, lidocaine, and calcium channel blockers may be effective for muscle cramps. Research has also shown that pickle "juice" can be an effective remedy based on its high sodium and electrolyte content. Cyclobenzaprine (Flexeril) has proven effective in preventing muscle cramps, although data suggests that effectiveness decreases when taken for more than several weeks.

Prevention

Adequate conditioning, stretching, mental preparation, hydration, and electrolyte balance are likely helpful in preventing muscle cramps.

Bruise

A contusion, commonly known as a bruise, is a type of hematoma of tissue in which capillaries and sometimes venules are damaged by trauma, allowing blood to seep, hemorrhage, or extravasate into the surrounding interstitial tissues. Bruises, which do not blanch under pressure, can involve capillaries at the level of skin, subcutaneous tissue, muscle, or bone. Bruises are not to be confused with other similar-looking lesions primarily distinguished by their diameter or causation. These lesions include petechia (< 3 mm result from numerous and diverse etiologies such as adverse reactions from medications such as warfarin, straining, asphyxiation, platelet disorders and diseases such as cytomegalovirus), purpura (3 mm to 1 cm, classified as palpable purpura or non-palpable purpura and indicates various pathologic conditions such as thrombocytopenia), and ecchymosis (>1 cm caused blood dissecting through tissue planes and settled in an area remote from the site of trauma or pathology such as periorbital ecchymosis, i.e.,"raccoon eyes" , arising from a basilar skull fracture or from a neuroblastoma).

As a type of hematoma, a bruise is always caused by internal bleeding into the interstitial tissues which does not break through the skin, usually initiated by blunt trauma, which causes damage through physical compression and deceleration forces. Trauma sufficient to cause bruising can occur from a wide variety of situations including accidents, falls, and surgeries. Disease states such as insufficient or malfunctioning platelets, other coagulation deficiencies, or vascular disorders, such as venous blockage associated with severe allergies can lead to the formation of purpura which is not to be confused with trauma-related bruising/contusion. If the trauma is sufficient to break the skin and allow blood to escape the interstitial tissues, the injury is not a bruise but instead a different variety of hemorrhage called bleeding. However, such injuries may be accompanied by bruising elsewhere.

Bruises often induce pain, but small bruises are not normally dangerous alone. Sometimes bruises can be serious, leading to other more life-threatening forms of hematoma, such as when associated with serious injuries, including fractures and more severe internal bleeding. The likelihood and severity of bruising depends on many factors, including type and healthiness of affected tissues. Minor bruises may be easily recognized in people with light skin color by characteristic blue or purple appearance (idiomatically described as "black and blue") in the days following the injury.

Cause

The presence of bruises may be seen in patients with platelet or coagulation disorders. Unexplained bruising may be a warning sign of child abuse, domestic abuse, or serious medical problems such as leukemia or meningoccocal infection. Unexplained bruising can also indicate internal bleeding or certain types of cancer. Long-term glucocorticoid therapy can cause easy bruising. Bruising present around the navel (belly button) with severe abdominal pain suggests acute pancreatitis. Connective tissue disorders such as Ehlers-Danlos syndrome may cause relatively easy or spontaneous bruising depending on the severity.

During an autopsy, bruises accompanying abrasions indicate the abrasions occurred while the individual was alive, as opposed to damage incurred post mortem.

Size and Shape

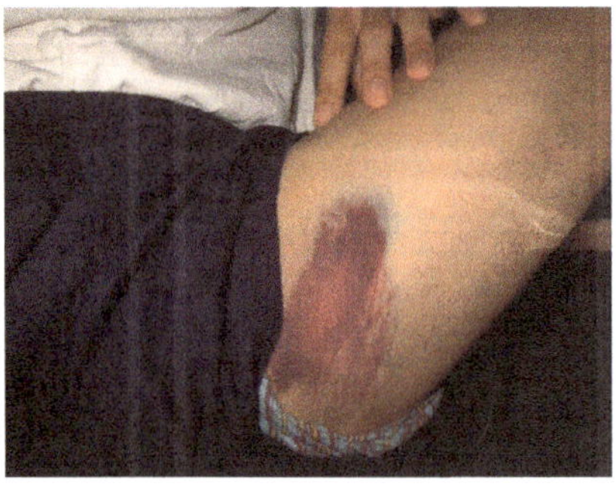

Bruise caused by a handrail, typical of extreme sports

Bruise shapes may correspond directly to the instrument of injury or be modified by additional factors. Bruises often become more prominent as time lapses, resulting in additional size and swelling, and may grow to a large size over the course of the hours after the injury that caused the bruise was inflicted. As stated above, bruising present in a different location than the site of impact is called *ecchymosis* and generally occurs when the tissue at the site of injury is loose, allowing blood to travel under the skin to another location due to gravity or other forces, such as in a black eye.

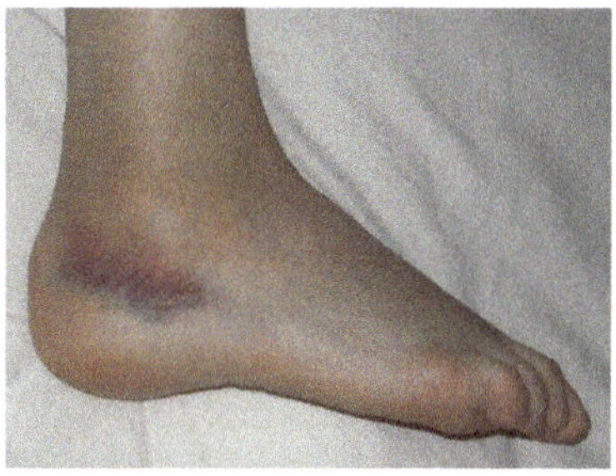

Bruise caused by a sprained ankle

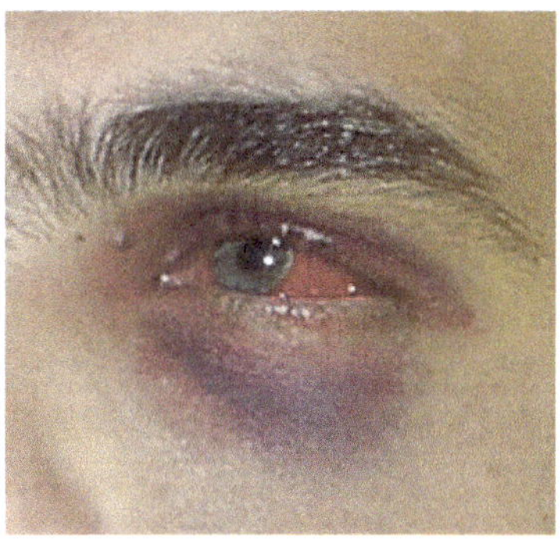

Black eye and subconjunctival hemorrhage after a punch to the face

- Condition and type of tissue: In soft tissues, a larger area is bruised than would be in firmer tissue due to ease of blood to invade tissue.
- Age: elderly skin and other tissues are often thinner and less elastic and thus more prone to bruising.
- Gender: More bruising occurs in females due to increased subcutaneous fat.
- Skin tone: Discoloration caused by bruises is more prominent in lighter complexions.
- Diseases: Coagulation, platelet and blood vessel diseases or deficiencies can increase bruising due to more bleeding.
- Location: More extensive vascularity causes more bleeding. Areas such as the arms, knees, shins and the facial area are especially common bruise sites.
- Forces: Greater striking forces cause greater bruising.

- Genetics: Despite having completely normal coagulation factors, natural redheads have been shown to bruise more, although this may just be due to greater visibility on commonly associated lighter complexion.

Severity

Bruises can be scored on a scale from 0-5 to categorize the severity and danger of the injury.

Bruise harm score		
Harm score	**Severity level**	**Notes**
0	Light bruise	No damage
1	Mild bruise	Little damage
2	Moderate bruise	Some damage
3	Serious bruise	Dangerous
4	Extremely serious bruise	Dangerous
5	Critical bruise	Risk of death

The harm score is determined by the extent and severity of the fractures to the organs and tissues causing the bruising, in turn depending on multiple factors. For example, a contracted muscle will bruise more severely, as will tissues crushed against underlying bone. Capillaries vary in strength, stiffness and toughness, which can also vary by age and medical conditions.

An alternate bruise severity ranking system called the Chien Intensity Scale is slowly growing in popularity in some research circles. Although not widely used, the Chien Intensity Scale is used by institutes including the Ryan Mackey Memorial Research Institute and the Sydney Medical Center.

Low levels of damaging forces produce small bruises and generally cause the individual to feel minor pain straight away. Repeated impacts worsen bruises, increasing the harm level. Normally, light bruises heal nearly completely within two weeks, although duration is affected by variation in severity and individual healing processes; generally, more severe or deeper bruises take somewhat longer.

Severe bruising (harm score 2-3) may be dangerous or cause serious complications. Further bleeding and excess fluid may accumulate causing a hard, fluctuating lump or swelling hematoma. This has the potential to cause compartment syndrome as the swelling cuts off blood flow to the tissues. The trauma that induced the bruise may also have caused other severe and potentially fatal harm to internal organs. For example, impacts to the head can cause traumatic brain injury: bleeding, bruising and massive swelling of the brain with the potential to cause concussion, coma and death. Treatment for brain bruising may involve emergency surgery to relieve the pressure on the brain.

Damage that causes bruising can also cause bones to be broken, tendons or muscles to be strained, ligaments to be sprained, or other tissue to be damaged. The symptoms and signs of these injuries may initially appear to be those of simple bruising. Abdominal bruising or severe injuries that cause difficulty in moving a limb or the feeling of liquid under the skin may indicate life-threatening injury and require the attention of a physician.

Mechanism

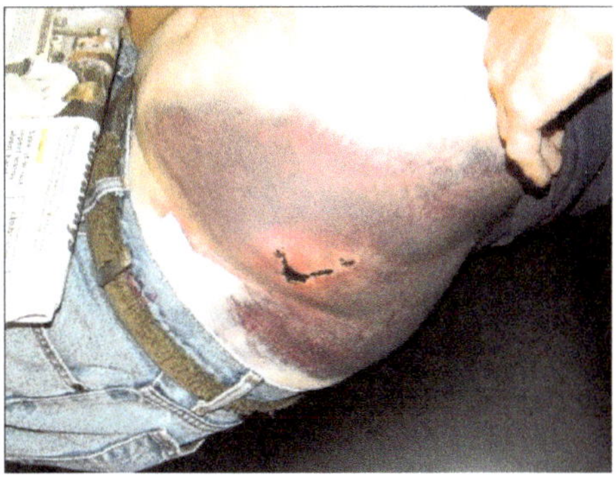

Severe bruising resulting from yard work injury

Increased distress to tissue causes capillaries to break under the skin, allowing blood to escape and build up. As time progresses, blood seeps into the surrounding tissues, causing the bruise to darken and spread. Nerve endings within the affected tissue detect the increased pressure, which, depending on severity and location, may be perceived as pain or pressure or be asymptomatic. The damaged capillary endothelium releases endothelin, a hormone that causes narrowing of the blood vessel to minimize bleeding. As the endothelium is destroyed, the underlying von Willebrand factor is exposed and initiates coagulation, which creates a temporary clot to plug the wound and eventually leads to restoration of normal tissue.

During this time, larger bruises may change color due to the breakdown of hemoglobin from within escaped red blood cells in the extracellular space. The striking colors of a bruise are caused by the phagocytosis and sequential degradation of hemoglobin to biliverdin to bilirubin to hemosiderin, with hemoglobin itself producing a red-blue color, biliverdin producing a green color, bilirubin producing a yellow color, and hemosiderin producing a golden-brown color. As these products are cleared from the area, the bruise disappears. Often the underlying tissue damage has been repaired long before this process is complete.

Treatment

Treatment for light bruises is minimal and may include RICE (rest, ice, compression, elevation), painkillers (particularly NSAIDs) and, later in recovery, light stretching exercises. Particularly, immediate application of ice while elevating the area may reduce or completely prevent swelling by restricting blood flow to the area and preventing internal bleeding. Rest and preventing re-injury is essential for rapid recovery. Applying a medicated cream containing mucopolysaccharide polysulfuric acid (e.g., Hirudoid) may also speed the healing process. Other topical creams containing skin-fortifying ingredients, including but not limited to retinol or alpha hydroxy acids, such as Der-Mend, can improve the appearance of bruising faster than if left to heal on its own.

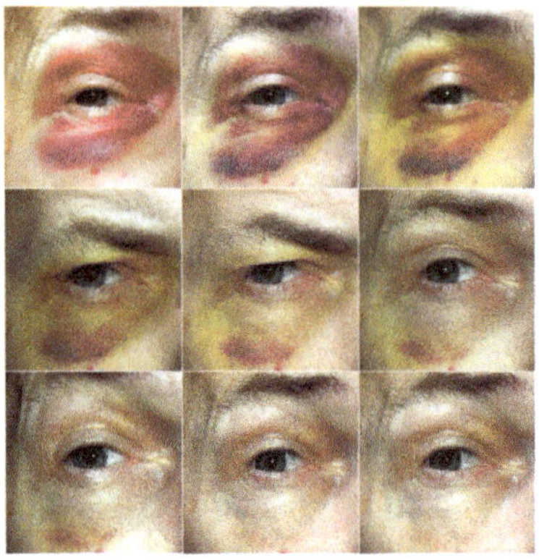

Healing of a black eye over a 9-day period caused by a wisdom tooth extraction

Very gently massaging the area and applying heat may encourage blood flow and relieve pain according to the gate control theory of pain, although causing additional pain may indicate the massage is exacerbating the injury. As for most injuries, these techniques should not be applied until at least three days following the initial damage to ensure all internal bleeding has stopped, because although increasing blood flow will allow more healing factors into the area and encourage drainage, if the injury is still bleeding this will allow more blood to seep out of the wound and cause the bruise to become worse.

In most cases hematomas spontaneously revert, but in cases of large hematomas or those localized in certain organs (*e.g.*, the brain), the physician may optionally perform a puncture of the hematoma to allow the blood to exit.

History

Folk medicine, including ancient medicine of Egyptians, Greeks, Celts, Turks, Slavs, Mayans, Aztecs and Chinese, has used bruising as a treatment for some health problems. The methods vary widely and include cupping, scraping, and slapping. Fire cupping uses suction which causes bruising in patients. Scraping (Gua Sha) uses a small hand device with a rounded edge to gently scrape the scalp or the skin. Another ancient device that creates mild bruising is a strigil, used by Greeks and Romans in the bath. Archaeologically there is no precedent for scraping tools before Greek archaeological evidence, not Chinese or Egyptian.

References

- McCaffrey RJ (1997). "Special Issues in the Evaluation of Mild Traumatic Brain Injury". The Practice of Forensic Neuropsychology: Meeting Challenges in the Courtroom. New York: Plenum

Press. pp. 71–75. ISBN 0-306-45256-1.

- Carlson, Neil R. (2013). “Physiology of Behavior”. In Campanella, Craig. Neurological Disorders. Pearson Education, Inc. pp. 526–527. ISBN 0-205-23939-0.
- Macfarlane, Robert; Hardy, David G. (1997). Outcome after Head, Neck and Spinal Trauma: a medicolegal guide. Oxford: Reed Educational and Professional Publishing Ltd. ISBN 0 7506 2178 8.
- Powell, Trevor (2004). Head Injury: A Practical Guide (2nd ed.). United Kingdom: Speech mark publishing Ltd. ISBN 0863884512.
- Seidenwurm DI (2007). “Introduction to brain imaging”. In Brant WE, Helms CA. Fundamentals of Diagnostic Radiology. Philadelphia: Lippincott, Williams & Wilkins. p. 53. ISBN 0-7817-6135-2. Retrieved 2008-11-17.
- Science and Racket Sports Edited by: T. Reilly, M. Hughes and A.Lees. Published by E & FN Spon ISBN 0-419-18500-3.
- Rüedi, etc. all; Thomas P. Rüedi; Richard E. Buckley; Christopher G. Moran (2007). AO principles of fracture management, Volume 1. Thieme. p. Page 96. ISBN 3-13-117442-0.
- Kumar, Vinay; Abbas, Abul K.; Fausto, Nelson; & Mitchell, Richard N. (2007). Robbins Basic Pathology (8th ed.). Saunders Elsevier. p. 86 ISBN 978-1-4160-2973-1
- “Head Injury: Description”. Seattle Children’s Hospital, Seattle, WA, USA. 2016. Retrieved 19 October 2016.
- Debas, H. T.; Donkor, P.; Gawande, A.; Jamison, D. T.; Kruk, M. E.; Mock, C. N., eds. (2015). Essential Surgery. Disease Control Priorities. 1 (3rd ed.). Washington, DC: World Bank. doi:10.1596/978-1-4648-0346-8.
- Kinnaman, Karen; Binder, William; Nadel, Eric; Brown, David (2015). “Petechiae, anemia, and throbocytopenia”. The Journal of Emergency Medicine.

Permissions

All chapters in this book are published with permission under the Creative Commons Attribution Share Alike License or equivalent. Every chapter published in this book has been scrutinized by our experts. Their significance has been extensively debated. The topics covered herein carry significant information for a comprehensive understanding. They may even be implemented as practical applications or may be referred to as a beginning point for further studies.

We would like to thank the editorial team for lending their expertise to make the book truly unique. They have played a crucial role in the development of this book. Without their invaluable contributions this book wouldn't have been possible. They have made vital efforts to compile up to date information on the varied aspects of this subject to make this book a valuable addition to the collection of many professionals and students.

This book was conceptualized with the vision of imparting up-to-date and integrated information in this field. To ensure the same, a matchless editorial board was set up. Every individual on the board went through rigorous rounds of assessment to prove their worth. After which they invested a large part of their time researching and compiling the most relevant data for our readers.

The editorial board has been involved in producing this book since its inception. They have spent rigorous hours researching and exploring the diverse topics which have resulted in the successful publishing of this book. They have passed on their knowledge of decades through this book. To expedite this challenging task, the publisher supported the team at every step. A small team of assistant editors was also appointed to further simplify the editing procedure and attain best results for the readers.

Apart from the editorial board, the designing team has also invested a significant amount of their time in understanding the subject and creating the most relevant covers. They scrutinized every image to scout for the most suitable representation of the subject and create an appropriate cover for the book.

The publishing team has been an ardent support to the editorial, designing and production team. Their endless efforts to recruit the best for this project, has resulted in the accomplishment of this book. They are a veteran in the field of academics and their pool of knowledge is as vast as their experience in printing. Their expertise and guidance has proved useful at every step. Their uncompromising quality standards have made this book an exceptional effort. Their encouragement from time to time has been an inspiration for everyone.

The publisher and the editorial board hope that this book will prove to be a valuable piece of knowledge for students, practitioners and scholars across the globe.

Index